Y0-AFY-542

Progress in Drug Research

Vol. 58

Edited by Ernst Jucker, Basel

Board of Advisors
Joseph M. Colacino
Pushkar N. Kaul
Vera M. Kolb
J. Mark Treherne
Q. May Wang

Authors
Jay A. Glasel
Vera M. Kolb
Paul L. Skatrud
John W. Ford, Edward B. Stevens,
J. Mark Treherne, Jeremy Packer and
Mark Bushfield
David T. Wong and Frank P. Bymaster
Satya P. Gupta

Birkhäuser Verlag
Basel · Boston · Berlin

Editor

Dr. E. Jucker
Steinweg 28
CH-4107 Ettingen
Switzerland
e-mail: jucker.pdr@bluewin.ch

Visit our PDR homepage: http://www.birkhauser.ch/books/biosc/pdr

.

ISBN 3-7643-6624-9 Birkhäuser Verlag, Basel – Boston – Berlin

© 2002 Birkhäuser Verlag, P.O. Box 133, CH-4010 Basel, Switzerland
Member of the BertelsmannSpringer Publishing Group
Printed on acid-free paper produced from chlorine-free pulp. TCF ∞
Cover design and layout: Gröflin Graphic Design, Basel
Printed in Germany

ISBN 3-7643-6624-9
9 8 7 6 5 4 3 2 1

Contents

Foreword by the Editor

This 58th volume of the series *Progress in Drug Research* contains six reviews which all highlight latest insights and discoveries in drug research and application. The first article is devoted to problems associated with individual-based medicine. One of the consequences of the "genomic revolution" is the recognition that individuals differ from one another in sequence variations in their genomes. This led to the optimistic assumption that an individual's pattern of sequence variations could lead to drugs that target that individual's variant proteins and make individual-based medicine possible. Jay Glasel examines these possibilities, and comes to the conclusion that the human genome is only one of the elements serving to maintain an organism's inter-action with its environment. The next article is very much in line with efforts to make use of natural sources as valuable addition to the modern agents in the instrumentarium of today's therapeutic methods. This masterly review by Vera Kolb is a valuable addendum to a number of reviews published in *PDR*, e.g. on Chinese Medicine, on herbal drugs and on drugs of maritime origin. Vera Kolb is in full agreement with the Editor, believing that alternative medicine offers more possibilities than is recognised today.

The next review deals with multiple drug resistance proteins. Bacterial and viral infections, as well as infections with fungi and/or parasites, increasingly pose problems or even unsurmountable barriers towards successful chemotherapy. On the other hand, multiple drug resistance proteins also present several positive opportunities, and Paul Skatrud highlights in this excellent review both sides of the problem. Existing drugs that modulate ion channels represent a key class of pharmaceutical agents across many therapeutic areas and there is considerable further potential for potassium channel drug discovery. In this respect, it is of utmost importance to identify lead compounds that can provide tractable starting points for medicinal chemistry. Several potassium channel screening platforms are described in the fourth review by John W. Ford et al., and particular emphasis is placed on the mechanistic basis of drug-target interaction in potassium channel discovery.

Improvement of existing and creation of new antidepressant drugs is still of great importance for the treatment of major depressive disorder. It has been recognized that promotion of serotonergic and noradrenergic transmission by inhibiting simultaneously the uptake of serotonin and noradrenaline could potentially result in improved antidepressant agents.

In this fifth review, David Wong and Frank P. Bymaster demonstrate the latest achievements in this field of research and provide new impulse for studies which can lead to new, potent antidepressants. Finally, in the last review, Satya Gupta continues with his extensive studies of QSAR analysis and surveys latest results with HIV-1 reverse transcriptase inhibitors, making an important addition to reviews on this subject previously published in PDR. The topicality and importance of such studies need not be stressed anymore.

All these six reviews contain extensive bibliographies, thus enabling the interested reader and the active researcher to have easy access to the original literature. The various indices facilitate the use of these monographs and also help to use PDR as an encyclopedic source of information in the complex and fast growing field of drug research.

The series *Progress in Drug Research* was founded in 1958/59. In the 43 years of its existence, drug research has undergone drastic changes, but the original purpose of these monographs remains unchanged: dissemination of information on trends and developments, discussion of crucial points and creation of new prospects on future drug design. The Editor is anxious to maintain the high standard of *PDR* and is grateful to the authors for their willingness to undertake the hard work of writing comprehensive review articles for the benefit of all involved with drug research. It is their high qualification and experience on which the success of these monographs is based.

In ending this Foreword, I would like to thank the authors for their contributions, the Members of the Board of Advisors foir their active help and advice and the reviewers for improving these monographs. Last but not least, I am greatly indebted to Birkhäuser Publishers and in particular to Beatrice Menz and Gabriele Fertöszögi, Editorial Department BioSciences, for their active participation with editing and producing this new volume. Hans-Peter Ebneter, Bernd Luchner, Eduard Mazenauer and Gregor Messmer have contributed their vast experience and intimate knowledge. My sincere thanks are due also for their personal engagement and for the rewarding, harmonious cooperation.

My very special thanks go to Mr. Hans-Peter Thür, Birkhäuser Publishing's CEO. For the many decades of our close cooperation Mr. Thür gave PDR and its Editor his full support and never ceased to give this series impulses which go far beyond his function as CEO. I would like to acknowledge that some of the most valuable review articles have been a result of Mr. Thür's suggestion, and it is also due to his encouragement that I continue with great enthusiam with the editorship of this series of monographs.

Basel, April 2002

Dr. E. Jucker

Progress in Drug Research, Vol. 58 (E. Jucker, Ed.)
©2002 Birkhäuser Verlag, Basel (Switzerland)

Drugs, the human genome, and individual-based medicine

By Jay A. Glasel

Global Scientific Consulting LLC
15 Colton St.
Farmington, CT 06032, USA
<jaglasel@consult-globalsci.com>

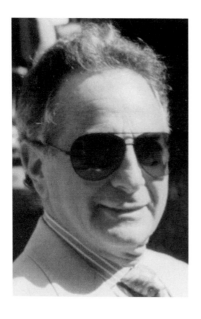

Jay A. Glasel

studied Chemistry and Physics at the California Institute of Technology and received his Ph.D. in Chemical Physics at the University of Chicago. He is managing member of Global Scientific Consulting LLC in Farmington, Connecticut and Professor Emeritus of Biochemistry at the University of Connecticut Medical-Dental School. He is senior author of an extensive list of research articles in scientific publications.

Summary

The so-called "Genomic Revolution" has made possible the high-resolution sequencing of the DNA making up the human genome. One of the main conclusions of the currently available sequencing data is that individuals differ genetically from one another *via* sequence variations in their genomes. When affected genes are transcribed and translated, some of these sequence variations result in protein products that may affect the functioning of the proteins. This has led to widespread optimism that information on an individual's pattern of sequence variations will lead to drugs that target that individual's variant proteins and make "individual-based medicine" possible. In this chapter some of the assumptions underlying the proposed production of individual drug treatments are examined. The assumptions are viewed in the light of very recent experimental evidence about the sequence patterns found in humans. Also discussed are ancillary ethical problems in cataloging and using databases containing individuals' sequence data, what human genomic sequences are revealing about the use of animal models in developing drugs, and how evidence is mounting that the human genome is only one element serving to maintain an organism's interaction with its environment.

Contents

Jay A. Glasel

Key words

Pharmacogenetics, pharmacogenomics, epigenetics, human genome, single nucleotide polymorphisms, molecular genetics, individual medicine, drug development.

Glossary of abbreviations

Anchored re-sequencing strategy: An expensive approach to obtaining a large number of SNPs using short sequences of DNA from individuals of different ethnic groups that are derived from a plasmid library. These sequences are then compared to the genome draft sequence to obtain a large number of SNPs in a very short amount of time.

Annotation (annotated sequence): A term used with very little consistency among researchers working on genome-related projects. As commonly used, annotation entails assembling information of several distinctive types, starting with refined DNA sequence data but extending beyond that level to varying degrees of complexity. For example, completed DNA sequence information may be segmented into distinct intervals that may be demarcated in terms of their encoding specific types of product, such as proteins. Next, a particular gene may be annotated in such terms as its protein coding region, its transcript, promoter region, and so forth. At a higher level of annotation, a protein that is encoded by a particular gene may be annotated in terms of its physical attributes, such as molecular weight, membrane spanning regions, structural domains, or three-dimensional structure. Annotation at the level of comparative biology may include information linking a particular protein from a specific organism to similar proteins from other organisms or to members of similar protein families. Genes may also be annotated at a functional level, in terms of their respective roles in cellular metabolism, a particular systematic enzyme number (EC) designation, protein-protein interactions, and expression profiles.

Contigs (contig map): Overlapping (contiguous) DNA segments assembled from sequenced fragments of a chromosome. A contig map is the sequence of DNA in a chromosome constructed by isolating contigs.

Epigenetics: The study of heritable changes in gene expression that occur without a change in DNA sequence.

EST: Expressed sequence tag, several hundred base pairs of known cDNA sequence flanked by PCR primers. Because they are derived from cDNA libraries (i.e., from reverse transcription of cellular mRNAs), ESTs represent portions of expressed genes. ESTs are useful for identifying full-length genes and a landmark for mapping.

Finished sequence: Complete sequence of a clone or of a genome with an accuracy of at least 99.99% and no gaps.

Functional genomics: The study of genomes to determine the biological function of all the genes and their products.

Genetic map: The ordering of genes on chromosomes according to their recombination frequency during meiosis. The unit of distance is centimorgans (cM) which corresponds to a 1%

chance of recombination. Genetic mapping preceded physical mapping and when a genome is completely sequenced, the genetic map becomes redundant.

Genetic linkage map: A map of the relative positions of genes and other regions on a chromosome, determined by how often loci are inherited together.

Genome draft sequence: The sequence produced by combining information from individual overlapping sequenced pieces of DNA with linkage information and positioning the sequence along the physical map of the chromosomes.

Haplotype: Long stretches of DNA (lengths as long as 100,000 bases have been found) at a given location on a chromosome. Also, a specific pattern of alleles or sequence variations that are closely linked (i.e., likely to be inherited together) on the same chromosome. Recently, it has been found that many such blocks come in a few different versions.

Linkage equilibrium, disequilibrium: When there is no preferential association of alleles at linked loci, they are said to be in equilibrium; when there is a nonrandom association of alleles at linked loci in a population, the population is said to be in linkage disequilibrium. As sometimes stated oppositely: at 0% disequilibrium, there is no association between alleles, at 100% disequilibrium, alleles are always found in association.

Microsatellite: A type of satellite DNA that consists of small repeat units (usually two, three, four, or five base pairs) that occur in tandem.

Minisatellite: A type of satellite DNA that consists of tandem repeat units that are each about 20 to 70 base pairs in length.

Missense (mutation): A DNA sequence change that results in a single amino acid change in the translated gene product.

Neutral hypothesis and neutral model: The hypothesis is that the large majority of polymorphisms within species and fixed substitutions between species are the result of the random drift of neutral mutations and not natural selection. Deleterious mutations are assumed to occur, but are quickly eliminated. The model assumes a random-mating population of constant size where new mutations occur at sites not previously mutated (a good approximation when mutation rates at all sites are relatively low).

Nonsense (mutation): A DNA sequence in which an mRNA stop codon is produced or removed, thus resulting in a premature termination of translation or an elongation of the protein product.

π (Pi): A measure of nucleotide diversity (per-site heterozygosity) in the sequences of single strands of DNA. It is the probability that a pair of chromosomes drawn from a population will differ at a nucleotide site.

Pseudogene: A nonfunctional sequence of DNA similar to a functional one. Pseudogenes are probably remnants of once-functional genes that accumulated mutations.

Radical (change in an amino acid residue): A commonly used, somewhat arbitrarily defined description of an amino acid substitution in a protein that is predicted to, or does, change the protein's observed properties. As discussed in this chapter, the concept has been given a more quantitative form.

Recombination frequency: The proportion of meioses in which recombinants between two loci are seen. The proportion rises the farther apart the recombining loci are. The recombination frequency is used to estimate genetic distances between loci.

RFLP: Restriction fragment length polymorphism; genetic variation in the length of DNA fragments produced by restriction enzymes. RFLPs are useful as markers on maps.

Satellite DNA: A portion of the DNA that differs enough in base composition that it is physically separable from other DNAs by its different density; usually contains highly repetitive DNA sequences.

Silent (mutation): A DNA sequence change that does not change the amino acid sequence in the translated protein product due to the degeneracy of the genetic code.

SNP: Single-nucleotide polymorphism; common DNA sequence variations that occur when a single nucleotide (A, T, C, or G) in the genome sequence is altered. Other types of polymorphisms include VNTRs (variable number of tandem repeats; a type of polymorphism created by variations in the number of minisatellite repeats in a defined region of the sequence) and MRPs (microsatellite repeat polymorphism; a type of genetic variation in populations consisting of differing numbers of microsatellite repeat units at a locus).

SNP map: A collection of SNPs that can be superimposed over the existing genome map, creating greater detail, and facilitating further genetic studies.

STS: Sequence tagged site, a unique stretch of DNA whose location is known. STSs serve as landmarks for mapping and assembly.

Trans-splicing: A process whereby a transcript, translatable into a protein, is produced from both the sense and antisense strands of a DNA double helix. Previously observed in viruses, trans-splicing has now been found in a eukaryote (*Drosophila*) and may take place in humans.

1   Introduction

This chapter presents a critical look at the practical impact that increasing knowledge of human molecular genetics will have on drug development in the next 5–10 years. Biotechnological advances are taking place with such rapidity that longer-term projections are worthless guesswork.

Many of the terms used to describe human molecular genetics have not yet entered into common use in pharmacological/pharmaceutical literature. Therefore, a glossary has been included at the start of the chapter. It is hoped that the glossary will be useful in guiding some readers through this chapter, the references quoted therein, and the developing literature on drugs and genetics.

1.1   Drugs, the genome, proposals for "individual medicine"

Within the last five years, the pharmacological literature has been flooded with publications hailing what is usually taken for granted: determining single nucleotide polymorphisms (SNPs) in an individual's genes will soon become a reality, and will inevitably result in what some have called "individual medicine." That is, drug and other clinical treatments will begin to be targeted to individuals on the basis of these individuals' own specific genetic variations. An examination of this widespread belief forms the basis for this chapter.

1.1.1 The genetic basis for the concept of individual medicine

The fundamental information upon which any practical application of individual medicine is based has been assumed to be the identification of genetic loci and functional significance of SNPs in an individual's genome.

The human genome is diploid, but the SNP information that is sought is haplotypic. In the most familiar conventional analyses of genomic DNA variation, both strands on each chromosome are analyzed together so that at every position in the DNA sequence where a variation occurs, the DNA sequence is heterozygous (two bases are identified instead of one). If multiple variant loci are present, there will be multiple heterozygous positions and the information of which variant is present on which DNA molecule is lost in these analyses. For example, if one allele is dominant (the most frequent case) it has been assumed that it will be the drugs directed against it, or its product, that are important to develop.

In conventional human genetic studies, the pattern of inheritance provides key information that allows most or all of the haplotypes to be reconstructed because, except for very rare recombination events, DNA molecules are inherited intact from parents. This allows the determination of which particular variant alleles have been coinherited from one parent and thus must lie on the same DNA molecule. The kinds of multi-generation linkage studies traditionally used in human genetics provide sufficient haplotype information that disease genes can be located based on the pattern of inheritance of nearby markers. It should be noted that such experiments are not the typical design used in clinical studies. Instead, case-control data are the norm, and this dramatically increases the difficulty of reconstructing haplotype information, because without this information, the statistical power of association of a particular DNA marker with a nearby phenotype becomes much weaker.

However, over several decades, studies of both types have resulted in the discovery of many variant genes whose products, or lack of products, are believed to cause disease in humans and animal models. These are the so-called "monogenic" diseases.

The technical ability to obtain gene sequence information from large numbers of chromosomes from large numbers of individuals' DNA has been recognized as the stumbling block to obtaining enough SNP information to be used for developing individual medicine. The background to this problem has been reviewed [1, 2] as have been technological advances to solve it [3].

At present, the practical situation is that technologies exist to obtain detailed SNP information for a limited number of genes from a relatively large population of individuals, or limited information from a large number of genes from a relatively small population of individuals. The information now available on both these types of studies will be discussed later in this chapter. The greatest effort now being made is an attempt to define all the SNPs in the human genome as obtained from DNA obtained from a few individuals.

1.1.2 Present progress in obtaining genomic SNP information

To the end of finding all SNPs in the human genome, the expensive anchored re-sequencing approach is the only strategy known that is rigorous enough to find the number of SNPs necessary to completely specify individual genetic variations. This strategy has been adapted cooperatively by a number of pharmaceutical firms along with public research facilities in a venture called the "SNP Consortium." The Consortium began pilot studies in January of 1999 and hopes to locate and map more than 150,000 SNPS by the end of 2001. All information collected by the groups involved is being published on The Consortium web site (http://snp.cshl.org).

1.1.3 Will genomics have an impact on clinical and pharmaceutical medicine?

At present, published opinions concerning the success of applying genomic sequencing data to produce new drugs – indeed how important the data will be to clinical medicine in general – range from deep scepticism [4] to a call to "wake up and get ready" [1], with a heavy emphasis on the latter position.

1.2   The need for new ideas in drug development

Both ends of this scientific opinion spectrum agree on one basic fact: there is a need for new ideas in pharmaceutical development. Despite the increasing intensity of drug development efforts throughout the world, some challenges must be faced concerning the efficacy of established drugs and the development of efficacious new ones. The facts are these:

- On average, for each specific drug treatment, less than 50% of patients experience a benefit (for example, it has been stated that 35% of people do not respond to β-blockers and as many as 50% do not respond to tricyclic antidepressants).
- Although accurate quantitative figures are controversial [5–9] there is general agreement that a large number of patients who take prescribed drugs have severe adverse drug reactions (ADRs) [10, 11].
- According to one estimate [5], drug-related side-effects were between the fourth and sixth leading cause of death in the United States in 1997–about 106,000 deaths that year–and nothing has reduced these figures since.
- It has been reported that 30–50% of pharmacies dispense drugs with interactions that could be life-threatening or life-altering without warning to patient or prescriber.
- ADRs are a major cause for removing prescribed drugs from the market [12]. In developing new drugs, costs per compound typically run at $7 million in phase I, but jump to $43 million in phase III; abandoning an unpromising or dangerous compound at the earlier phase of development could save a pharmaceutical company $36 million per drug.

Not all directions are negative in bringing efficacious drugs to market and having them stay there:

- Many technical developments (e.g., combinatorial libraries, computer docking models, high-throughput screening, etc.) have led to an increase in the number of compounds under development for drug use. For exam-

9

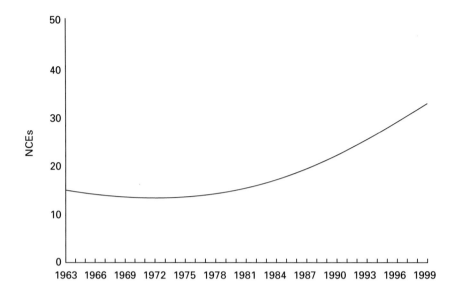

Fig. 1
New chemical entity (NCE) approvals in the United States from 1963 to 1999 as a quadratic fit to raw annual approval data. Adapted from [14].

ple, between 1995 and 1999, the number of compounds increased by 35% to 7434 [13].

- In the United States, several years following the 1962 Amendments to the Federal Food, Drug and Cosmetic Act of 1938, the number of NCEs (New Chemical Entities) approvals began to rise (Fig. 1). This upturn is likely to be due to a combination of the technical developments, such as those just cited, with governmental and economic changes [14].
- Following the Prescription Drug User Fee Act (PUDFA) of 1992 in the United States, drug approval times have fallen (Fig. 2) [15].
- Viewed by therapeutic classes, there is a variation in clinical phase times between the first half of the 1990s to the second half [15] (Fig. 3) with significant drops in the times for AIDS antiviral, antiinfective, anticancer, and respiratory classes, respectively, along with modest increases for CNS, endocrine, anesthetic/analgesic and cardiovascular classes, respectively.

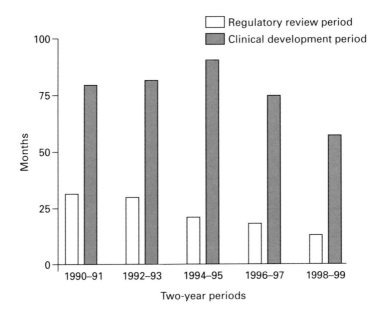

Fig. 2
Mean clinical development period [time from the date of investigational new drug application (IND) file to the date of new drug application (NDA)] and the mean regulatory review period [time from NDA submission to approval] after the PUDFA in five two-year periods. Adapted from [15].

On balance, despite these positive developments, the rate at which approved new drugs are entering clinical use is falling, and has been for some time: during the period 1995–99, the number of new product launches declined 22% to 56, and at an estimated cost of $500 million Research and Development cost per drug [13]. Between 1961 and 1995, 131 approved drugs were withdrawn from the market in western European countries and the United States because of severe ADRs [16]. This is in the face of the fact that, compared to 20 years ago, a growing proportion of drugs is being prescribed and used long-term for treating chronic conditions, thus requiring the drugs to be free of side-effects [13].

To accomplish the aims of this chapter, recent results bearing on a few important medical areas – asthma and its treatment, the responses of humans to glucocorticoids, and the roles of drug-clearing enzymes – will be used as illustrations of some of the opportunities and some of the problems associ-

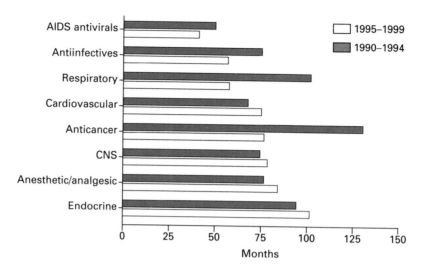

Fig. 3
Mean clinical phase for NCEs approved in 1990–94 and 1995–99, grouped by therapeutic class. Adapted from [15].

ated with producing individual medicine. However, it will be useful to begin by briefly reviewing how the relation between genes and health or disease are currently regarded in biomedical science.

2   Viewpoints on health and disease

2.1   Theoretical basis for "individual medicine"

The underlying reason why the belief in the future of individual medicine has taken such a hold on projections about the future of drug research is what may be termed a "genetocentric" viewpoint of human biology – one that permeates contemporary biological and medical thinking.

This genetocentric viewpoint is bolstered by a belief that the increasingly powerful technological tools becoming available to molecular geneticists will solve all technical problems. In this chapter, the further development of these tools is taken for granted. However, the genetocentric viewpoint is not taken for granted and its background, basis, and implications for development of individual medicine is examined using some specific recent examples.

2.1.1 The genetocentric viewpoint of health and disease

The genetocentric viewpoint is based on the reductionist concept of an organism as an automatic control entity. This idea, that organisms are controlled by instructions encoded into their genomes, has been a powerful influence in the explosive development of molecular biology and, up to now, on hopes for decisive clinical applications of genetic discoveries. According to a strict interpretation of this viewpoint, organisms are no different from subtle machines: the whole is the sum of its parts (in physical terms, organisms are "linear systems") which are arranged in such a way that an internal energy source can move them in accordance with a built-in program of purposeful action – a program encoded in the genome of each individual organism.

From the genetocentric viewpoint, prediction of health, diagnosis of disease, and targeting of drugs should largely be attainable from genomic information.

In an influential article about the Human Genome Project, the Head of the National Institutes of Health's effort, Francis Collins, stated the genetocentric case succinctly, "Largely, but not entirely, at the behest of our genes, we fare better or worse." [17].

Yet, it is a universally acknowledged fact that life expectancy in wealthy countries has increased greatly in the past century, and clearly this increase could not be due to genetic factors. This fact has led many to speculate that environmental factors are of equal or greater importance to human health than is genetic makeup. Despite some dissenting arguments of this sort, it is widely accepted in both the scientific and lay communities that advances in molecular biology corroborate Collins's claim: the idea that, in principle, organisms are no more than complicated physical systems and therefore biological principles can be reduced to physical and chemical laws.

Probably many (if not most) scientists, physical and biological alike, regard philosophical concepts like reductionism as woolly-minded and having little application to their work or to the practical implications of molecular genetics, especially in medicine. The immense outpouring of literature within the last two years on the implications of the results of current genetic research – particularly those stemming from the human genome projects – for the future of drug development and treatment largely assumes that it will be based on the genetic diversity of individuals as revealed by their individual genomic sequences.

But there is an alternate view of the nature of organisms that, while accepting the importance of the information contained in their genomes, looks at health and disease differently.

2.1.2 The epigenetic viewpoint of health and disease

This is an anti-reductionist viewpoint and contends that molecular genetics cannot explain all, or even the most important, aspects of living forms. Leaving aside the faith-based aspects of this view, there is increasing evidence and awareness that living processes all take place in a cellular environment and that this fact may largely influence the applications of ideas based strictly on genetic results.

Recently, this viewpoint – that living systems are non-linear ones – has come to be expressed with increasing frequency [18, 19] as new evidence mounts indicating that reductionism is not adequate to describe their health or diseases. Pertinent to the present topic, this viewpoint questions whether analysis of disease on the basis of single SNP, or even single gene, causality can be expected to help in the development of new drugs [19].

As discussed in the next section, evidence of this nature was first noticed by cell biologists but has recently been advanced in another context.

2.2 Cytoplasmic inheritance and epigenetics

As a background to understanding the consequences of the assumption that individualized drug treatments will be a necessary outcome of accurate sequencing of the human genome, this section includes a brief discussion of some often overlooked experiments in cell biology.

2.2.1 Cytoplasmic inheritance

In an elegant series of experiments performed over 30 years ago on ciliated paramecia, Sonneborn and collaborators first showed that the form and arrangement of preexisting parental cilia determine the form and arrangement of the new cilia on their progeny [20]. The cilia are small "hairs" that are the locomotive organelles for the cells (mostly, they use them to swim toward food). On a molecular level, cilia are structurally complex although constructed mainly from proteins. The distribution of cilia on a cell varies among different taxonomic groups.

The architectural complexity of ciliates sets them apart from mammalian cells because besides being cells, they are complete, independent organisms. Adaptations to particular habitats over evolutionary time have resulted in both intracellular and extracellular structures seldom, if ever, found in higher eukaryotic cells. On the other hand, the metabolic pathways known for these animals are essentially no different from those found in other eukaryotic cells and they have been studied as good models for higher eukaryotic cells.

Asexual reproduction is the norm for ciliates: it involves nuclear division followed by binary fission of the cell that produces two identical daughter cells that each share some of the parental cytoplasm.

Work by Frankel on the ciliate *Tetrahymena pyriformis* [21] has given the most easily illustrated experimental results on the nongenetic inheritance of structural forms. *Tetrahymena* has its cilia arranged in rows that have a definite orientation along the longitudinal axis of the cell (Fig. 4). The motion of these cilia allow the cells to swim in more or less straight lines. Frankel used micromanipulation techniques on single cells to invert the orientation of one or more rows of their cilia by 180° with respect to the rest of the rows. After the operation, their swimming patterns were changed but the altered *Tetrahymena* could survive perfectly well and were allowed to divide normally.

In typical experiments, the swimming and ciliary patterns of the progeny *Tetrahymena* were observed over hundreds of cell divisions. These experiments showed that the inverted rows were perpetuated over those generations and passed on to all progeny, directly demonstrating the stability and determinism of a structural intracellular rearrangement in the absence of differences in genes or gene action. Occasionally, the "mutant" cells' cilial patterns reverted to normal after some generations, but the fastest reversions took 30–40 cell generations, during which they transmitted the variant organization of their cilia to a billion to a trillion progeny cells.

These cell biological experiments do not mean that genes play an unimportant role in cell organization: genes are, of course, needed to make the macromolecules that make the altered structures that are perpetuated. But the

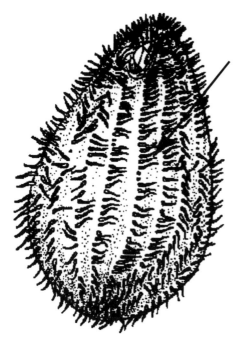

Normally, the rows of cilia work together to rhythmically propel the cell in one direction. When one or more rows are reoriented 180 degrees from normal, the cell's swimming pattern is altered. This allows easy visual detection of cells with reoriented rows.

Fig. 4
Sketch of cilia in *Tetrahymena pyriformis*. Adapted from [21].

experiments raise some important points about cell replication in higher organisms – points that are often forgotten in genetocentric thinking.

The main point is that subcellular structures and organelles are not assembled in a vacuum, but in a structured cellular environment, the molecules of which are an essential part of a cell's means for locating, orienting and patterning new molecular structures or assemblies of molecules. The experiments just described show that physical interactions between existing structures and newly synthesized ones may result in hereditary extragenetic variations.

Thus, not only protein structures may be passed along to progeny extragenetically (as is the case for prions). The "blueprints" (i.e., information) for the cellular construction of complex structures made from multiple proteins can be passed to progeny as well.

The concept of non-genetically determined interacting signaling pathways has also been applied to human disease.

2.2.2 Epigenetics

The existence of non-genomic interactive networks in cells such as those described in the previous section is at the core of the epigenetic viewpoint. This viewpoint has recently been reviewed [19, 22]. Epigenetic ideas about regulation in cells and organisms emphasize the dependency of organisms on environments and the adaptive variations possible when are respond to environmental changes. Recently, an entire issue of the journal *Science* was devoted to a review of epigenetics. The electronic edition of the journal (http://www.sciencemag.org/feature/plus/sfg/resources/res_epigenetics.shtml) contains many connecting links to sites offering publications and information on epigenetics.

In epigenetic regulation, large networks of intracellular genes, gene products and groups of cells such as tissues and organs all absorb environmental signals and are active in producing adaptive behavior. These networks may seek out new pathways of response to varying inputs. The process is analogous to what is found in cell populations, in neural network activity, and in physiological organ system feedback interactions of diverse descriptions. It is a concept of organism based on past, conserved genetic adaptation coupled with current epigenetic regulation. Most importantly, it is a concept that attempts to integrate biology with molecular biology.

In epigenetics, genetic and higher-order networks operating within environmental limits defined during evolution determine healthy behavioral outcome, not single genes. On the other hand, when the world presents epigenetic information for which the genome and its interactive epigenetic network have no adequate response – for example, an overly oxidative environment – the result is maladaptation, regressive-state change in cell behavior and, finally, end-state disease. In this viewpoint, disease is a result of the organism's frustrated attempts to adapt phenotypically to a hostile environment or set of elements for which there is no adequate response basis.

In epigenetics, responses to environmental change may be seen as analogous to the functioning of the world-wide web (the Internet). The original intention in the development of the Internet was to allow military information transfer in the United States to take place even when some information relay points had been destroyed by enemy attack. The Internet was designed to allow packets, containing parts of the total message, to be transferred over varying routes and to be re-directed when some "nodes" (computer relay points) are overloaded or non-functional. The packets are reassembled into the whole message at their final destination. Only in the cases of massive overload or destruction of the web does the system irreversibly break down.

Further underlying the epigenetic viewpoint is a model that predates molecular biology. It holds that evolution selects not single genes but genetic interaction [18, 23]. In this model, it is the physiological product of many genes interacting with one another, with many gene products and with environmental and developmental signals that provides advantage in, and is selected during, evolution.

In the epigenetic viewpoint, it would be very difficult, in cases where phenotype is clearly polygenic, to identify a particular single gene or even a set of genes that would always produce the same outcome, even under identical environmental circumstances. If one or a few genes, each with small effect, were deleted in an interactive network, one would expect multiple rearrangements of the entire network. In slightly differing circumstances, therefore, these rearrangements have some ability to produce adaptive phenotypes.

If there is even partial validity to the epigenetic viewpoint, there are broad implications concerning drug development. The main implication is that even in the case of monogenic diseases, targeting even the most efficacious drug to one gene or one gene product, may not suffice to either alleviate the disease or prevent ADRs. So the question immediately arises: Is there evidence for the validity of the epigenetic viewpoint of the organism in human disease?

2.2.3 Single- and multi-genic disease

Contemporary genetic research has been extremely successful in identifying the mutated genes for monogenic diseases and familial hypercholesteremia was one of the first to be identified. It furnishes a good example of the possible role of epigenetic concepts in how disease should be regarded.

Familial hypercholesterolemia arises from mutations in the low density lipoprotein receptor gene, carries an increased risk of coronary heart disease, and is one of the commonest autosomal dominant disorders with over 600 known genetic variants. But even for this monogenic disease, the relation between genotype and phenotype appears to be modified both by other genes and environmental effects. In a recent study [24] carried out in the

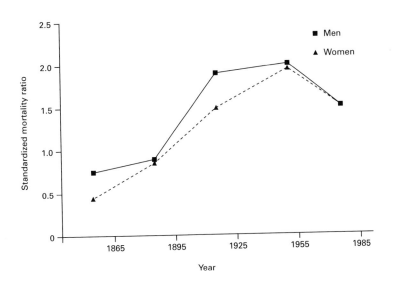

Fig. 5
Mortality from familial hypercholesterolemia according to sex and time. Adapted from [24].

Netherlands using historical records and designed to estimate all-cause mortality from untreated familial hypercholesterolemia free from selection for coronary artery disease, it was found that risk of death varies significantly among patients with the disease. The study concluded that the large variability in risk of mortality over time and between branches of the pedigree points to a strong interaction with environmental factors (Fig. 5). In fact, the mortality in the pedigree did not differ significantly from national rates until early in the 20th century. The importance of environmental factors in familial hypercholesterolemia has been found in other studies from the United States [25] and Finland [26].

The overall conclusion from these studies is that even in monogenic disease, other genes and the environment can be important and must be taken into account in risk analysis and clinical treatment of patients.

Furthermore, while new monogenic diseases are being discovered with increasing frequency and reported with much publicity, they affect only small segments of the population – altogether they have a frequency of about 2% of live births [27]. Also, there is no evidence that major diseases like cancers, diabetes and cardiovascular disease result from either single-gene mutations or any other unitary cause. On the contrary, it is believed that the major human diseases are polygenic, have environmental determinants, and that the mechanisms of these diseases cannot be analyzed by a strictly genetic approach [18, 28].

Reductionism as currently applied to medicine asserts that, while they may have an environmental component, monogenic diseases such as hypercholesterolemia and more complex ones all have separate genetic components that can be discovered and used to pursue treatment strategies. This linear view of gene-disease causality thus finds itself in serious debate with a significant amount of evidence supporting the epigenetic viewpoint which sees complex traits, including disease, as highly interactive and impossible to separate into genetic components.

To understand how interactive networks may affect drug developments and treatments, we need to review what is currently known about drugs and the genome.

3 Drugs and human genomics

Under most current proposals to implement individual medicine, drug developers would apply SNP data for the human genome to identify affected genes and their variant proteins as drug targets. Thus, global attention has been forcefully directed toward building SNP databases and developing cost-effective haplotyping strategies for humans. The complexities associated with SNP-based drug development are just beginning to be realized.

3.1 An abbreviated history of pharmacogenomics

In the published literature, two terms describing individual responses to drugs – "pharmacogenetics" and "pharmacogenomics" – have often been used interchangeably or in confusing ways. Traditionally, pharmacogenetics has been defined as the study of the linkage between an individual's genotype and his or her ability to metabolize a foreign compound, while pharmacogenomics is a broader study of the identity of the genes or loci responsible for different individuals' different responses to a drug. Since the two studies are growing closer together and their molecular basis – genetic variation – is the same, it seems redundant to use them both. In this chapter we will use pharmacogenomics as the umbrella term covering both genetic variations that affect drug metabolism and drug targeting.

3.1.1 Drugs and ethnicity

At the start of the discussion a social-political problem needs to be addressed.

Some opinions concerning the applications of human genetics to individual medicine have attempted to draw a clear distinction between genetic studies that identify ethnic groups who are at risk for specific diseases and genetic studies that identify individuals who may respond differently to the same drug used to treat their disease [29]. As will be described below, this ignores the fact that individual responses to drug treatments were first observed and reported on the basis of ethnicity [30]. The quality of recent quantitative studies [31] of human genetic variation indicates that a good description of the structure of human variation across populations and genomic regions could be available in the short term. However, the same studies emphasize that ethnic variations in genetic diversity are large and cannot be accounted for by the neutral model [32, 33]. The question is whether or not worldwide public opinion will allow these differences to be uncovered on a large scale and used as a basis for clinical treatments.

Attempts to dissociate ethnicity from drug development and treatment are understandable but unrealistic. Genetic testing has become highly controversial because of its social, economic and political implications. Altruistically, one would hope that this would not complicate the use of human genetics to develop healing treatments. Unfortunately, the political history of the last part of the twentieth century and continuing to the present tells us that all ethnically linked medicine becomes controversial and pharmacogenomics will be no exception.

3.1.2 Ethical considerations

Nor should the ethical problems associated with gathering data for pharmacogenomic purposes be ignored [34]. For example, the controversy resulting from the proposed formation and uses of the Icelandic Health Sector Database has been reviewed [35–37] and similar databases have been proposed for the United Kingdom [38, 39]. Development and use of databases consisting of individuals' genetic data may seem logical to drug researchers and pharmaceutical firms [40], but may not seem so even to individuals who might ultimately benefit from the use of the data.

3.2   Metabolic pharmacogenomics

In humans, variations in clinical responses to drugs began to be observed in the 1950s. These included:

- inherited ethnic differences in hemolysis after average primaquine doses used in antimalarial therapy [30] where the differences are associated with differences in erythrocyte glucose-6-phosphate dehydrogenase activities [41];
- inherited differences in rates of acetylation of the drug isoniazid [42];
- the association of prolonged apnea that sometimes occurred after administration of the muscle relaxant, suxamethonium chloride (succinyl chloride), with levels of plasma pseudocholinesterase [43].

In retrospect, these results are not terribly surprising in light of data from the late 1930s showing that sometimes different strains of animals of the same species differ enormously in their responses to drugs [44].

At about the same time as human variations in drug responses were first observed – that is, at the dawning of the molecular genetic age – drug-metabolizing enzymes, present in all eukaryotic cells (but first identified in hepatocytes) began to be identified. Genetically derived variations in these enzymes' activities were soon suggested to be the cause of some ADRs [45].

Cytochromes P450 (members of the CYP superfamily) came to be identified as "detoxification" proteins and the study of P450 enzymes and their genetic variations became central to what was called "pharmacogenetics" [46–48].

From results of rapid advances in the technology of gene sequencing, it is now clear that SNPs exist in most, if not all, CYP isozymes, but that the majority of the polymorphisms exist in four CYPs and that these four are responsible for about 40% of all drug metabolism mediated by CYP isozymes. We will return to this subject later.

3.3 What is the extent of human genomic heterozygosity?

As more genes have been sequenced, it has become apparent that genomic DNA polymorphisms in individuals are far more common than was believed even 10 years ago. In effect, this has blurred the distinction between mutations and polymorphisms. Because of the redundancy of the genetic code, many of these SNPs result in no primary sequence alterations in the proteins the genes encode. However, some SNPs (missense variants) do result in changes in protein primary sequences that may increase, decrease, abolish, or have no effect upon the protein's function. The structures of these proteins would have to be determined or predicted accurately for them to furnish potential drug targets. Even more recently, it has become clear that many SNPs occur in promoter regions where they affect expression levels of gene products.

We now summarize and compare the available data on heterozygosity estimates for the human genome.

3.3.1 Results from the human genome projects

Before actual sequencing results were available, widely quoted estimates of human genome-wide nucleotide diversity were about one SNP for every 1000 base-pairs [31, 49]. A standard estimate for the average size of a human protein is 300–400 amino acids. This corresponds to a total transcript length of approximately 1.2–1.5 kb and leads to a prediction of 1–2 SNPs per total exon content of an average human gene.

Using statistical methods, an estimation of nucleotide diversity from ascertained SNPs has been made from the private draft sequence of the human genome [50]. Several features were reported:

- Agreement with the previous estimates of nucleotide diversity of about 1 SNP per 1000 base-pairs.

- 75% of the SNPs found are intergenic.
- Considerable unexplainable variability of SNP density across the human genome exists and G + C content accounts for only a small part of the variation.
- Based on sequences of 10,239 known genes, missense SNPs are only about 0.12% of the total SNP count and of these, only 47% are radical protein changes (the meaning of radical changes is discussed below in Section 3.2.3).
- The results from the National Institutes of Health draft sequence [51] are in qualitative agreement with those from the private study, at least for estimates of nucleotide diversity. However, the authors don't make estimates of the frequency of potential protein structural changes.
- A total of about 35,000 protein-encoding genes in humans was predicted.

Some of these observations would be likely to have a significant impact on the use of drugs to treat disease.

- The variable SNP density makes it important to identify "hot-spots" in DNA encoding proteins involved in drug-responsiveness because the particular proteins will be the most likely to vary in a population.
- The low frequency of differences in protein activities due to SNPs seemingly presents the possibilities of favorable practical outcomes from pharmacogenomics developments as much more promising because of the decreased likelihood of multiple protein activity changes in drug response and metabolic pathways.
- Optimism about the promise of individual medicine is also based on reasoning that the smaller number of protein differences defining individual responses to drugs may also mean that targeting drugs to non-variable proteins could result in more uniform responses in populations.

In summary, drawing high-resolution conclusions on the basis of the draft sequences is currently risky [52]. Even the number of genes encoded by the human genome – one of the most widely publicized original conclusions – is in dispute [53] at the time of writing.

The primary reason for not weighting the results of the draft sequences of the whole genome too heavily when discussing SNPs is one that has not been widely commented on: both draft sequences are based on DNA obtained from only a few anonymous subjects (< 10 in each case). In the private project, the selected donors were two males and three females, including one African-American, one Asian (Chinese), one "Hispanic-Mexican," and two Caucasians. For the NIH Project, the eight libraries used all derived from male DNA, ethnic mix not stated. Indeed, it is widely believed that, because of political considerations, the NIH is very reluctant to deal with the ethnic component of genomic diversity.

These facts are important because conclusions drawn concerning human genetic diversity on the basis of such small samples are statistically unreliable. Also, as discussed in the next section, the results from the Genome Projects do not agree well in some important details with the results of a recent but smaller-scale sequencing project that was specifically designed to investigate the impact of ethnicity on genomic diversity [54].

3.3.2 SNP evidence from direct sequencing

The result of a project of significance to future efforts in the pharmacogenomics area of drug development has been recently reported. This study [54] undertook a systematic discovery of gene-based sequence variation in 82 unrelated individuals, whose ancestors were from various geographical origins. The sample size and composition were sufficient to detect, with high certainty, globally distributed variants present at a frequency of at least 2% and population-specific variants present at a frequency of at least 5%. The population sample, using the definitions of the U.S. Census Bureau, included an approximately equal number of self-described Caucasians, African-Americans, Asians, and Hispanic-Latinos. The project's goal was to identify SNPs and to organize them into their gene-specific allelic haplotypes.

The exons (coding regions, 5'UTR and 3'UTR), up to 100 bases into the introns from the exon-intron boundaries (including the splice junctions), and the 5' upstream genomic regions were sequenced for 313 genes. These genes were chosen from ones for which complete genomic organization is publicly available. To assist in assessing the quality of the sequence information and to validate the construction of haplotypes, a three-generation Caucasian family and a two-generation African-American family were included. For evolutionary comparisons, the corresponding genomic regions from a chimpanzee were sequenced but will not be discussed here.

Table 1.
Nucleotide diversity estimates from the Human Genome Project draft sequences and a previous estimate.

Source	$\pi_{av} \times 10^4$	SNP/kb
[50]	8.98	1113
[51]	7.51	1331
[54]	5.8	1724
prev. estimate [31]	8	1250

Nucleotide sequence variation is conventionally estimated using a normalized measure of heterozygosity (π), representing the likelihood that a nucleotide position will be heterozygous when compared across two chromosomes selected randomly from a population. Table 1 gives the results from the three sequencing efforts discussed here [50, 51, 54] and a previous estimate [31].

For π, the results from the three recent sequencing studies agree reasonably well with previous estimates of about 1 SNP for every 1000 kb surveyed in two human chromosomes.

However, more detailed analysis of the results available from sequencing in the study of 313 human genes [54] reveals another scenario. This may be taken to be predictive of the results for similar analyses of the whole genomes of different individuals. Figures 6 A, B summarize some of these detailed results.

Figure 6 (A) shows that about 33% of the SNPs found were found in all four populations and that the number of population-specific SNPs for the African-American population was almost three times higher than the next highest figure (for Asians). Figure 6 (B) shows that the population distribution of haplotypes was similar to the population distribution of SNPs.

Other highly significant genetic conclusions from this study were:

- An average of about 12.7 SNPs and 14 different haplotypes per gene were observed.
- A significant fraction (48%) of population-specific haplotypes was seen only in the African-American sample.
- Many genes did not have one predominant haplotype and for 35% of the genes, no single haplotype had a frequency $\geq$ 50%. This indicates that the idea that there is one predominant "wild-type" form of a gene and various

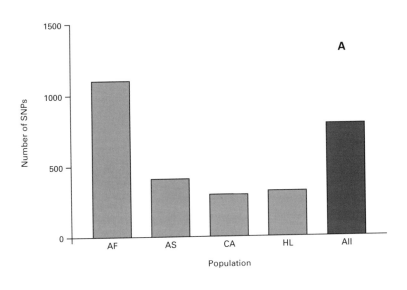

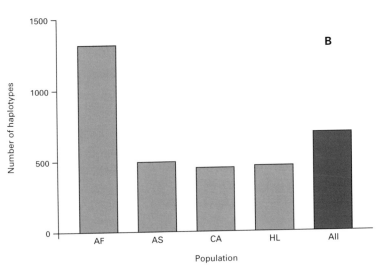

Fig. 6
(A) The distribution of total SNPs in 313 genes among population samples. The gray bars show the number of SNPs that are variable in each population, the black bar shows the number of SNPs that are variable in all four populations(B) The distribution of total haplotypes in 313 genes among population samples. The gray bars show the number of haplotypes that are variable in each population, the black bar shows the number of haplotypes variable in all four populations. Population codes are AF, African-American; AS, Asian; CA, Caucasian; HL, Hispanic-Latino; All, all four populations. Adapted from [54].

27

other rare or "mutant" forms is misleading. Instead, there are multiple haplotypes, each of which are observed in multiple populations and which account for a large fraction of human variability.

- Complex or unknown patterns of human migration and evolution complicate the distribution and interpretation of human genomic variation.
- The average number of polymorphic sites per kilobase of DNA found was 3.4 in the coding regions, 5.3 in the 5'UTR, 5.9 in the 5' upstream region, 6.5 in the exon-intron boundaries, and 7.0 in the 3'UTR, results that also differ from those found from the Human Genome Project data.
- The pattern of variation reflects the recent expansion of the human population.

Focusing on the impact these conclusions will have on pharmacogenomics:

- On average, there are many more SNPs and haplotypes per gene than previously predicted or estimated from the draft sequences of the human genome.
- There are large ethnic variations in genomic diversity.
- There is no "wild-type" human genome.
- The changes in population and distribution of individuals are changing the patterns of genetic diversity.
- Haplotypes generally supply more information on heterozygosity than individual SNPs.
- Of the polymorphic sites within the coding regions (about 30% of the total sites found), about 50% coded for an amino acid change of which 42% were essentially conservative, and 12% essentially radical.

3.3.3 Conservative and radical changes in polypeptides

Predictions of functional changes in proteins due to amino acid substitutions are currently more an art than a science. This situation stems from a lack of experimental structural data on substituted proteins to back up the predictions. In an attempt to determine which substitutions could be important, an integration of several chemical properties of residues – their chemical properties, polarities, and molecular volumes – has been made [55]. This integration comprises one of the few tools currently available to predict structural variations in residue-substituted proteins. Table 2 summarizes this effort: the

Table 2.
Chemical "distances" between amino acid pairs used in predicting conservative to radical changes in protein structures due to amino acid substitutions of one member of a pair by another. Adapted from [55].

	Arg	Leu	Pro	Thr	Ala	Val	Gly	Ile	Phe	Tyr	Cys	His	Gln	Asn	Lys	Asp	Glu	Met	Trp
Ser	110	145	74	58	99	124	56	142	155	144	112	89	68	46	121	65	80	135	177
Arg		102	103	71	112	96	125	97	97	77	180	29	43	86	26	96	54	91	101
Leu			98	92	96	32	138	5	22	36	198	99	113	153	107	172	138	15	61
Pro				38	27	68	42	95	114	110	169	77	76	91	103	108	93	87	147
Thr					58	69	59	89	103	92	149	47	42	65	78	85	65	81	128
Ala						64	60	94	113	112	195	86	91	111	106	126	107	84	148
Val							109	29	50	55	192	84	96	133	97	152	121	21	88
Gly								135	153	147	159	98	87	80	127	94	98	127	184
Ile									21	33	198	94	109	149	102	168	134	10	61
Phe										22	205	100	116	158	102	177	140	28	40
Tyr											194	83	99	143	85	160	122	36	37
Cys												174	154	139	202	154	170	196	215
His													24	68	32	81	40	87	115
Gln														46	53	61	29	101	130
Asn															94	23	42	142	174
Lys																101	56	95	110
Asp																	45	160	181
Glu																		126	152
Met																			67

Table 3.

Categories of amino acid substitutions based on chemical distances, D, between pairs of residues. Adapted from [56].

Descriptor of structural effect	D value (Tab. 2)
Conservative	$0 < D \leq 50$
Moderately conservative	$51 < D \leq 100$
Moderately radical	$101 < D \leq 150$
Radical	$D > 151$

Table presents values of a parameter (D) for amino acid pairs and D is interpreted as a "chemical distance" between pairs. The D values have been further broken down somewhat arbitrarily into categories that express in words the dissimilarities between the chemical characteristics at each substitution site [56]. Table 3 gives these categories.

This categorization is, at best, only moderately convincing. For example, the SNP which converts hemoglobin A (HbA) to hemoglobin S (HbS, Gluβ6 → Val), resulting in a medically significant change in the properties of the blood containing large amounts of HbS (sickle cell hemoglobin) instead of HbA, would be classified as "moderately radical" according to Table 3. On the other hand, many HbA variants resulting from single amino acid substitutions are functionally unchanged, even though the substitution is in the same moderately radical category. The conclusion is that it is currently very difficult to predict functional changes in proteins from missense codon substitutions.

The result of applying these amino acid classifications to the proteins encoded by the 313 genes is shown in Table 4.

Clearly, there is a greater frequency of SNP-encoded amino acid substitutions that might lead to variant protein functions than were found from preliminary analyses of the draft sequences of the genome. This means that more quantitative structural and biochemical functional analyses than previously estimated would have to be performed before variant proteins could be regarded as drug targets.

3.3.4 Summary of preliminary SNP work

Problems associated with pharmacogenomics based purely on SNP data are just beginning to be realized. Much effort is being expended on building SNP

Table 4.
Coding region SNP consequences on amino acid substitutions.

Type of amino acid change	(%)
None	44.4
Conservative/moderately conservative	42.8
Moderately radical/radical	11.9
To stop codon	0.9

None means a silent nucleotide substitution. Change types categorized according to Grantham [55] values as: conservative/moderately conservative < 100, moderately radical/radical > 101. Adapted from [54].

databases and developing cost-effective genotyping strategies, while little regard is given to the matters of complexity, functionality, utility, and ethnic diversity of genetic associations revealed in patient populations.

By focusing on diversity in one gene – the one encoding the β_2-adrenergic receptor (β_2-AR) – instead of 313 different genes, a recent study [57] illustrates what efforts may be needed to uncover associations between genetic variants and drug response. Preceded by background on the clinical problem, we turn to a discussion of that study in the next section.

4 The molecular genetics of asthma

4.1 Asthma, the disease

In light of the discussion just presented, asthma serves as a good exemplar of the problems facing the application of pharmacogenomics to clinical medicine:

- Asthma affects 5 to 7 percent of the population of North America and may affect 150 million or more individuals worldwide [58, 59]. It is one of the most common and economically burdensome chronic diseases. However, a clear definition of the disease is lacking and no single symptom, physical finding or laboratory test serves to diagnose asthma.
- Only a few new therapeutic agents based on novel mechanisms of action have been developed over the last two decades. In addition, there is no evidence that morbidity and mortality are decreasing.

- Since asthma is often triggered by an allergic response, the environmental milieu of patient populations can play a significant role in expression of the disease.
- The varied clinical presentations of asthma have led to the concept that there may be multiple asthmatic phenotypes, which adds to the complexity of genetic studies.
- The varied clinical presentations of asthma have led to the belief that there may well be a multigenic component to the disease.
- Even though asthma has long been recognized as having a significant heritable component, genetic studies have been difficult to perform and the results have been difficult to interpret, although an increasingly large amount of conventional genetic data is now being accumulated.

4.2 Drug treatment for asthma

Ephedrine, obtainable from plants of the genus *Ephedra*, particularly the Chinese species *E. sinica*, has been used in China for more than 5,000 years to treat asthma and hay fever. This drug initiates its actions on cells by binding to the β_2-AR.

About 60 to 70 percent of patients diagnosed with asthma have mild disease for which a variety of synthetic agonists to the β_2-AR, introduced over 35 years ago and which revolutionized the treatment of asthma, suffice today. However, that leaves the treatment of millions of patients with more severe asthma subject to ongoing controversy about treatment with agonists which sometimes have very adverse effects [60].

The β_2-AR is a member of the G protein-coupled receptor superfamily that mediate the actions of catecholamines in many tissues. The β_2-AR expressed on bronchial smooth muscle acts to relax contracted muscle, resulting in bronchodilation, and beta agonists are the most effective acute treatment for reversal of bronchospasm in asthma. The bronchodilating response to beta agonists is known to exhibit significant inter-individual variation [58] and reports have been recently been published reporting on, and speculating on, the role of SNPs in responses of the β_2-AR to agonists used in asthma treatments [61, 62].

For future reference in section 6 of this chapter: much of the research on asthma has involved traditional animal models of asthma, inbred animal models of hyperreactivity, and genetically altered mice. Most researchers in this area regard transgenic and gene-knockout mice as powerful tools for probing the mechanisms of disease. The strategy has been to use mouse models, when candidate genes for asthma are identified, in assessing the role of a given pathway in the pathogenesis of asthma.

As a major clinical problem and the object of intense past drug development efforts, asthma affords a good example of how molecular genetics might affect future efforts. A recent landmark paper [57] describes the haplotypes in the gene encoding the β_2-AR.

4.3 The genome and asthma

4.3.1 SNPs in the β_2-AR gene

The sequence variations in the gene were studied in a multiethnic population consisting of Caucasian, African-American, Asian, and Hispanic-Latino groups, and associations of the haplotypes found with bronchodilating responses to the agonist, albuterol, in asthmatics were studied [57].

The control sequencing data were gathered from an index repository of apparently normal individuals. This repository consisted of 23 Caucasians, 19 African-Americans, 20 Asians, and 15 Hispanic/Latinos. This number of individuals in each ethnic group provided for a > 90% probability of detecting a SNP with an allele frequency between 0.05 (Caucasian group) and 0.08 (Hispanic-Latino group). To determine whether haplotypes of the β_2-AR gene were associated with the bronchodilatory response to the agonist albuterol, 121 Caucasian patients with asthma, enrolled from an outpatient facility, were used.

From sequencing, 13 SNPs organized into 12 haplotypes within a span of 1.6 kb were identified in the β_2-AR gene. Taken at face value, this is a promising result with respect to drug targeting: if SNPs were distributed randomly in individuals at a frequency of one SNP per kb of DNA, the number of different SNP combinations over a haplotype could be large – $2^{\#SNPs}$ – which in this case corresponds to $2^{13} = 8,192$ possible combinations. The actual number of haplotypes comprise only a fraction of this – a result that seems to be the general pattern for genes that have been investigated so far. This has been used as evidence to predict that haplotype blocks may be at least 10 times longer than

Table 5.
Localization of SNPs and identification of haplotypes of the β_2-AR. Adapted from [57].

SNP Position	–1023	–709	–654	–468	–406	–367	–47	–20	46	79	252	491	523
Alleles:	G/A	C/A	G/A	C/G	C/T	T/C	T/C	T/C	G/A	C/G	G/A	C/T	C/A
Haplotype													
1	A	C	G	C	C	T	T	T	A	C	G	C	C
2	A	C	G	G	C	C	C	C	G	G	G	C	C
3	G	A	A	C	C	T	T	T	A	C	G	C	C
4	G	C	A	C	C	T	T	T	A	C	G	C	C
5	G	C	A	C	C	T	T	T	G	C	G	C	C
6	G	C	G	C	C	T	T	T	G	C	A	C	A
7	G	C	G	C	C	T	T	T	G	C	A	T	A
8	G	C	A	C	C	T	T	T	A	C	A	C	C
9	A	C	G	C	T	T	T	T	A	C	G	C	C
10	G	C	G	C	C	T	T	T	G	C	A	C	C
11	G	C	G	C	C	T	T	T	G	C	G	C	C
12	A	C	G	G	C	T	T	T	A	C	G	C	C
Location:	5′	5′	5′	5′	5′	5′	*	5′	**	***	silent	****	silent

Nucleotide numbers are relative to the start codon at position + 1. Allele refers to the two nucleotide possibilities at each SNP position; 5′ means 5′ upstream of the β_2-AR open reading frame; *Cys/Arg substitution; **Gly/Arg substitution; ***Gln/Glu substitution; ****Thr/Ile substitution.

had been previously predicted, so that sequences as long as 50,000 bases may contain small numbers of haplotype blocks that would account for variations in these genes in 80–90% of the population [63]. The results of the study under discussion here are contrary to this expectation. For the β_2-AR gene, and by extension to other genes, the actual case is much more complicated.

Tables 5 and 6 show the haplotype blocks found and their frequencies. Examination of Table 5 shows that no individual SNP serves to adequately predict a haplotype. Thus, it would be hazardous to select an individual SNP as a marker for a haplotype in this case. That conclusion may hold true in general. This would enormously complicate identification of haplotypes.

4.3.2 SNPs in the β_2-AR gene; clinical correlates

Using a cohort of 121 Caucasians diagnosed with asthma, the work under discussion was extended to an examination of the predictive value of the SNPs

Table 6.
Five most common β_2-AR haplotype pairs found in an asthmatic cohort of 121 Caucasians. All other less common pairs total 12.2%. Adapted from [57].

Haplotype pair	%
2/4	30.6
2/2	20.7
2/6	18.2
4/4	11.6
4/6	6.6

and haplotypes in response to albuterol. No differences were found in the frequencies of the haplotypes between index and this asthmatic population. The five most common haplotype pairs in the asthmatic cohort and their frequencies are shown in Table 6.

From their sequencing work on the β_2-AR gene in the control group, the authors conclude:

- They identified 13 SNPs in a contiguous region of the 5′ upstream and coding sequence regions of the gene.
- 12 distinct haplotypes are represented in their population consisting of four major United States ethnic groups.
- A striking divergence in ethnic distribution exists for several haplotypes.

Their results are therefore in excellent agreement with the number of SNPs and haplotypes per gene observed in the study of 313 genes [54].

The results from albuterol treatment were:

- Five haplotype pairs were common in Caucasian asthmatics.
- Specific pairs of haplotypes were required to show maximum predictive value in treatments with albuterol (Fig. 7) and there are clear differences in the *in vivo* response to the drug based on these pairs.
- Individual haplotypes showed intermediate predictive value.
- None of the individual SNPs had any predictive value for response to the drug.

Examination of Figure 7 with reference to Table 5 indicates that differences in response to albuterol for the three most common haplotype pairs (present

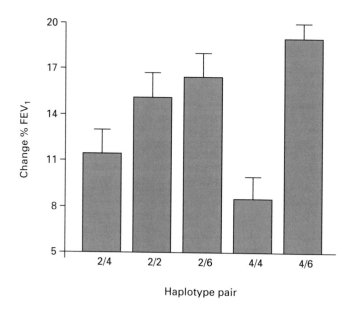

Fig. 7
In vivo responses to albuterol distinguished by haplotype pairs. Data from 121 Caucasian subjects diagnosed with asthma. FEV_1 = forced expiratory volume in 1 second. Adapted from [57].

in 69.5% of the patient population) varied minimally. The maximum differences in response for the most common haplotype pairs was a 50% better response for patients with the 2/4 pair than with the 4/4 pair and about a 120% better response for patients with the 4/6 pair than with the 4/4 pair. Using a cultured human embryonic kidney cell line that expresses β_2-AR, it was then shown that haplotype 2 significantly increased expression of β_2-AR protein and β_2-AR mRNA compared to haplotype 4, results consistent with the *in vivo* results.

4.3.3 Conclusions from this study

Although it was not discussed in these terms, the authors present an overall summary that is in agreement with the epigenetic viewpoint: their results indicate that the unique interactions of multiple SNPs within a haplotype ultimately affect biological and therapeutic phenotypes and that individual SNPs may have poor predictive value for patient responsiveness to drugs.

Their results also highlight some other clinical problems in applying SNP data to drug development and treatment. With respect to treatments:

- The difference in efficacy between the most and least responsive pairs of haplotypes to treatment with albuterol was found to be significant but comprises only about 20% of the asthmatic Caucasian population used in this study. This leaves 80% of patients whose responses range between poor and good; what are to be recommended treatments for these patients?
- The very large differences in haplotype frequencies (> 20-fold) between the important United States ethnic groups described here have been found in all similar investigations so far. This study did not look at whether or not identical haplotypes from different ethnic groups exhibit the same responses to albuterol *in vivo* or whether or not the same correlations with *in vitro* studies exist. If they don't, it is possible that other factors that interact with the β_2-AR haplotypes may exist.
- The results send no clear signals as to how individual drug development might proceed. In fact, the data show that although its impact may be limited, haplotyping may be useful mainly for predicting individual responses to currently used drugs in individuals.
- Clearly, the results from β_2-AR haplotype analysis would have to be used in conjunction with haplotype analysis of drug-metabolizing enzymes before it could apply to a clinical scenario. As has been remarked, "The mantra of pharmacogenomics has been 'one drug may not fit all'. It might be the case that one pharmacogenomic test might not fit all" [64].

Obviously, major conclusions cannot be made with certainty on the basis of one study, landmark that it may be. However, because of its basic agreement with the later study on 313 genes [54], it seems likely that outcomes from studies of SNP organization in many other genes will be similar to the β_2-AR gene results. Recent studies on sequence-based haplotype analysis of the interleukin-11 (IL-11), tissue-type plasminogen activator (t-PA), and angiotensin genes [65–67] certainly show that individual SNPs have little predictive value in clinical correlations.

We now turn to a case of a gene of major importance in health and disease – the gene encoding the glucocorticoid receptor – where haplotype maps have not yet been reported in the open literature, but where consideration of non-genomic pathways must be a major consideration when such maps become available.

5 Genomic and non-genomic effects mediated by the glucocorticoid receptor

5.1 Genomic effects

Glucocorticoids exert a strong influence on human metabolism and especially on mesenchymally derived tissues such as the hematopoietic system, the lymphatic system, and the thymus. In lymphoblastic leukemia cells, glucocorticoid treatment leads to cell cycle arrest and subsequent apoptosis. The molecular sequence of events leading to these phenotypic changes is unknown, but they depend on a functional glucocorticoid receptor (GCR).

Glucocorticoids are also involved in a variety of human functions including behavior, cardiovascular status, regulation of blood pressure, inflammation and metabolism. A common medical dilemma is the identification of those individuals with a strong family history of high blood pressure and associated diseases, such as diabetes, heart disease and stroke, that require very close monitoring and early drug treatment or lifestyle changes.

Specific for glucocorticoid hormones, the GCR was the first steroid hormone receptor to be highly purified and shown to be a DNA-binding protein.

Gene transcription is affected by these hormones in several steps as follows: (1) glucocorticoids bind to GCR complexes located in the cytoplasm; (2) the GCR complexes release associated (mainly heat-shock) proteins upon binding the ligand; (3) the GCR-ligand complex translocates to the nucleus and binds to specific recognition sites; (4) gene transcription is enhanced or inhibited depending on the type of the GCR and the specific genomic site.

The characteristic nucleotide sequences of the DNA sites, called response elements, that bind several major hormone receptors have been determined. The sequences of the consensus response elements for the glucocorticoid and estrogen receptors are 6-bp inverted repeats separated by any 3 base-pairs.

Essential hypertension is a complex multifactorial disorder in which genetic predisposition interacts with environment to yield the ultimate phenotype. In turn, hypertension acts as a risk factor for the development of ischaemic heart disease and stroke. It is now accepted that several loci contribute to the genetic component of hypertension. Although the field is complicated by numerous unconfirmed or contradictory findings, the evidence that genes are involved in renal sodium handling or aspects of corticosteroid production and action is remarkably consistent.

As an example of the commercial interest in studying the GCR gene for commercial development, Gemini Genomics has been issued a patent (U.S. Pat. No. 6,156,510) for its method of diagnosing a predisposition to hypertension or sustained high blood pressure. The hope is that diagnostic tests based on this patent will enable the early detection of those at risk, allowing physicians to recommend treatments that will minimize the consequences of high blood pressure disease, such as stroke, kidney disease, and cardiovascular disease. The patent covers proprietary methods of detecting mutations in a GCR gene.

Gemini's patent is based on their study which revealed an apparent association between certain SNPs in the glucocorticoid receptor gene and hypertension. The study compared the glucocorticoid receptor genes of individuals who had high blood pressure, who were taking anti-hypertensive medication, and who had two parents with hypertension, with those of individuals whose blood pressure was normal, who were not taking anti-hypertensive medication, and who had two parents with normal blood pressures.

While the diagnostic uses of SNPs in GCR-encoding genes may be important, the existence of important non-genomic effects of glucocorticoids will impede pharmacogenomic studies of these hormones.

5.2 Non-genomic effects

The presence of non-genomic effects of glucocorticoids can be experimentally tested:

- The genomic actions take place on a long time-scale compared to non-genomic effects. The fastest genomic effects take place on the order of min-

39

utes, but many actions take place on a time-scale of days. Rapid non-genomic effects can be determined by washout experiments.

- The genomic actions are mediated by the GCR. Non-genomic effects may be determined by blockading the receptor with antagonists.
- The genomic actions result in protein synthesis. Non-genomic effects may be determined by inhibitors of protein synthesis.

The slowness of genomic effects from these hormones may be partly characteristic of glucocorticoids because they require translocation of the ligand-bound receptors to the nucleus (requiring 10–30 min). However, in general all genomic effects require time for transcription and protein synthesis to take place. Drug effects that have very rapid actions should always be suspected of having non-genomic interactions.

Although these transcriptional effects of glucocorticoids are well known, there is growing evidence suggesting that hormonal steroids use multiple transduction pathways, either genomic or non-genomic or both. In particular, glucocorticoids affect neural function also *via* mechanisms that do not involve a genomic component. Non-genomic mechanisms appear to be activated by a series of other steroids as well (progesterone, estrogens, testosterone, aldosterone, vitamin D3, and neurosteroids) [68].

Evidence has accumulated suggesting that non-genomic mechanisms activated by glucocorticoids involve various brain areas, neurotransmitter, and second messenger systems as well as behaviors. The non-genomic effects of glucocorticoids may be one of the major keys to understanding the role of these hormones in controlling brain function.

Nevertheless, non-genomic effects of glucocorticoids are still poorly understood. Moreover, discriminating between genomic and non-genomic mechanisms is difficult in some cases.

From animal model and human studies, glucocorticoids have been implicated in non-genomic early stress responses. It appears that specific changes induced by glucocorticoids in early phases of the stress reaction are especially important. The meaning and consequences of stress may be different in early and late phases. While the early response often needs an active response, chronic stressors lead to behavioral depression. Non-genomic mechanisms appear to be crucial for the active phase of the stress response.

The targets of glucocorticoid hormones and pharmacological agents present in the central nervous system overlap. The GABAergic, cholinergic, serotonergic and other systems are important targets of drug action, and all these systems appear to be influenced by glucocorticoids *via* both genomic and non-genomic mechanisms. Disparate data suggest that stress in general and glucocorticoids in particular affect both the desired and adverse effects of pharmacological agents. For example:

- The anxiolytic efficacy of benzodiazepines is affected by experiential background .
- The effects of serotonergic drugs were affected by the intrinsic HPA-axis-stimulating effects of some drugs, housing and testing conditions, handling history, and stress.
- Amphetamine increased locomotor activity of subordinate squirrel monkeys, but caused hypoactivity in dominant group members. Desipramine has antidepressant-like effects in the Porsolt test in rats previously exposed to forced swimming only. Uncontrollable, but not controllable, stress was shown to potentiate morphine's rewarding properties. The behavioral effects of kainate and bicuculline applied to the hypothalamic attack area (subfornical intermediate hypothalamus) depend on the previous aggressive experience of subjects. Some human observations indicate that the interaction between stress and the efficacy of drugs is clinically meaningful.

All the above manipulations affect acute stress responsiveness. The effect of isolation and handling history on pharmacological efficacy might be especially relevant, because they do not change background levels of glucocorticoids but change the reactivity of the HPA-axis. Therefore, it has been hypothesized [68] that non-genomic glucocorticoid effects may have contributed to the interaction between stress and the efficacy of drugs. This assumption is supported by the fact that some effects of glucocorticoids on drug efficacy were expressed rather quickly. The anxiolytic effect of buspirone in the social interaction test was abolished by corticosterone applied 10 min before testing. In addition, acute glucocorticoid treatments decrease, while a chronic elevation in plasma glucocorticoids increases anxiety, i.e., acute and long-term effects of glucocorticoids appear to be opposite.

The non-genomic mechanisms of glucocorticoids interact with genomic mechanisms. They (1) prepare the field for genomic mechanisms, (2) contribute to the early occurrence of effects supported later by genomic mechanisms, and (3) induce early adaptive changes that are opposite to the delayed genomic effects. Such opposing ways of interaction can be reconciled only by assuming that the nature of the interaction depends on the nature of the challenge and/or on the brain sites involved. It is noteworthy that opposing ways of interaction are not always contradictory. One can hypothesize that preparing the field for delayed responses may be useful when the early response proved inefficient (i.e., there is a need for activating additional mechanisms).

Clearly, the development of specific agonists and antagonists for non-genomic glucocorticoid actions – drugs unavailable now – would be of major clinical importance. Some evidence suggests that some unknown molecular properties may make steroids effective or non-effective in triggering non-genomic effects: for example, triggering could be initiated by glucocorticoids specifically binding to proteins other than the GCR [68]. However, whatever the mechanisms are for the non-genomic actions of these hormones, the actions themselves will have to be taken into account in developing drugs that alter the genomic actions.

In conclusion, the actions of glucocorticoid hormones, once believed to be a classic case of a small signalling molecule acting directly on the genome, are now known to have a non-genomic component. These multiple modes of interaction are in accord with the epigenetic viewpoint. Since some genomic effects of the hormones counter the non-genomic effects [68], especially in the central nervous system, taking both into account in treatments involving these hormones or their antagonists is needed.

6   Animal models in the genomic era of drug research

The sequencing of the human genome and growing awareness of human genomic diversity has brought another problem into the drug development process: the differences in diversity between the genomes of inbred animal strains and humans. In this chapter emphasis has been placed on the need to consider ethnic diversity and epigenetic mechanisms to understand genomic sequence data in humans. We now turn to how human genomic data may affect drug research involving animal models.

Preclinical drug development relies heavily on animal models – typically inbred strains of mice and rats – for drug-target validation. This strategy increases data reproducibility due to the small genetic heterogeneity of the animals. However, this advantage is often offset by the failure of later clinical trials on humans, which must be partly due to the failure of the inbred animals to adequately model human genetic diversity [69]. Furthermore, as discussed earlier in this chapter, results already obtained for the human genome reveal that there is no such thing as a human wild-type genome. It would be foolish to expect that this won't be true for other animal genomes as well.

It is not known, nor is it presently feasible to determine, what fraction of human and mouse or rat genomes contain similar haplotypic patterns [69]. Thus, drug efficacy trials using a disease model in a single inbred mouse strain are analogous to a similar trial on a small inbred population of humans – such trials throw away diversity information now known to be important in connecting haplotype to phenotype. In general, the knockout and transgenic models suffer the same problem of not accurately reflecting the human genome because these strains are typically produced from an inbred background.

For example, the paternally expressed gene 3 (PEG3 gene), common to humans and mice, plays an important role in mouse maternal behavior. In the knockout model when the PEG3 gene is removed from the mouse genome, mothers ignore their offspring and let them die. This must be associated with the fact that in mice, the gene product is expressed primarily in the brain while, in humans, expression is mainly in the ovaries and placenta. The same gene is clearly acting in different ways in the two organisms.

In September 1999, the NIH in the United States announced that it was setting up a Mouse Genome Sequencing *Network* (as distinct from a well-financed Project), which aims to sequence the mouse genome in draft form by the year 2003. This network includes several research groups who are working at sequencing a variety of mouse chromosomes. In 2000, The Celera Corporation announced that they had begun a private mouse genome project of their own based on the methods they used in their human genome sequencing project [50]. Both these projects will presumably be based on DNA obtained from one, or a few, inbred strains.

An annotated mouse cDNA project [70] that is based on sequencing every transcript encoded by the C57BL/6J inbred strain of mice, is the project furthest along. However, it suffers not only from being confined to sequences from an inbred strain, but also, because of the use of cDNA, from exclusion of promoter and intron sequence data.

So far as characterizing mouse SNPs and haplotypes are concerned, nothing like the human SNP Consortium exists and the discovery and genotyping of mouse SNPs lags far behind the human project [71]. Thus, application of human SNP and haplotypic data to mouse models will remain uncertain for many years. Suggestions for interim solutions to this problem include:

- If the relevant mouse and human genes are found to exhibit comparable variation, the new drug target should be studied, preferably, in parallel in several mice strains that could partially resemble the genetic polymorphism of humans in analogy to studying drug efficacy in parallel in patients from different ethnic origins.
- Transgenic mice expressing the spectrum of the human allele repertoire could be prepared.
- Increase the use in drug trials of mouse strains showing higher levels of natural polymorphism compared with classical inbred strains, such as the PWD/Ph and PWK/Ph strains that are more closely related to wild mice.

7   Conclusions and future directions

7.1   Metabolic pharmacogenomics

It seems clear that this branch of pharmacogenomics will continue to develop at a rapid pace. Its impact is already being felt in isolated cases. For example, about 2,400 children are diagnosed with acute lymphoblastic leukemia (ALL) each year in the United States. Treatment of ALL usually involves a combination of chemotherapeutic drugs including 6-mercaptopurine. Children presenting with an inherited deficiency in thiopurine methyltransferase (TMPT, the drug that metabolizes 6-mercaptopurine and other thiopurine drugs), need to be treated with lower concentrations of the drug. About one in 300 children are homozygotes in the deficient enzyme, and one in ten are heterozygotes. These patients are at risk with standard doses of 6-mercaptopurine. A DNA-based test has been developed to identify them so that they may be treated with lower doses of the drug [72].

Technological advances in testing for polymorphisms have led to a test for all the known 18 polymorphisms in the cytochrome p450 2D6 (CYP2D6) enzyme. Polymorphisms in CYP2D6, resulting in deficiencies in enzymatic activity, occur in about 7–10 percent of the population with wide ethnic variations. The enzyme is responsible for metabolizing about 25% of all drugs, including many of the top 100 best-selling ones, including tricyclic antidepressants and the antidepressant Prozac. Research versions of the test currently cost in the neighborhood of $100 in the United States and prices will surely drop [72]. This is certainly inexpensive for a test that predicts individual responses to such a wide variety of drugs.

Because the effects of deficiencies in metabolizing drugs are relatively easy for patients and physicians to understand, because it will have positive impact on both physicians' and patients' insurance premiums, and because data from an individual's test do not have to be entered into a large database, it seems likely that testing individuals for cytochrome p450 and some other metabolizing enzyme polymorphism patterns will shortly become standard.

7.2 Personalized drugs

As more data on the human genome and its roles in human life are analyzed, the epigenetic viewpoint of human biology and medicine appears to be growing stronger. Even in its present unfinished form, the human genome sequence, accompanied by increasing data from a variety of sources, is showing genetic interactions that were previously unknown. For example, in all of the cases below, polymorphisms in a given gene will produce protein targets potentially having multiple functional roles:

- The one-gene/one-polypeptide concept is dead. Gene interactions are now recognized as more important than gene numbers. Many discontinuous genes can encode more than one protein by splicing together alternate exon combinations [73]. On the basis of a draft sequence of the human genome, it has been estimated that at least 10,000 human genes take part in this process [51].
- Introns sometimes take part in protein production. For example, the gene for prostate-specific antigen (PSA) has five exons and four introns but encodes a second protein (called PSA-linked molecule) which is partly encoded by the fourth intron of the PSA gene [74].

- Although the frequency of occurrence is not yet known, some transcripts are translated into precursor proteins which are then differentially cleaved into proteins of different functions [75, 76].
- Trans-splicing takes place (although with as yet unknown frequency in humans) and can be vital to a eukaryotic organism. For example, a gene in *Drosophila* that controls chromatin structure in early development, transcribes RNA from four exons on one strand and two exons in the opposite orientation on the opposing strand in a process that eventually yields four proteins with different functions [75, 76].
- The frequency of overlapping genes is also not currently known in humans although, since many eukaryotes use this mechanism for producing different proteins, it is difficult to believe that this mechanism is not employed in humans.
- The concept that data currently being consolidated by the SNP consortium will inevitably lead to new drug developments has not been borne out by data reviewed in this chapter. The concept may need to be folded into one that might be called the "Haplotype consortium."

In conclusion, much more evidence needs to be gathered before it can be stated unequivocally that personalized drug treatments are even theoretically possible. What is presently known about haplotype variations lends little confidence to the idea that SNP data will clearly lead the way to new drug development.

There are no adequate structural data available on what variant proteins produced by particular haplotypes might form attractive drug targets. It is surprising that more effort is not being put into systematic, quantitative studies of structural modifications to proteins due to missense substitutions. Structural data are going to be at least as important as raw SNP data in determining if there are drug targets with any advantages.

7.3 Animal models

Pharmaceutical development now depends, and will depend as far as can be seen into the future, on use of animal models. However, firm genomic data are rapidly emerging, showing how inadequate are the inbred, knockout, and transgenic animal models for developing efficacious drugs for humans. It is therefore somewhat surprising that a higher priority in the form of international collaborations has not been placed on completing the mouse genome project. Furthermore, as the epigenetic viewpoint of human biochemistry and physiology takes hold, questions immediately arise as to whether the same interaction networks that occur in humans are the same as those occurring in animals.

7.4   Ethical considerations

As we have seen, as more data on the human genome is brought forth, epigenetic thinking and considerations have become more important in foreseeing future drug development and treatments. We know that single genes do not determine most of the effects of medications and not all responses have inherited roots. We know that some drug responses are caused by environmental factors such as age or diet, and teasing out this nature-*versus*-nurture difference may prove difficult. We know from actual cases that amassing databases of human genetic profiles creates enormous ethical and privacy problems. Among the basic questions in dealing with these problems are: do the benefits outweigh the complications? If they do, can the public be convinced of this?

Not the least part of the problem would be the development of adequate quality assurance of individual sequence data. The general case of quality control in molecular genetic testing has been recently reviewed [77]. Some features of genetic testing are worth mentioning here: (1) unlike other forms of laboratory tests, genetic composition of an individual remains unaltered through life so the results of a single test can stay with them for life, including false positives and false negatives, (2) because of the present perception that genetic predisposition is an all-or-none proposition, genetic test results can have profound psychological implications for individuals and their supporting family members, (3) if genetic test databases are ever to enter mainstream medical practice, there must be absolute public confidence in the accuracy of the results.

The worldwide status of the art is nowhere near achieving a high enough level of confidence in genotyping, much less haplotyping. For example, Figure 8 shows the status in Europe for well-established genotyping for cystic fibrosis. The apparent asymptotic approach to 90% correctness as the number of laboratories grows larger is not impressive.

Jay A. Glasel

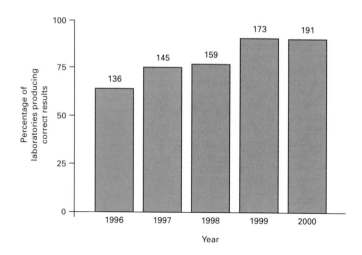

Fig. 8
Errors in European laboratories during the five years of European external quality assessment schemes for cystic fibrosis. Numbers across the tope indicate the total number of participating laboratories. Adapted from [77].

References

1   C.R. Cantor: Mol. Diagn. *4*, 287 (1999).
2   A.D. Roses: Novartis Found. Symp. *229*, 63 (2000).
3   M.M. Shi, M.R. Bleavins and F.A. de la Iglesia: Mol. Diagn. *4*, 343 (1999).
4   S. Jones: Genetics in Medicine: Real Promises, Unreal Expectations. Milbank Memorial Fund, New York 2000.
5   J. Lazarou, B.H. Pomeranz and P.N. Corey: JAMA *279*, 1200 (1998).
6   M. Kvasz, I.E. Allen, M.J. Gordon, E.Y. Ro, R. Estok, I. Olkin and S.D. Ross: Med. Gen. Med. E3 (2000).
7   T.R. Einarson: Ann. Pharmacother. *27*, 832 (1993).
8   D.W. Bates, D.J. Cullen, N. Laird, L.A. Petersen, S.D. Small, D. Servi, G. Laffel, B.J. Sweitzer, B.F. Shea, R. Hallisey et al.: JAMA *274*, 29 (1995).
9   D.W. Bates, N. Spell, D.J. Cullen, E. Burdick, N. Laird, L.A. Petersen, S.D. Small, B.J. Sweitzer and L.L. Leape: JAMA *277*, 307 (1997).
10   I.R. Edwards and J.K. Aronson: Lancet *356*, 1255 (2000).
11   I.R. Edwards: J. R. Coll. Physicians Lond. *34*, 48 (2000).
12   D.B. Jefferys, D. Leakey, J.A. Lewis, S. Payne and M.D. Rawlins: Br. J. Clin. Pharmacol. *45*, 151 (1998).
13   J.K. Borchardt: Mod. Drug Disc. *4*, 35 (2001).
14   J.A. DiMasi: Drug Inf. J. *34*, 1169 (2000).
15   K.I. Kaitin and J.A. DiMasi: Drug Inf. J. *34*, 673 (2000).

16   S. Aldridge: Gen. Eng. News *21*, 29 (2001).

17   F.S. Collins: N. Engl. J. Med. *341*, 28 (1999).

18   R.C. Strohman: Perspect. Biol. Med. *37*, 112 (1993).

19   R.C. Strohman: Toward an Epigenetic Biology & Medicine, http://www.mentalhelp.net/perspectives/articles/art05963.htm.

20   J. Beisson and T.M. Sonneborn: Proc. Natl. Acad. Sci. USA *53*, 275 (1965).

21   S.F. Ng and R.J. Williams: J. Protozool. *24*, 257 (1977).

22   A.P. Wolffe and M.A. Matzke: Science *286*, 481 (1999).

23   S. Wright: Phys. Rev. *21*, 487 (1941).

24   E.J. Sijbrands, R.G. Westendorp, J.C. Defesche, P.H. de Meier, A.H. Smelt and J.J. Kastelein: BMJ *322*, 1019 (2001).

25   R.R. Williams, S.J. Hasstedt, D.E. Wilson, K.O. Ash, F.F. Yanowitz, G.E. Reiber and H. Kuida: JAMA *255*, 219 (1986).

26   A.F. Vuorio, H. Turtola, K.M. Piilahti, P. Repo, T. Kanninen and K. Kontula: Arterioscler. Thromb. Vasc. Biol. *17*, 3127 (1997).

27   T. McKeown: The Role of Medicine: Dream, Mirage or Nemesis? Princeton University Press, Princeton 1979.

28   T. McKeown: The Origins of Human Disease. Basil Blackwell, Inc., New York 1988.

29   A.D. Roses: Lancet *355*, 1358 (2000).

30   R.S. Hockwald, J. Arnold, C.B. Clayman and A.S. Alving: JAMA *149*, 1568 (1952).

31   M. Przeworski, R.R. Hudson and A. Di Rienzo: Trends Genet. *16*, 296 (2000).

32   M. Kimura: Proc. Natl. Acad. Sci. USA *63*, 1181 (1969).

33   M. Kimura: Nature *217*, 624 (1968).

34   A.M. Issa: Trends Pharmacol. Sci. *21*, 247 (2000).

35   H. Rose: The Commodification of Bioinformation: The Icelandic Health Sector Database, Wellcome Trust, London 2000.

36   G.J. Annas: N. Engl. J. Med. *342*, 1830 (2000).

37   D. Winickoff: N. Engl. J. Med. *343*, 1734; discussion 1735 (2000).

38   R. Fears and G. Poste: Science *284*, 267 (1999).

39   R. Fears, D. Roberts and G. Poste: BMJ *320*, 933 (2000).

40   K.Y. Kreeger: The Scientist *15*, 32 (2001).

41   P.E. Carson, C.L. Flanagan, C.E. Ickes and S. Alving: Science *124*, 484 (1956).

42   H.B. Hughes, J.P. Biehl, A.P. Jones and L.H. Schmidt: Am. Rev. Tuberc. *70*, 266 (1954).

43   H. Lehmann and E. Ryan: Lancet *211*, 124 (1956).

44   F. Bernheim and M.L.C. Bernheim: J. Pharm. Exp. Ther. *64*, 209 (1938).

45   A.G. Motulsky: JAMA *165*, 835 (1957).

46   E.S. Vesell: Pharmacol. *61*, 118 (2000).

47   E.S. Vesell: J. Clin. Pharmacol. *40*, 930 (2000).

48   D.W. Nebert: Clin. Genet. *56*, 247 (1999).

49   A. Chakravarti: Nat. Genet. *19*, 216 (1998).

50   J.C. Venter, M.D. Adams, E.W. Myers, P.W. Li, R.J. Mural, G.G. Sutton, H.O. Smith, M. Yandell, C.A. Evans, R.A. Holt et al.: Science *291*, 1304 (2001).

51   E.S. Lander, L.M. Linton, B. Birren, C. Nusbaum, M.C. Zody, J. Baldwin, K. Devon, K. Dewar, M. Doyle, W. FitzHugh et al.: Nature *409*, 860 (2001).

52   N. Katsanis, K.C. Worley and J.R. Lupski: Nature Genetics *29*, 88 (2001).

53   J.B. Hogenesch, K.A. Ching, S. Batalov, A.I. Su, J.R. Walker, Y. Zhou, S.A. Kay, P.G. Schultz and M.P. Cooke: Cell *106*, 413 (2001).

54   J.C. Stephens, J.A. Schneider, D.A. Tanguay, J. Choi, T. Acharya, S.E. Stanley, R. Jiang, C.J. Messer, A. Chew, J.-H. Han et al.: Science *293*, 489 (2001).

55   R. Grantham: Science *185*, 862 (1974).

56   W.H. Li, C.I. Wu and C.C. Luo: J. Mol. Evol. *21*, 58 (1984).

57   C.M. Drysdale, D.W. McGraw, C.B. Stack, J.C. Stephens, R.S. Judson, K. Nandabalan, K. Arnold, G. Ruano and S.B. Liggett: Proc. Natl. Acad. Sci. USA *97*, 10483 (2000).

58   J.M. Drazen, E. Israel, H.A. Boushey, V.M. Chinchilli, J.V. Fahy, J.E. Fish, S.C. Lazarus, R.F. Lemanske, R.J. Martin, S.P. Peters et al.: N. Engl. J. Med. *335*, 841 (1996).

59   S.B. Liggett and D.A. Meyers (eds): The Genetics of Asthma. Marcel Dekker, Inc., New York 1996.

60   P.M. O'Byrne and H.A. Kerstjens: N. Engl. J. Med. *335*, 886 (1996).

61   S.B. Liggett: Am. J. Respir. Crit. Care Med. *156*, S156 (1997).

62   E. Israel, J.M. Drazen, S.B. Liggett, H.A. Boushey, R.M. Cherniack, V.M. Chinchilli, D.M. Cooper, J.V. Fahy, J.E. Fish, J.G. Ford et al.: Int. Arch. Allergy Immunol. *124*, 183 (2001).

63   L. Helmuth: Science *293*, 583 (2001).

64   J. McCarthy: Trends Pharma. Sci. *21*, 461 (2000).

65   Y. Shinohara, Y. Ezura, H. Iwasaki, I. Nakazawa, R. Ishida, M. Kodaira, M. Kajita, T. Shiba and M. Emi: J. Hum. Genet. *46*, 494 (2001).

66   I. Nakazawa, T. Nakajima, T. Ishigami, S. Umemura and M. Emi: J. Hum. Genet. *46*, 367 (2001).

67   N. Sato, T. Katsuya, T. Nakagawa, K. Ishikawa, Y. Fu, T. Asai, M. Fukuda, F. Suzuki, Y. Nakamura, J. Higaki et al.: Life Sci. *68*, 259 (2000).

68   G.B. Makara and J. Haller: Prog. Neurobiol. *65*, 367 (2001).

69   D. Gurwitz and A. Weizman: Drug Discov. Today *6*, 766 (2001).

70   J. Kawai, A. Shinagawa, K. Shibata, M. Yoshino, M. Itoh, Y. Ishii, T. Arakawa, A. Hara, Y. Fukunishi, H. Konno et al.: Nature *409*, 685 (2001).

71   K. Lindblad-Toh, E. Winchester, M.J. Daly, D.G. Wang, J.N. Hirschhorn, J.P. Laviolette, K. Ardlie, D.E. Reich, E. Robinson, P. Sklar et al.: Nat. Genet. *24*, 381 (2000).

72   J. Wallace: The Scientist *15*, 10 (2001).

73   W. Gilbert: Nature *271*, 501 (1978).

74   N. Heuze, S. Olayat, N. Gutman, M.L. Zani and Y. Courty: Cancer Res. *59*, 2820 (1999).

75   X. Zhang, J. Zhao, C. Li, S. Gao, C. Qiu, P. Liu, G. Wu, B. Qiang, W.H. Lo and Y. Shen: Nat. Genet. *27*, 151 (2001).

76   S. Xiao, C. Yu, X. Chou, W. Yuan, Y. Wang, L. Bu, G. Fu, M. Qian, J. Yang, Y. Shi et al.: Nat. Genet. *27*, 201 (2001).

77   E. Dequeker, S. Ramsden, W.W. Grody, T.T. Stenzel and D.E. Barton: Nature Rev. Gen. *2*, (2001).

Progress in Drug Research, Vol. 58 (E. Jucker, Ed.)
©2002 Birkhäuser Verlag, Basel (Switzerland)

Herbal medicine of Wisconsin Indians

By Vera M. Kolb

Department of Chemistry
University of Wisconsin-Parkside
Kenosha, WI 53141, USA

<kolb@uwp.edu>

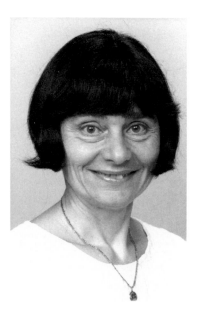

Vera M. Kolb

*received a Chemical Engineering degree in 1971 and
an MS in Chemistry in 1973, both from Belgrade University. In 1973 she was awarded a Fulbright grant to
pursue her chemistry studies at Southern Illinois University at Carbondale. After obtaining her Ph.D. in
1976, she continued her career in Carbondale until
1985, when she moved to Wisconsin. She is currently
Professor of Chemistry at University of Wisconsin-Parkside. Her research contributions, which comprise
over 80 publications, including 3 patents, are in the
fields of organic reactions and mechanisms, morphine-type opiates and their receptors, estrogens, nucleosides,
teratogens and, since 1992, prebiotic chemistry,
including alternative genetic systems. She was a visiting scientist at Uppsala University in 1982 and at the
Salk Institute for Biological Sciences from 1992–1994.
Her major hobby is violin playing.
Vera M. Kolb's interest in American Indians developed
in her childhood. She was greatly inspired by a book
about the Okefenokee Swamp and the use of its plants
as medicines by the Seminole Indians. The book was
given to her brother Vladimir by their beloved grade
school teacher Zivka Blagojevic, to whom this chapter
is dedicated.*

Summary

In this chapter we will familiarize the reader with selected aspects of the
herbal medicine of Wisconsin Indians. We will concentrate on the Menominee, Potawatomi, Ojibwe and Meskwaki tribes. We will address the following topics: (1) selected methods for research in the existing literature to reveal
both the identity and the chemical composition of plants which Indians used
for medicinal purposes; (2) some aspects of Indian medicine, such as the
mode of delivery of herbal drugs, extensive use of plant mixtures, and other
practices; (3) selected literature resources on comparison of uses of medicinal plants among different North American Indian tribes and contemporary
white men.

Contents

Key words

Wisconsin Indians, Menominee, Potawatomi, Ojibwe, Meskwaki, North American Indians, ethnobotany, ethnopharmacology, phytochemistry.

1 Introduction and objectives

The need for new drugs is still an urgent matter for the pharmaceutical industry despite tremendous advances in the field in recent decades. Many more drugs are needed to combat new diseases such as AIDS, to deal with drug resistance developed by the pathogens that cause infections, to address chronic diseases, including those of aging populations, to conquer cancer, to alleviate anxieties, depressions and more severe mental conditions, just to name a few. Thus, it is not surprising that a multi-pronged approach to drug discovery and development is pursued by the investigators in the field. It is felt, and rightfully so, that no stone should be left unturned in the search for a successful drug.

For this reason, one can see a rather interesting mix of recent publications in scientific journals, books and magazines. On the one hand we find publications on rational drug design. An example is a recent account of the newest approaches using combinatorial chemistry, evolutionary algorithms, computer-based evaluations of binding affinities of drugs to the receptors, and other advanced computational methods [1, 2]. On the other hand, we find very recent titles, such as "Tapping traditional healer's treasures" in *Modern Drug Discovery* [3] and "Shamans vs. Synthetics" in *The Scientist* [4]. Popular books on the latter subjects, such as Plotkin's *Tales of a Shaman's Apprentice* [5] and *Medicine Quest* [6], are as fascinating to the general public as they are to the scientists.

The role of ethnopharmacology in drug discovery and development is well documented [7]. Continuing interest in this subject is reflected in many recent articles and reviews. Some examples are: "Phytomedicines: Back to the Future", by Tyler [8], "Old Yet New – Pharmaceuticals from Plants", by Houghton [9], "Ethnobotany: The Chemist's Source for the Identification of Useful Natural Products", by Hosler and Mikita [10], "Recent Natural Products-Based Drug Development: A Pharmaceutical Industry Perspective", by Shu [11] and "Search for New Drugs of Plant Origin", by Hamburger et al. [12].

Our main interest resides with the pharmacology of the medicinal plants used by the Native Americans, often referred to as Indians, from the present state of Wisconsin. These Indians were discovered rather late (in 1634) by Europeans [13] and, due to their relative isolation, their cultural development until then was original and unique. Their uses of medicinal plants may likewise be original and unique. In addition, the ethnobotany of Wisconsin Indians was studied and recorded in great detail by Smith in the 1920s and 1930s [14, 16–18]. Since that time, however, the pharmacopoeia of Wisconsin Indians has not been updated or studied in a comprehensive manner. It is our objective to bring Smith's work to the attention of readers, with a hope that it will spark new research efforts. There is a great deal that can be still learned from the Indians. Much information is actually available in old sources, when used in conjunction with new databases.

For the benefit of readers who are not specialized in the field, we describe first some general tools for researching the literature on ethnomedicine and on the chemical composition and the biological properties of any particular plant.

2   General method for literature research

2.1   Identification of plants

An important goal is to find the chemical composition of the plants used by the Native Americans for medicinal purposes and to verify that these chemicals exhibit pharmacological properties in line with their claimed ethnomedicinal use. One must start by finding information about the medicinal plants. While some plants may be part of the tribal secret lore, others are not.

One needs to identify the plants first by their common names, by which they would be referred to in the literature about the Native Americans. To find these common names, one needs to consult all available sources on the subject, including encyclopedias, history and anthropology books and other references, scholarly and popular. Museum publications are usually valuable resources, as they are typically written by the experts. Such publications are usually not widely distributed and may not be easily available.

After learning the common name, one needs to further identify the medicinal plant by a proper phylum, order and family. One way to accomplish this task is with the help of the following two references: (1) *CRC Ethnobotany Desk Reference* by Johnson [19]. This reference contains an inventory of ca. 30,000 plant species and historical uses by the cultures throughout the world, including the current uses. This book includes the three largest U.S. Government ethnobotany databases and the U.S. National Park Service plant inventory list, among other sources. (2) A 3-volume book set entitled *The Cross Name Index to Medicinal Plants*, by Torkelson [20], which provides 28,000 common names of 4,000 species of medicinal plants, as well as their scientific names, taxonomic classification, and a cross index. The common names originate from 41 countries or regions. Twenty-six languages are cited in this index. Therefore the value of this reference is truly global.

It is, then, possible for readers who are not botanists to read the ethnobotanical and other literature without confusion about the variety of the common names given to the same plant, and the matching scientific names.

To find out if the chemical composition of the plant has been studied and if any medicinally important compounds have been identified, the reader may consult various electronic databases in addition to the traditional literary sources. We present here examples of the searches to illustrate the use of references 19 and 20 in conjunction with some selected electronic databases.

2.2   Chemical Abstracts

Let us suppose that we are interested in the plant commonly known as blood root (also spelled bloodroot), or Indian red paint. We can find its proper species name from Torkelson [20] to be *Sanguinaria canadensis*, from the Papaveraceae family. We also discover that this plant is known by many other common names, such as tetterwort, red puccoon, blutwurzel in German, and sanguinaire in French. In Johnson [19] we find the proper species and family name, the common names in English, and a wealth of additional information. For example, numerous geographic locations where this plant can be found are listed. They include national parks, nature preserves, historic sites and various scenic routes, such as Great Smoky Mountains National Park, Cyahoga Valley National Recreation Area, Big Thicket Nature Preserve, Manassas National Battlefield and Ozark National Riverways, to name a few. Further, we find a listing of numerous medicinal activities associated with this plant, for a total of 23, and 24 diseases and ailments known to be treated by this plant. We learn that the blood root is good for bronchitis, pneumonia, whooping cough and croup, and, as a tincture, to clear up ringworm. It has also been used for sores, eczema and other skin problems. Most importantly for our study, we find that this plant was used by various American Indian tribes, for example, Appalachian, Cherokee, Chippewa, Delaware, Fox, Iroquois, Monominee, Ojibwa, Potawatomi, Mohegan and some others.

At this point we wish to find out if the chemical composition of blood root has been studied, and if some medicinally active ingredients have been found. We can find this information quickly by a computer search of the electronic database of Chemical Abstracts, from its beginning (1967) to the present (January 5, 2001). (The search of the CA entries prior to 1967 would need to be done manually). We find only five hits if we use "bloodroot" and only three hits with "blood root". However, we find 60 hits for "*Sanguinaria canadensis*". The total number of hits, accounting for some overlap between the files generated by using these three names, is 62. This example illustrates not only the need to use the proper species name, but also the value of trying the search under the common name (extra two references). One should include both names, since the ratio of the hits obtained solely by the proper species name vs. that for the common name varies from plant to plant. The following two examples illustrate the point. If one uses the common name "Mayapple", one gets 38 hits. "May apple" gives 12 hits. The proper species name, "*Podophyllum peltatum*", gives 27 hits. The total number of the unique hits (i.e., taking care of the overlap of the files) is 49. We see here that it did pay to enter the common names, since we got an extra 22 references. In another example, that of "deadly nightshade", we get only six hits, while the use of the proper name, "*Atropa belladonna*", gives 202 hits. The total number of unique hits is 205. Here, it was essential to use the proper name. Still, one could get an extra three references from the use of the common names.

We return now to the results of the Chemical Abstracts (CA) search for blood root. Just by surveying the titles of the published papers, dissertations and patents, one can quickly find out that the blood root contains benzophenanthridine alkaloids, the specific compounds oxysanguinarine, sanguinarine, sanguidimerine and others, and that the extracts from the blood root are currently used in toothpaste as an anti-plaque agent and for general oral health. We also find a title: "Herbal Remedies of the Maritime Indians: Phytosterols and Triterpenes of 67 Plants", published in the *Journal of Ethnopharmacology* in 1984 [21]. The follow-up on this article will reveal additional articles which were published previously on the herbal remedies of the Maritime Indians from Canada [22–27].

The type of the literature search described in this section could be performed easily by chemists, who are typically well versed in the use of the CA. Since many chemists work in drug discovery teams, the knowledge gained could be used as an inspiration for drug design.

Other electronic databases and Web sites exist which are relevant to our task. We describe below some selected sources, some of which are commercial. The reader would need to pick and choose among them.

2.3 Other electronic databases and Web sites

2.3.1 NAPRALERT

NAPRALERT is an acronym for NAtural PRoducts ALERT and stands for a database which is compiled by the University of Illinois at the Chicago School of Pharmacy. It provides information on chemistry, activities of extracts, and taxonomy. It describes the ethnomedical and traditional uses of plants. It covers information from the global literature mostly since 1975, but also earlier. Some references go back to the year 1650. This database is updated monthly. It can be reached in the following ways:
- In Europe: http://stneasy.fiz-karsruhe.de
- In Japan: http://stneasy-japan.cas.org
- In North America and elsewhere: http://stneasy.cas.org

We provide here a couple of examples of the NAPRALERT search.

The search for May apple/Mayapple/*Podophyllum peltatum* covered the years 1650 to present. The search resulted in 25 references, which included books, journal articles and a dissertation. The printout from the search was ca. 200 pages long, since it listed information about many other plants, in addition to the one sought (May apple). This occurred in all but one book references (for one book we counted 419 entries, out of which only three were relevant to May apple) and some journals (for one journal article we counted 125 entries, again mostly for plants different from May apple). We found this somewhat distracting, but some people may find information on the additional plants useful. The search revealed an interesting mixture of useful references, but it did not pick up the references on the use of May apple by Wisconsin Indians, which we have discovered by research into the museum publications. The NAPRALERT search for bloodroot/blood root/*Sanguinaria canadensis* provided 59 entries.

2.3.2 Agricultural Research Service/Dr. Duke's Phytochemical and Ethnobotanical Databases

The address for this site is: http://www.ars-grin.gov.duke/

This site enables the following specific queries of the phytochemical database:
- Plant searches: chemicals and activities in a particular plant, high-concentration chemicals, chemicals with one activity, ethnobotanical uses;
- Chemical searches: plants with a chosen chemical, activities of a chosen chemical;
- Activity searches: plants with a specific activity, search for plants with several activities, chemicals with a specific activity, chemicals with a lethal dose value;
- Ethnobotany searches: ethnobotanical uses for a particular plant, plants with a particular ethnobotanical use;
- Database references: reference citation.

We have found this site easy to use and rich in information. We give here a couple of examples for illustrative purposes. A search for chemicals and their biological activities for May apple reveals 27 non-ubiquitous chemicals. (Ubiquitous chemicals are not included in the analysis.) For example, desoxypodophyllotoxin is listed. Concentration of this chemical in the root is given at 1000 ppm. The biological activities such as anticarcinomic, antiherpetic, antitumor of nasopharynx, antiviral, hepatoprotective, insecticide, larvicide and pesticide are listed, together with the references. For some of the 27 chemicals listed, e.g., alphapeltatin-glucoside, no activity is reported. Some other chemicals, such as berberine, have a very large number (93) or activities reported, including abortifacient, antiarrythmic, anticirrhotic, antidysenteric, antigonorrhea, antiviral, diuretic, hypoglycemic and antifungicide, among many others. Activities such as a reverse-transcriptase inhibitor, prostaglandin-synthesis-inhibitor, RNA–depressant, topoisomerase-II-inhibitor and others linked to the biochemical investigations of the foundation of the activity are also listed.

A similar search for blood root gave 24 chemicals and 149 activities. More pertinent to the objectives of this chapter is a specialized search done *via* this site for "Ethnobotanic uses" of bloodroot. We find here just 25 uses listed, such as aphrodisiac, against burns, cancer, as a laxative, against rheumatism, as a tonic and as a vermifuge, among others.

An attractive feature of this database is that we can also search for plants which contain particular chemicals. For example, we find that the female hormone estradiol is found in the hops fruit, ginseng and the pomegrante seed. Chaste-tree contains progesterone and testosterone. If we search for chemicals that are found more commonly in plants, we can chose an option to view, for example, only the top 40 plants with quantitative data. For example, the search for morphine will give us various poppy plants as expected, but it will give us also the quantity of morphine in various parts of the plant. In the opium poppy we find 100, 000 ppm in the latex exudate, 3, 900 ppm in the root, and only 30 ppm in the stem. Similar information for another plant of ethobotanical interest may justify the native's use of a selected part of a plant for medicinal purposes.

We have easily found detailed and very valuable information about the following plants the Native Americans used for medicinal purposes: Slippery elm, Lady slipper, Skunk cabbage, Wintergreen, Bearberry and Black cohosh, among others.

2.3.3 Other Web sites

Other Web sites, such as the "Native American Ethnobotany" site by Dr. Daniel E. Moerman (http://www.umd.umich.edu/database/herb/about_ ethnobot.html), with many good links, exist. Many excellent Web sites are based on NAPRALERT and can be discovered by searching the key word NAPRALERT. One such site is "Plant Constituents" (http://chili:rt66.com/ hrbmoore/Constituents/Constituents.htms).

Numerous other sites exist. We consulted about 300 of them, and still many more are available.

3   About Wisconsin Indians

The largest number of Native American tribes and bands east of the Mississippi River can be found today in the State of Wisconsin [28]. There are eleven reservations and many other settlements occupied by the Indian Nations of Chippewa, Ho-Chunk, Menominee, Mohicans, Oneida and Potawatomi [28].

There are several bands of the Lake Superior Chippewas: St. Croix, Lac Court Oreilles, Red Cliff, Bad River, Lac du Flambeau and Sokaogon, located in the northwest, north, and north-central parts of the state. Chippewas are also known as Ojibwe. The Indians of the Ho-Chunk Nation, previously called Winnebago, can be found in the central and west-central parts of the state. The Indians of the Menominee Nation have a reservation in the central-northeast region of Wisconsin. The Stockbridge-Munsee tribe of Wisconsin is a band of Mohican Indians. It is located in the central part of the state. The Indians of the Oneida Nation now live in east-central Wisconsin. The Forest County Potawatomi are in the northeast [28].

Some of the present-day Indians in Wisconsin were relocated from the northeast part of North America during their turbulent history. For example, the Stockbridge band of Mohicans (also called Mahicans) was relocated from the state of New York in 1822 [29, 30]. In 1856 they were given a reservation in Wisconsin along with the Munsee band of Delawares, which were also relocated from the northeast. A group of Oneidas, one of the original Iroquois tribes from the northeast, resettled in Wisconsin on land they purchased in 1938 from the Menominees [29–31].

Throughout their modern history Wisconsin Indians were involved in complex and often turbulent interactions with white men. The French were the first explorers (since 1634) and rulers of Wisconsin, followed by the British (1761) and then by U.S. domination (1815). Superimposed on this history is an entangling web of inter-tribal conflicts [13].

Due to the interaction with white men, the Wisconsin Indians' herbal medicine cannot be assumed to be pristine. However, the cultural and language barriers probably impeded ethnobotanical exchange.

Since different Indian tribes belong to different language groups, a language barrier existed between them also. For example, while the Menominee, Potawatomi and Chippewa belong to the Algonkian language group, the Winnebago are members of the Siouan group, and the Oneida speak the

Iroquoian language. It is said that the differences between these language groups are as large as, for example, the difference between English and Chinese [13].

4 Herbal medicine of the Wisconsin Indians

4.1 Menominee Indians

The main source on the topic of herbal medicine of the Menominee Indians is Huron H. Smith [18].

The Menominee Indians, which are of the Algonkian stock, named themselves "wild rice men". The Menominee word for wild rice is "Manoman". During Huron Smith's study of the tribe (in 1921 and 1922) there were only about 1745 people. Smith observed that because of the sanctity of most of their medicinal knowledge, it was difficult to obtain full information on the uses of plants as medicines. The history of the Menominee medicinal lore is entangled with their religion, which is briefly reviewed in [18]. The Menominee were taught that the plant medicines were very valuable, and that it would offend the various spirits to value them lightly. Thus, the Indians guarded the lore jealously. The knowledge about the medicinal plants included the proper season for collecting the plants, which, in some instances, was of only two to three days' duration. Apparently, Indians learned to recognize the periods during which the drug properties are the best, such as, for instance, just before the plant blossoms, or when the sap is first moving. Smith acknowledged that while the success of many of the Indian plants as remedies is mythical, there are plants of definitive medicinal values "which the white man has acquired from his Indian brother" [18, p. 18].

One aspect of the Menominee (and other) Indians' medicine we found fascinating and worth further exploration is their use of combinations of remedies.

Smith classified the Menominee Indians' medicinal plants by both the common English names and the proper botanical names. In addition, he provided the Indian names for the plants, the phonetic key for their pronunciation, and the literal translation. He obtained these with the help of Indian guides, interpreters and informants. Smith gave the details of the preparation of the Indian medicinal remedies, such as boiling the plant's root, bark, or flower to make a tea, pounding the plant's root or bark to make a poultice, etc. He also recorded the use of many of the Menominee Indians' medicinal plants by the white man at that time. The latter use was sometimes parallel to, and sometimes different from that of the Indians. Smith used the same format in his work on the Forest Potawatomi [16], Ojibwe [14] and Meskwaki Indians [17].

We cite here the medicinal uses of selected plants and plant mixtures, out of ca. 100 recorded by Smith, to illustrate the range of medical conditions that Indians treated. We also list some interesting and less common modes of drug delivery. We use common English names; the Latin names are used only for the families.

In describing Smith's account of the medicinal plants and their uses by the Menominee and other tribes (*vide infra*), we tried to stick to his original language. Such language may be archaic in some cases. Some terms are obsolete; some may be offensive. All are typical of the language used in his time, not ours. For example, he uses words like physic, dropsy, flux, consumption and ptomaine poisoning, among others. His descriptions of the diseases, such as craziness, lunacy, fits, female troubles, etc., may not be appropriate today. However, our desire was to preserve the true meaning of Smith's descriptions, which could be altered in an attempt to rephrase him, and to provide the flavor of his times. Also, as a sign of those times, he used "he", rather than today's "he or she". We have not attempted to update his language. We have also largely omitted the numerous descriptions of the use of the Indian herbal plants by the white men contemporary to Smith, mostly for lack of space.

Anacardiaceae; Sumac Family
- Staghorn Sumac
  This tree yields three different types of medicines, from the root bark, the inner bark, and from the twigs. The latter was used for treatment of various female diseases. The berries were used in combination with other herbs for consumption and pulmonary troubles.

Araceae; Arum Family
- Sweet Flag

The root of this plant was used to cure stomach cramps. A dose was the length of a finger joint. It was known to the white man as the drug "Calamus".

- Dragon Root

This was used for female disorders.

- Skunk Cabbage

Skunk root was one of the ingredients of the tattooing set. The Menominee tattooed medicines in over the seat of the pain. The medicines were moistened and tattooed into the flesh with the teeth of the gar pike, which was dipped in the medicine. The various colors stayed and presumably acted as a talisman against the return of the disease. Skunk root was used by the white man as the drug "Dracontium".

Asclepiadaceae; Milkweed Family
- Butterfly Weed

This was one of the most important Menominee medicines. The root was used for cuts, wounds and bruises. It was also used in mixtures with other remedies. The white man used it under the name "pleurisy root".

Berberidaceae; Barberry Family
- Mandrake (Mayapple)

The entire plant was boiled. The liquid thus obtained was used to kill potato bugs. The white man in Smith's time used this plant for slow purging, to excite the flow of bile, and to treat children's diarrhea. The drug was used by the white men and was known as "Podophyllum".

Betulaceae; Birch Family
- Hoary Alder

Its inner bark and the root bark were used as poultices to reduce swelling. The infusion was used against sores and to cure saddle gall in horses.

Caprifoliaceae; Honeysuckle Family
- Red Elderberry

By a very careful and measured procedure, a tea was made out of the inner bark. It was used as a last-resort purgative and as a very powerful emetic.

Compositae; Composite Family
- Yarrow

  This plant had multiple uses, such as against fever (hot tea made from the leaves), to cure eczema sores (by rubbing with the fresh plant tops), and against children's rashes (as a poultice made from the leaves).
- Canada Wormwood

  This herb was used as a leaf medicine in combination with angelica root to treat suppressed menstruation. This plant was used by the white man as "Artemisia".
- Joe-pye Weed

  This plant was used in diseases of the genito-urinary canal. The white man used it for its diuretic properties.

Cornaceae; Dogwood Family
- Alternate-leaved Dogwood

  The liquid made out of the bark of this shrub was the source of a pile remedy. The tepid liquid was placed in a special syringe, made out of the bladder of the deer or bear. The neck of the syringe was a two-inch hollow duck bone. The two pieces of the syringe were tied with sinew. The bladder was compressed to force the liquid into the rectum where it was retained for half an hour for each application.

Cruciferae; Mustard Family
- Shepherd's Purse
- Virginia Peppergrass

  Shepherd's purse and Virginia peppergrass were used as a cure for poison ivy. These plants were steeped and the water was used as a wash.

Cucurbitaceae; Gourd Family
- Balsam Apple

  It was described as being the greatest of all medicines and useful in any medicinal combinations. The pulverized root was used as a poultice for headache. A decoction was used as a bitter tonic and in love potions.

Equisetaceae; Horsetail Family
- Scouring Rush

The plant was boiled in water which was then used against kidney troubles, and "to clear the system" after childbirth.
- Wood Rush
The tea from the stems was used to cure dropsy, while the pulverized stems were applied in a poultice to stop the flow of blood.

Ericaceae; Heath Family
- Bearberry
- Prince's Pine
Bearberry and prince's pine were valuable remedies in female troubles. They were also used as seasoners to make other female remedies taste good. The white man used bearberry for many conditions, including female ones, as the drug known as "Uva Ursa".
- Wintergreen
The leaf of this plant was steeped with the berry to make a tea, which was used against rheumatism. This was the same as the white man's use. It was known in Smith's time that the wintergreen contains methyl salicylate, an active principle closely related to aspirin.

Hamamelidaceae; Witch-Hazel Family
- Witch Hazel
A decoction of this plant was used by the participants in the games, who rubbed it on their legs to keep them limbered up. The Menominee learned about this use from their neighbors, the Stockbridge Indians.

Hypericaceae; St. John's Wort Family
- Great St. John's Wort
This was a very important remedy, which was also used in mixtures. For example, it was a remedy for kidney diseases (in a mixture with blackcap raspberry root).

Labiatae; Mint Family
- Wild Mint
- Peppermint
- Wild Bergamot
This was a universal remedy for catarrh.

Liliaceae; Lily Family
- Solomon's Seal

  The root of this plant was dried, pulverized, mixed with cedar balm and burned as a smudge. The smoke was blown into the nostrils of an unconscious person close to death. This treatment was supposed to revive the patient. The white man used it as a less powerful substitute for digitalis.
- Large-flowered Trillium

  Its root was used to make a poultice to reduce swelling of the eye, to make a tea for cramps, for irregularity of menses, and to remove the defilement entailed by intercourse with one during the menstrual period.

Myricaceae; Bayberry Family
- Sweet Fern

  A tea made of this plant was used in childbirth.

Orchidaceae; Orchid Family
- Stemless Ladies' Slipper

  The root was used in male disorders.
- Yellow Ladies' Slipper

  This plant was used in female disorders.

Papaveraceae; Poppy Family
- Bloodroot

  It was often added to other medicines to strengthen their effect. It was used by the white man as the drug "Sanguinaria".

Pinaceae; Pine Family
- Balsam Fir

  The liquid balsam was used for colds and pulmonary troubles. The tea made from the inner bark was used for pains in the chest. The fresh inner bark was used for poultices.
- Tamarack

  The bark was used as a poultice when fresh and as a tea when steeped. The tea was used against inflammation and was also given to horses to improve their condition from distemper.
- Arbor-vitae

The inner bark was used as a tea to treat suppressed menstruation. The leaves were used as a smudge to revive lost consciousness.

Plantaginaceae; Plantain Family
- Rugel's Plantain
  The fresh leaf was heated and applied to swellings with the top of the leaf towards the flesh. Smith tried this remedy and found that it reduced his badly swollen hand to normal in one afternoon. He reported that the binding of the plantain leaves to the hand caused profuse perspiration.

Polygonaceae; Buckwheat Family
- Pennsylvania Persicaria
  The tea from this bitter leaf was used against hemorrhage of blood from the mouth and, in a mixture with other herbs, to heal women internally after childbirth.

Polypodiaceae; Polypody or Fern Family
- Maidenhair Fern
  This plant was used in the treatment of female diseases.
- Brake
  The root of this fern was boiled to make a drink to relieve caked breast. A dog whisker was used to pierce a hole in the teat.

Ranunculaceae; Crowfoot Family
- Gold Thread
  From the roots a mouthwash was prepared, which was used for sore throat of babies, for teething babies, and to cure cankers of the mouth. The white man used it for the same purpose and, according to Smith, had probably learned about these uses from Indians.

Rhamnaceae; Buckthorn Family
- New Jersey Tea
  The tea from the roots was used as a cure-all for stomach troubles.

Rubiaceae; Madder Family
- Partridge Berry
  A tea made out of the leaves was used to cure insomnia.

Rutaceae; Rue Family
- Three-leaved Hop Tree
  This was a valuable source of a sacred medicine. A piece of the white bark of the root, about the size of the index finger, was worth a pony, or one or two blankets. This medicine was called a great leader among all medicines. It was used principally as an addition to other known remedies to make them more potent. No specific examples of medicinal uses were given, however.
- Prickly Ash
  The root bark was used in poultices, often with other medicines. An example of a treatment of swelling was given. The poultice was applied by a special method by the medicine man. The teeth of the gar fish were moistened with the medicine, the swelling was punctured to make it bleed, so that the pulverized or liquid medicine may enter the flesh. The swelling was then punctured a few more times, and a poultice of the medicine was kept on for four days, by which time the healing should be completed.

Salicaceae; Willow Family
- Balm of Gilead
  The buds, which are resinous, were boiled in fat to make a salve for dressing wounds and to put up the nostrils to cure a head cold.
- Dwarf Willow
  The root was used for the medicinal purposes. It was taken only from the plants which had insect galls. Such a root was used to stop colic, dysentery and diarrhea.

Scrophulariaceae; Figwort Family
- Great Mullen
  The root was used in pulmonary diseases, while the leaf was smoked as an Indian tobacco. The white man smoked the leaf for the relief of asthma and bronchitis.

Taxaceae; Yew Family
- American Yew or Ground Hemlock
  It was used in a form of a sudatory to treat rheumatism, numbness and paralysis.

Thymeleaceae; Mezereum Family
- Leatherwood

   The roots were steeped to make a tea, which was used as a diuretic and against kidney troubles.

Umbelliferae; Parsley Family
- Angelica

   The roots were cooked, pounded to a pulp, covered with some bruised leaves, enclosed in a piece of cloth, and made into a hot plaster. The latter was good for any pain in the chest or body.

Valerianaceae; Valerian Family
- Edible Valerian

   The root was used for many purposes, such as for cuts, wounds, in poultices for boils, and also as a tapeworm medicine.
- Swamp Valerian

   The identity of this important medicine was jealously guarded. It had multiple medicinal uses, such as against cramps and disorders of the head. Also, if one chews it and spits the juice on the hook and bait, it will lure fish.

4.2   Potawatomi Indians

We first provide a brief history of the Potawatomi Indians, mostly based on references [16, 29, 32–33].

   The Potawatomi Indians belong to the Algonkian tribes and are related to the Ojibwe and Ottawa Indians. According to the tradition, the Potawatomi kept a perpetual fire. Thus, they were known as the "keepers of the fire", which is also the meaning of their tribal name. The Potawatomi originally lived in the northeast part of America, but were driven out westward by their hereditary enemies, the Iroquois. The Potawatomi eventually migrated to Wisconsin. They were found established in 1637 and 1638 on the Green Bay shores, at the time of the first visits by the white men. The Potawatomi were directly in the path of the French-Jesuit missionaries and voyagers. Thus, it is possible that the contact with these white men had influence on the Potawatomi Indians' use of the medicinal plants. The Potawatomi Indians in Wisconsin were represented by two branches, which differ both in their language and ethnology, the Forest branch and the Prairie branch. The latter was also known as the Mascoutens. According to Smith, the Mascoutens have disappeared from Wisconsin's history. The Potawatomi were sent by the U.S. government to Kansas in 1835. Some remained in the Wisconsin woods (thus the name "Forest" Potawatomi), and of those who went to Kansas, about 350 returned to Wisconsin. During this exile the Potawatomi's knowledge about the medicinal plants may have been further influenced by the white men or by some other Indian tribes.

Smith studied the Forest Potawatomi Indians' use of plants during a three-month period, June–September 1925 [16]. At the time of Smith's study, there were only about 850 Forest Potawatomi left. They were living in Forest County, in the northeast of Wisconsin. In 1954 there were 350 members [13], and in 1998 there were 999 tribal members [28].

Forest Potawatomi were generally difficult to approach and were secretive about their medicinal use of plants. They were most unwilling informants. Smith found fewer principal informants among the Forest Potawatomi than among other tribes he had studied. There were in total total six main informants. One of them was Mrs. Spoon, a medicine woman, who often traveled great distances to get the desired plants.

Smith followed the same format for the classification of the plants, use of the Indian names, and the medicinal uses, as he did in the previously described work on the Menominee [18]. The religious and general medicinal customs, including the ceremonial forms in acquiring the medicinal plants, are covered by Smith [16] and Landes [33]. Most of the Potawatomi medicine men had a special bowl and pestle in which they ground the roots or other parts of the medicinal plants. They often used the mixtures of the medicinal ingredients, sometimes as many as fifteen. In addition to the treatments with plants, other, more drastic treatments existed. For example, a patient was made to walk barefoot over a live smoldering fire. The rationale was that the greater suffering somehow produced cure, or induced unconsciousness, in which no pain would be felt.

It was interesting that both the medicine man and the patient believed that the medicine had no value unless it was properly paid for. However, the payment by the patient or by his family entitled them not only to the cure, but also to the medicinal knowledge which was responsible for the cure. This knowledge would then become the property of the family for all time to come. The family, in turn, would not disclose this knowledge to others suffering from a similar disease without charging a fee. These practices made it very difficult for Smith to get the actual formulas for treatment. Smith noticed that the Potawatomi would talk about different medicinal plants only in general, but were reluctant to talk about the quantities used and the complete set of ingredients which went into a medicine ready for administration.

We list here just some of ca. 160 plants which Smith described as medicinal. Some medicinal applications are similar to those by the Menominee Indians, and some are different. We list below some examples of the Potawatomi medicinal plants and their applications.

Aceraceae; Maple Family
- Red Maple
  The inner bark was boiled and used as an eye wash. It was used for the same purpose by the whites.
- Sugar Maple
  The inner bark was used as an expectorant.
- Mountain Maple
  The inner bark was used in a mixture with other medicinal materials as a cough syrup.

Alismaceae; Water-Plantain Family
- Broad-leaved Arrowhead
  A pulp made from the lateral rootlets was used for poulticing wounds and sores. It was used similarly by the white man.

Anacardiaceae; Sumac Family
- Poison Ivy
  The Forest Potawatomi considered this plant to be poisonous. The Prairie Potawatomi, according to the earlier sources quoted by Smith, made a poultice out of pounded root and used it on swellings to make them open.
- Staghorn Sumac
  The root bark was used as a hemostatic. The leaves were made into a tea, which was used against sore throat.

Apocynaceae; Dogbane Family
- Spreading Dogbane

The root was used as a diuretic and as urinary, kidney and heart medicine. The white men used a closely related plant for similar purposes.

Araliaceae; Ginseng Family
- Indian Spikenard
  The root of this plant had different uses among the different tribes. The Forest Potawatomi pounded the root into a pulp and used it as a hot poultice on inflammations. The Menominee used the root against blood poisoning. The Meskwaki used it as seasoner for other medicines.

Balsaminaceae; Touch-me-not Family
- Spotted Touch-me-not
  The Forest Potawatomi used the fresh juice of the plant to wash nettle stings or poison ivy itching and infections. Smith gave himself instant relief from the stinging nettle by use of this juice.

Berberidaceae; Barberry Family
- Blue Cohosh
  This is known to the Forest Potawatomi as the Squaw Root. It was universally used by the Wisconsin Indian tribes to furnish a tea which suppresses profuse menstruation and aids in childbirth.

Betulaceae; Birch Family
- Speckled Alder
  A bark tea was applied with a form of syringe to the rectal area to cure piles.

Caprifoliaceae; Honeysuckle Family
- Bush Honeysuckle
  A tea from the root was used as a diuretic. It was used by the white men for the same purpose.

Chenopodiaceae; Goosefoot Family
- Lamb's Quarters
  It was used as a medicinal food to cure or prevent scurvy. The same use was reported for the white man.

Compositae; Composite Family
- Yarrow

The flowers were placed on a plate of live coals to create a smudge. This smudge was supposed to revive a patient who might be in a state of coma.
- Forking Aster
  The basal leaves were steeped and the solution was rubbed on the head to cure a severe headache.
- Several Goldenrods (Canada-, Fragrant-, Broad-leaved and Late-)
  The flowering part was used to make a tea against fever.
- Field Sow Thistle
  The fresh leaves were made into a tea, which was used for the treatment of caked breasts.

Cornaceae; Dogwood Family
- Alternate-leaved Dogwood
  The bark was made into an infusion and was used as an eye-wash, to cure granulation of the eyelids.
- Red Osier Dogwood
  The root bark provided the most efficacious remedy the Potawatomi had against diarrhea.

Fagaceae; Beech Family
- Beech
  Smith quoted early records by Captain J. Carver, who traveled among the Forest Potawatomi in 1796, that a decoction made from the leaves was used to cure wounds arising from scalding and burning, and also frost-bites.

Hamamelidaceae; Witch-Hazel Family
- Witch-hazel
  The twigs were placed in water and with hot rocks created steam in the Potawatomi sweat baths. This steam was supposed to help sore muscles.

Hypericaceae; St. John's Wort Family
- Marsh St. John's Wort
  A tea made from the leaves was used to cure fevers.

Iridaceae; Iris Family
- Blue Flag
  The root was used to make poultices against inflammation.

Liliaceae; Lily Family
- Indian Spikenard
  The smoke or smudge from the root burning on a pan of live coals was fanned towards the nostrils of the patient. A paper cone was placed over the nose to ensure that the fumes reached the nostrils. This treatment was supposed to revive a patient who had sunk into a coma.
- Large-flowered White Trillium
  An infusion of the root was used to treat sore nipples. The medicine man would speed up the action of the medicine by piercing the teats with a dog whisker.
- Large-flowered Bellwort
  An infusion of the root was used to cure a backache. Also, the infusion was boiled down and mixed with lard. This was used as a salve to massage sore muscles and tendons.

Nymphaeaceae; Water Lily Family
- Yellow Pond Lily
  Smith went with Mrs. Spoon to collect this plant. The root was pounded into a pulp and it was used as a poultice against inflammatory diseases.

Papaveraceae; Poppy Family
- Bloodroot
  An infusion from the root was used against diphtheria, which the Potawatomi believed was a disease of the throat. They also made throat lozenges for mild cases of sore throat, by squeezing out drops of the bloodroot juice on maple sugar.

Pinaceae; Pine Family
- Balsam Fir
  Resinous exudate from the blisters on the trunk was swallowed fresh to cure colds. Also, the exudate was collected in a bottle for use as a salve to heal sores.
- Jack Pine
  The resin obtained from boiling the cone of the tree was used as a basis for an ointment. The leaves were used as a fumigant to revive patients who were in a coma, or to clear congested lungs.
- Hemlock

A tea brewed from the leaves causes the patient to perspire profusely and is valuable for breaking up a cold.

Plantaginaceae; Plantain Family
- Common Plantain
  The Indian name for this plant means "choke weed", which also indicates its use. The root was boiled to furnish a slippery liquid. The fluid was given to a patient who was choking on a bone in the throat. When the patient would drink the liquid, the bone would either pass on down the throat or be coughed up.

Rosaceae; Rose Family
- Agrimony
  The Prairie Potawatomi used the plant as a styptic to stop the nose-bleed.

Salicaceae; Willow Family
- Balsam Poplar
  The winter buds were melted with mutton or bear tallow to form an ointment for persistent sores and eczema.

Saxifragaceae; Saxifrage Family
- Prickly Gooseberry
  The Prairie Potawatomi used root bark to prepare a uterine remedy, while the Forest Potawatomi made a tea of the root and used it to treat sore eyes.

Scrophulariaceae; Figwort Family
- Common Mullein
  The dried leaves were smoked in a pipe to get relief from asthma.

Typhaceae; Cat-Tail Family
  The fresh roots were pounded and made into poultices for various inflammation.

Urticaceae; Nettle Family
- White Elm
  The bark was used for cramps and diarrhea.
- Slippery Elm

The inner bark was chewed and the mass applied to the eye for fast relief of inflammation. A splinter of the inner bark was sharpened and inserted into a boil, a poultice was placed around the splinter, and the splinter pulled out when the boil came to a head. A complete recovery was expected.

Violaceae; Violet Family
- Downy Yellow Violet
  A medicine made from the root was used for treating various heart diseases.

4.3 Ojibwe Indians

The Ojibwe, also known as the Chippewa, is one of the largest tribes in the United States and Canada. They originally inhabited the Western Great Lakes area, especially near Lake Superior [29], and lived as far west as Turtle Mountains, North Dakota [14]. Today they live on reservations in Michigan, Wisconsin, Minnesota, North Dakota, Montana, Ontario and Manitoba, and are populous in the cities of the Midwest and central Canada [29].

The Ojibwe Indians are the most numerous of the Wisconsin tribes. They live in the northern forest and lake districts of Wisconsin [14]. Their population in 1940 was 5,605 [13]. Today, the number is much larger. It includes 6,000 members of the Lac Court Oreilles band, 1,523 members of the Lac du Flambeau band, 2,000 members of the St. Croix band [28], 300 members of the Mole Lake band (Sokaogon) [34], in addition to the Red Cliff and Bad River bands.

We describe briefly the history of the Wisconsin Ojibwe, and some of their customs, mostly based on Smith [14]. However, much can be learned from the *History of the Ojibway People*, by William W. Warren [35], which was first published in 1885. Warren's mother was an Ojibwe and he got lots of information from the tribal elders. The Ojibwe customs and some aspects of their history are described beautifully by the German ethnologist, geographer and travel writer Johann Georg Kohl in his classic book *Kitchi-Gami, Life Among The Lake Superior Ojibway* [36], which was first published in 1859 in German. Kohl lived with the Wisconsin Ojibwe for four months in the summer of 1855.

The name "Ojibway" means "to roast until puckered up". It refers to the puckered seams on the moccasins [14, 29], or to the Ojibwe custom of torturing their enemy by fire [35]. However, Smith noticed that at least fifty names other than Ojibwe were given to this tribe. The name Ojibwe does not date far back. The Ojibwe people called themselves Anishinabe, meaning "first men" in Algonkian [29, 35].

The Ojibwe in Wisconsin resided in Ashland County near Lake Superior. They were discovered by the white men in the 1640s. The Ojibwe are Algonkian tribes. They were closely associated with the Ottawa and the Potawatomi, through Michigan and Minnesota. These three tribes were called the Three Fires Confederacy.

As with the other Indian tribes, there was a rich history of inter-tribal conflicts, which involved Sioux, Meskwaki and Sauk Indians. The Ojibwe took part in frontier settlement wars. They made a treaty with the U.S. Government in 1815 and remained peaceful. An exception was an uprising among the Pillager Band of Ojibwe on Leech Lake, Minnesota, which was over in 1898 [14].

Smith made three trips of six weeks' duration to study the Ojibwe ethnobotany. He visited the Lac du Flambeau reservation in Vilas County, Wisconsin, in June 1923 and again in the fall. In the spring of 1924 he made a trip to Leech Lake, Minnesota, where the remnants of the Pillager Band of the Ojibwe lived on Bear Island. In addition to these main trips, Smith visited Redcliff, Bayfield County, Odana, Iron County, Lac Court Oreilles, Clark County, and scattered bands in various parts of northern Wisconsin. His main work was performed at Lac du Flambeau and Leech Lake.

Smith collected every plant he could find in each region, since the Ojibwe, in contrast to other Wisconsin Indians, believed that every plant is some sort of medicine or is useful for something else. Based on Smith's judgement, about 65% of the Ojibwe herbal medicines are valuable medicinally, and the rest, he believed, was used in a shamanistic or superstitious manner. Smith, however, acknowledged the Ojibwe's great knowledge of plants.

Smith had more than thirty informants, some of whom were outstanding members of the tribe, including a medicine man, two Village Chiefs, and a Captain in the Civil War.

Frances Densmore [37], in a period from 1907 to 1925, studied the various uses of plants, including medicinal ones, among the Ojibwe. She researched the Ojibwe on the White Earth, Red Lake, Cass Lake, Leech Lake and Mille Lac reservations in Minnesota, the Lac Court Oreilles reservation in Wisconsin, and the Manitou Rapids reserve in Ontario, Canada. However, a majority of the plants she described were obtained on the White Earth reservation in Minnesota. The Ojibwe who lived on other reservations were accustomed to go to White Earth to get many of their medicinal plants.

Densmore listed 69 medicinal plants used by the Ojibwe which were recognized as medicinal by the white people. Like Smith, she used Indian, English and botanical names for the plants and the Latin names for the plants' families. She explained various routes of administration of the herbal remedies, as well as various medical appliances, including those for surgical treatment. She listed and referenced known uses of a particular plant by other tribes. Also, she gave medicinal constituents of the plants, such as pinene, bornyl acetate, tannic acid, gallic acid, alkaloid narceine, berberine, salicin, saponin, sanguinarin, etc. The latter information was limited by the medicinal chemistry knowledge of her time.

Both Densmore and Smith addressed the Ojibwe customs, especially the teaching of their Great Medicine Society or Midewiwin. Although the Midewiwin was a repository of knowledge of herbs, not all the knowledge was accessible to every member [37]. Thus, the individual members would know about their own medicines, but would not know about other people's medicines nor their uses of the same plants. Members of the Midewiwin were not taught many remedies at once, except when they were initiated. There was a process of instruction for advancement from one degree to another, which was more extensive for higher degrees [37].

There was great secrecy surrounding the herbal remedies. The medicine men frequently added an aromatic herb to their medicines to prevent their identification [37]. The Ojibwe did not disclose any knowledge of medicines, even to a member of their own family, without compensation [14, 37]. The medicinal uses of the plants described by Densmore and Smith were obtained from the informants. The latter had various motivations, from the desire to preserve the knowledge for posterity, to the trust in and respect for the white researchers [14, 37]. Thus, Smith was known among the Ojibwe from Lac du Flambeau and Lac Court Oreilles, as Shagashkandawe, meaning "Flying Squirrel", which was also the name of a famous old chief and medicine man.

Smith also noted that since 1924 some members of the tribe adopted the peyote lodge [14]. They learned about the peyote cult during their trips to the other tribes out of the state of Wisconsin.

Both Densmore and Smith pointed out that combinations of herbs were common. A mixture of nine to twelve, sometimes as many as twenty, was ground with a mortar and pestle, until it would be difficult to identify the ingredients of the prepared medicines.

The Ojibwe had knowledge of surgery. Various surgical appliances and treatments were described by Densmore [37]. They include: the letting of blood (also described by Smith [14]); making incisions to relieve swellings, various inflammations and headache; application of medicine with a set of needles; amputations; treatment of gangrenous wounds; lancing the gums in case of toothache; and dental surgery, including pulling teeth and insertion of an almost red-hot metal instrument into the hollow tooth. Detailed descriptions of these treatments and photographs of the surgical equipment were given [37].

We describe here an example of blood-letting by means of "tattooing outfits" [14]. The instrument consisted of sharp fish teeth, which were mounted at the end of a stick, four to five inches long. A quick stroke of this instrument on the upper part of the elbow effected a gush of blood. When the medicine man decided that enough blood was removed, a tourniquet was placed on the upper arm and the medicine man then sucked out the residue.

Since we are concentrating on the Wisconsin Indians, we use Smith [9] as a source for the ethnobotanical information.

He listed a total of ca. 160 medicinal plants, out of which ca. one-half was used only by the Flambeau band of Ojibwe (from Wisconsin), ca. one-third was used only by the Pillager band of Ojibwe (from Minnesota), and the rest was used by both bands. We provide below some examples of the medicinal plants and their uses, almost exclusively by the Flambeau Indians.

Anacardiaceae; Sumac Family
- Smooth Sumac
  Among many uses of the different parts of this plant, we note that the root bark tree was used as a hemostatic, and that the fruit was used as a throat cleanser.

Apocynaceae; Dogbane Family
- Spreading Dogbane
  The stalk and root were steeped to make a tea which was given to pregnant women to keep the kidneys "free".

Araliaceae; Ginseng Family
- Wild Sarsaparilla
  The fresh root was pounded and applied as a poultice to cure a boil or a car-buncle.

Betulaceae; Birch Family
- Speckled Alder
  When one passes blood in his stool, the root tea will act as a hemostat.
- Beaked Hazelnut
  The Flambeau Ojibwe boiled the bark and used it as a poultice to help close and heal cuts. The Pillager Ojibwe, however, used only the hairs of the hazelnut husk as a medicine to expel worms.

Boraginaceae; Borage Family
- Hound's Tongue
  The plant was burned on live coals, and the patient inhaled the fumes as a cure for headache.

Compositae; Composite Family
- Woolly Yarrow
  The leaves of this plant were used as a poultice to cure the bite of a spider.
- Pearly Everlasting
  The flowers were powdered and sprinkled on live coals. The fumes thus generated were inhaled by a stroke or paralysis patient to revive him.
- Large-leaved Aster
  Young roots were used to make a tea in which the patient's head was bathed to cure a headache.
- Tall Blue Lettuce
  A tea was made and given to women with caked breasts to make lactation easier. A dog whisker was used to pierce the teat.
- Indian Cup Plant
  A root tea was made for lumbago and other rheumatic pains in the back.

Cornaceae; Dogwood Family
- Bunchberry
  A tea from the root was used to cure babies of colic.

Cyperaceae; Sedge Family
- Hare's Tail
  The matted fuzz was used as a hemostatic.

Ericaceae; Heath Family
- Wintergreen
  The leaves were used to brew a tea against rheumatism and "to make one feel good".

Fagaceae; Beech Family
- Red Oak
  The bark provided a medicine for heart troubles and bronchial problems.

Gramineae; Grass Family
- Rattlesnake Grass
  The roots were used as a female remedy.

Labiatae; Mint Family
- Wild Mint
  The entire plant was brewed into a tea, which was used as a blood remedy. This plant was also used in the sweat bath.
- Catnip
  A tea made of catnip leaves was used as a blood purifier. The mint water obtained by steeping this plant in lukewarm water was used for bathing a patient for the purpose of raising his body temperature.

Liliaceae; Lily Family
- Northern Clintonia
  The root tea was used as a remedy to help parturition.

Onagraceae; Evening Primrose Family
- Great Willow-herb
  The outer rind of the root, which lathers in water, was pounded to make a poultice. This was used to draw out inflammation from a boil or a carbuncle.

Papaveraceae; Poppy Family
- Bloodroot

The Pillager Ojibwe squeezed the orange-red juice of this plant on a lump of maple sugar and retained it in the mouth until it had dissolved. This was the treatment for sore throat. They also used the juice to paint their faces for the medicine lodge ceremony or when at war.

Pinaceae; Pine Family
- Balsam Fir
  Among other uses, it was employed in the sweat bath . Other usual plants used for the same purpose were White Pine leaves, Hemlock leaves, Arbor Vitae leaves, Wild Bergamot plant, Balsam needles, Peppermint plants, etc. The sweat bath was taken in a small hemispherical wigwam, entirely covered with mats. The medicine was placed into large iron kettles, to which water and hot rocks were added. The steam thus produced was medicinal. The patient would sit naked in the wigwam, until there was no more steam, and his body was completely dry again. The patient would then put on all clean clothes, and would not wear the old clothes until they were washed.

Plantaginaceae; Plantain Family
- Common Plantain
  The leaves were soaked in warm water, and then used as a poultice on bruises, sprains, sores, burns, scalds, bee stings, or snake bites.

Ranunculaceae; Crowfoot Family
- Canada Anemone
  The Pillager Ojibwe eat the root to clear the throat to help them sing well in the medicine lodge ceremony.

Rosaceae; Rose Family
- Wild Strawberry
  A tea was made for stomach-ache, especially in babies.
- Marsh Five-finger
  This plant was used a cure for stomach cramps.
- Smooth Rose
  The powder of dried flowers was used to relieve heart-burn. The skin of the rose hips was used against indigestion.
- Steeple Bush

A tea made from the leaves and flowers was drunk to relieve the sickness of pregnancy and to act as an easy parturient.

Rubiaceae; Madder Family
- Small Bedstraw
  The Pillager Ojibwe made a tea for eczema, ringworm and scrofula.

Sarraceniaceae; Pitcher-Plant Family
- Pitcher-plant
  The root was made into a tea to help women in parturition.

Typhaceae; Cat-Tail Family
- Cat-tail
  The fuzz of the fruit was used as a "war medicine". The fuzz thrown into an enemy's face would blind him.

Umbelliferae; Parsley Family
- Black Snakeroot
  The root was pounded into a poultice to cure rattlesnake or other snake bites.

Urticaceae; Nettle Family
- Hop
  The Pillager Ojibwe made a tea to increase the flow of urine and reduce its acidity.
- Lyall's Nettle
  The leaves were soaked in warm water and used as a poultice for heat rashes. This was a procedure of "fighting fire with fire".

Violaceae; Violet Family
- American Dog Violet
  The whole plant was used to make a tea for heart trouble.

4.4   Meskwaki Indians

The Meskwaki Indians are another band of the Algonkians [17]. The name Meskwaki means "red-earth people", and reflects the belief that the first man of this tribe sprang from the red earth. The Meskwaki are also known as the Foxes. The Meskwaki are closely related to the Sauk Indians. The Sauk came to Wisconsin from Michigan, and were found on the Wolf River by the French (Father Allouez) in 1670. The Foxes lived around the Fox River and Lake Winnebago. A complex history of intertribal wars followed, in which the Foxes often made an alliance with the Sioux and Iroquois, and were fighting against the Ojibwe, Potawatomi and Menominee, and also against the Illinois tribes on the south. The Foxes were the only Algonkian tribe against whom the French made war [17]. As a consequence of these conflicts the Foxes were driven down the Wisconsin River. Eventually, in 1850, the Government assigned them a reservation in Kansas. But, without the water and trees the Meskwaki wanted, they did not like the site and eventually settled in Tama, Iowa. In Smith's time (1920s) there were only 342 Meskwaki left, out of the original population of at least five thousand.

The Meskwaki of Smith's time cherished a memory of their religion and regretted that they had to abandon the medicinal lodge. Some had taken the peyote cult.

Smith realized that the older tribal members who had knowledge of the tribal medicines were dying fast, and felt a sense of urgency to study this knowledge before it was gone. Thus, he made two field trips, each of one month's duration, in June and September of 1923, to the Meskwaki reservation in Tama, Iowa. Smith had as the main informant Mr. John McIntosh (Kepeosatok), a Prairie Potawatomi with a Meskwaki wife, who had spent most of his life with the Meskwaki. McIntosh was a famous medicine man, eighty-three years old, and well known in several states. He accompanied Smith and pointed out the plants under their Indian names. He had also loaned Smith his notebooks with the medicinal formulae, written in the Indian language, and expressed a wish that his knowledge be recorded in Smith's work for posterity. Smith had also used other informants from the Meskwaki reservation to corroborate McIntosh's recipes.

Smith also had access to the Meskwaki plant specimens collected in 1900 by Dr. William Jones, who was part Meskwaki. Dr. Jones collected these plants while a student at Columbia University, and performed an ethnobotanical study for the American Museum of Natural History in New York City. Smith studied 211 of Jones' specimens, many of which were mixtures, and included them in his work [17]. Dr. Jones died tragically in 1907, without completing his study, and thus Smith saved his work for posterity.

The Meskwaki Indians found in their Iowa reservation that many of the plants and trees were similar to those from Wisconsin. However, since there are no swamps on their reservation, they had to travel, often for many miles, to get certain plants, such as the skunk cabbage, that grow only in swamps.

Most Meskwaki medicines were mixtures. The Meskwaki believed that one plant is one power and as such has one unit of strength. They used as many as nine different plants in one mixture. Smith gave nineteen remedies of McIntosh, which he took directly from McIntosh's notebooks. These remedies were all mixtures. Some of the precious ingredients, which were not found in Iowa, had to be imported, for example from the Meskwaki's home land of Wisconsin. Smith commented on the rarity of such detailed descriptions of the remedies given to a white man by an Indian medicine man. Smith contrasted this with his inability to get a single complete remedy from the Menominee. McIntosh's recipes have not been further studied, but we hope that they will be in the future.

We present below selected examples of ca. 180 Meskwaki medicinal plants and their uses which were given by Smith. The format is the same as in the previous accounts.

Aceraceae; Maple Family
- Box-elder
  The inner bark was boiled and the liquid was drunk as an emetic.

Apocynaceae; Dogbane Family
- Indian Hemp
  The root was a universal medicine, but used especially in dropsy and ague.

Araceae; Arum Family
- Skunk Cabbage
  The fine rootlets or root hairs were used to cure toothache. The leaf bases were employed as a poultice to reduce swellings.
  It is interesting that the Meskwaki believed that if one had more than four roots of this plant in his possession, the snake spirit would make the rattlesnakes come to his home and bite the inhabitants. This belief was certainly useful in preserving a steady supply of this swamp plant by avoiding overexploitation.

Aristolochiaceae; Birthwort Family
- Wild Ginger
  The root had many uses. The cooked root was put into the ear for earache or sore ears. Spoiled meat was cooked with the root to avoid ptomaine poisoning.

Asclepiadaceae; Milkweed Family
- Swamp Milkweed
  The root tea was used to drive the tapeworms from a person, reportedly in one hour.

Caprifoliaceae; Honeysuckle Family
- Common Elder
  The bark tea was used only in very difficult cases of parturition, when the baby was stillborn.
- Wolfberry
  The root tea was drunk to cleanse the afterbirth and to speed up convalescence.

Caryophyllaceae; Pink Family
- Starry Campion
  The root was used on pus-discharging swellings to dry them up.

Celastraceae; Staff-tree Family
- Wahoo
  The Meskwaki call this tree "the weak-eye tree". The inner bark of the trunk is steeped into a tea with which the weak or sore eyes were bathed. However, a tea made from the root was especially powerful in curing sore eyes.

Compositae; Composite Family
- Yarrow
  Both leaves and flowers were used to make a tea which cured fever and ague.
- Lobed Cud-weed
  A tea from the leaves was used to cure tonsilitis and sore throat. A smudge of the leaves drove away mosquitoes. Thus, the Indian's name for this plant is "mosquito smoke".
- Starved of Calico Aster

The blossoms were smudged to cure a crazy person who had lost his mind.
- Narrow-leaved Purple Cone-flower
  The root was used to cure cramps in the stomach and also to cure fits.
- Naked Stemmed Hawksbeard
  The entire plant was used to make a poultice, which was applied to a carbuncle or cancer, so that they would open up. An excision would then be performed without fear of complications.
- Thin-leaved Sunflower
  The root was macerated and used to make poultices and heal sores of long standing.
- Dotted Button-Snakeroot
  An infusion made out of the root was used when the urine was bloody, and as a cure for bladder trouble of women.
- Blazing Star
  It was used as a remedy for bladder and kidney troubles.
- Compass Plant
  The gum that exudes from the stalks was chewed as a chewing-gum. The smaller roots were boiled and the tea thus obtained was drunk cold as an emetic.
- Indian Cup Plant
  The root was used to alleviate vomiting during pregnancy, and was also used to reduce menstrual flow in profuse menstruation.

Cornaceae; Dogwood Family
- Panicled Dogwood
  A tea made out of the bark was used to cure the flux. The tea was injected as an enema, using a pig's bladder as the syringe, and the hollow bone of a goose as the nozzle.
  This tea was also held in the mouth to stop the pain of sore teeth.

Crassulaceae; Orpine Family
- Ditch Stonecrop
  The seeds were used for making a cough syrup.

Cruciferae; Mustard Family
- Black Mustard
  The seeds were ground up and used as a snuff to cure cold in the head.

Dioscoreaceae; Yam Family
- Wild Yam
  The root was used by women to relieve pain of childbirth.

Geraniaceae; Geranium Family
- Wild Geranium
  The root infusion was used to cure sore gums and pyorrhea, aching teeth, and neuralgia. A poultice made of the pounded root was bound to the anus to cause protruding piles to recede.

Iridaceae; Iris Family
- Blue-eyed Grass
  A tea was made by boiling the whole plant and was used to cure hay fever.

Labiatae; Mint Family
- False Dragon-head
- Rough Hedge Nettle
  The leaves were used to make a tea for a bad cold.

Leguminosae; Bean Family
- Lead Plant
  A tea from the leaves was used to kill pinworms and other intestinal worms. The leaves when steeped gave a liquid which was used to cure eczema.
- Partridge Pea
  The seeds were soaked in water until they became mucilaginous. Then they were eaten for sore throat.
- Honey Locust
  The bark tea was used in measles, smallpox and fevers. The tea reportedly prevented pitting.
- Kentucky Coffee-tree
  The wax from the pods was given to a patient to cure him of lunacy.
- Purple Prairie Clover
  A root tea was drunk as a cure for measles.

Polemoniaceae; Phlox Family
- Downy Phlox
  A tea was made from the leaves and was used to wash the eczema.

Polygalaceae; Milkwort Family
- Senega Snakeroot
  This root was boiled and made into a drink which was used for heart trouble.

Polygonaceae; Buckwheat Family
- Swamp Persicaria
  The root was used for treating sores in the mouth. The leaves and stems were made into a tea, which was used for the treatment of flux in children. The plant parts were soaked without heat, since, the Indians claimed, the drug's active principle is destroyed by heat.

Ranunculaceae; Crowfoot Family
- Thimbleweed
  The root was made into a tea, and was used for headache, dizzy spells, and as a medicine for crazy people.

Rosaceae; Rose Family
- Queen of the Prairie
  The root provided a very important medicine for heart trouble.
- Wild Plum
  The bark of the root was used to cure canker in the mouth.

Rutaceae; Rue Family
- Prickly Ash
  The bark and berries were used to make cough syrup and medicine which acted as a strong expectorant. It was also used for tuberculosis.

Salicaceae; Willow Family
- Trembling Aspen
  The buds were boiled in fat to make a balm for nasal applications to cure colds and coughs.

Santalaceae; Sandalwood Family
- Bastard Toad Flax
  A tea was prepared from the leaves and was drunk for internal pains in the lungs.

Scrophulariaceae; Figwort Family
- Slender Gerardia
  A tea made of this plant was used against diarrhea.
- Lousewort
  The entire plant was boiled to make a tea, which reportedly reduced any internal swelling. The root was used to make a poultice against external swelling.

Typhaceae; Cat-tail Family
- Cat-tail
  Children born in the winter were wrapped in a quilt of the cat-tail fuzz to keep them warm. This fuzz was also used to pad old neck sores to help heal them.

Umbelliferae; Parsley Family
- Smooth Sweet Cicely
  This plant was used as an eye remedy. The grated root was mixed with salt and used as a horse medicine for distemper.

Verbenaceae; Vervain Family
- White Vervain
  The root tea was used against profuse menstruation.

Vitaceae; Vine Family
- Frost Grape
  The Meskwaki children made a tea from the twigs and used it when poisoned by eating Indian turnip. They held the tea in their mouths, until the element which caused the pain (calcium oxalate, according to Smith) dissolved.

4.5 Summary

From the accounts of Smith [14, 16–18] and Densmore [37] we have learned that the Wisconsin Indians used medicinal plants extensively. They had a great variety of treatments for various medical conditions. These include diseases and injuries, such as headache, "craziness", problems with the heart, lungs, kidneys, bladder, various colds, coughs, mouth sores, stomach problems, colic, cramps, menstrual disorders, pains and complications of childbirth, wounds, sores, eye problems, teeth and gum problems, rheumatism, ear ache, intestinal worms, skin conditions such as boils and eczema, bites of poisonous reptiles and insects, and others. These Indians had knowledge of both emetics and physics, sweat baths, and the use of plant smudges for revival purposes. They were competent in various modes of drug delivery, which included external and internal administrations, for example, tattooing the remedy into the skin with a set of needles, delivery by enema, smoking, snuffing or chewing, by steam or fumes, application of a salve made by boiling the herbs with grease, in addition to more common uses of teas, infusions and poultices. They were proficient in uses of herbal mixtures, and had an extraordinary knowledge about the location of the medicinal principles in different parts of the plant and the concentration of these during the plants' growth cycle. Many Indian medicinal plants were used by the white men of Smith's and earlier times. It is known that white men have learned a great deal about herbal medicine from the Indians.

Since Smith's time there have been no reports of comprehensive study of the Wisconsin Indians' medicinal plants. This makes Smith's original work even more important.

4.6   Herbal medicine of other North American Indian tribes

In this section we present selected literature sources on comparison of uses of medicinal plants among different North American Indian tribes. When different tribes used the same plant for medicinal purposes, the claim for the medicinal value of such a plant is strengthened. The use of Indian medicinal plants by the contemporary white men was often included in the studies.

There are several books which deal with this approach. One is *American Indian Medicine* by Vogel [38]. This is a true classic in the field, which addresses, among other topics, Indian theories of diseases, early observations by white men of Indian medicine, Indian therapeutic methods, and a valuable appendix on American Indian contribution to pharmacology. The appendix summarizes comparative uses of medicinal plants by different Indian tribes. The plants selected are those that were/are also the official drugs in the Pharmacopoeia of the United States of America or the National

Formulary. Vogel credits North American Indians with the discovery of at least 170 official drugs. Out of ca. 80 entries in the appendix, which often comprise several related plants, almost one-half refers to the Wisconsin Indians. The entries are listed in alphabetical order of common names of the representative plants. We revisit here some of the plants listed in the appendix, which were previously described by Smith, to illustrate the contribution of Wisconsin Indians to the medicine of white men: Alder, Anemone, Angelica, Arbor vitae, Balm of Gilead, Balsam fir, Bearberry, Birch trees, Butterfly weed, Cohosh (blue), Crowfoot, Dogwood, Elm, Goldenrod, Hops, Indian hemp, Joe Pye weed, May apple, Mint family, Mullen (or Mullein), Mustard, Partridge berry, Poison ivy, Puccoon (blood root), Purple coneflower, Sarsaparila (wild), Snakeroots, Skunk cabbage, Spikenard, Sumac, Sweet flag, Trillium, Violet, Wahoo, Wild geranium, Wild ginger, Wild yam, Wintergreen, Witch hazel and Yarrow, among others.

Another classic book is *Medicinal and Other Uses of North American Plants, A Historical Survey with Specific Reference to the Eastern Indian Tribes* by Erichsen-Brown [39]. The author, as the title indicates, provides a historical survey, but the end product is much more. Evidence from different historical sources amplifies the single claims for the medicinal activities of the plants. Uses of plants by different tribes and also by white men provide additional support to the medicinal value of the plant. The author brings up the fact that most Indian medicines were mixtures, usually of seven to nine plants, and points out that useful medical knowledge may be gained by exploration of such mixtures. This is also the point which we have brought up. Erichsen-Brown provided numerous examples in which the Indians' and white men's herbal medicines were compared. Often, Indian remedies were better and were subsequently adopted by the white men. For example, the use of medicinal plants in childbirth put Indian tribes ahead of contemporary European practice. For example, Blue cohosh facilitates delivery, since it provokes strong uterine contractions, which are more successful than those caused by ergot, the plant fungus used at that time by white physicians for the same purpose.

Another well-known book in the field is *Indian Herbalogy of North America* by Hutchens [40]. The author covers ca. 200 Indian medicinal plants and, where applicable, reports on their use in the old USSR, referred to as Russia. This adds an entirely new importance to the study of the Indian medicinal plants, as it becomes apparent that many of these plants grow in other geographic regions of the world (as local or imported flora), where their medicinal properties have also been exploited. The author lists twenty-five Russian publications and provides their summaries. Uses of the medicinal plants in other regions of the world, such as India, Pakistan and South Africa, are also mentioned, but to a much smaller extent. We list here some examples of Indian medicinal plants that were/are used in Russia: Alder, Angelica, Ash, Barberry, Bearberry, Beech, Birch, Snakeroot, Indian hemp, Blue cohosh, Purple coneflower, Elder, Ginger (wild), Golden rod, Hops, Horsetail, Liverwort, Indian tobacco, May apple, Mullein, Plantain, Sage, Snakeroot, Solomon's seal, Spikenard, St. John's wort, Sumac, Sweet flag, Wild Valerian, Violet, Witch hazel and Yarrow, among others. The author has written another, similar book [41].

Duke's *Handbook of Northeastern Indian Medicinal Plants* [42] is another true classic in the field. The plants are listed in the alphabetical order of their Latin names, their uses by different Indian tribes are described, and each statement is supported by a reference. An index section correlates common names of plants and medical terms for ailments to those in Latin and provides a list of the plants that were used to treat these ailments.

As just one illustration of multiple use of medicinal plants by different Indian tribes: Yarrow was used by Abenaki, Algonquin, Blackfoot Indians, Cherokee, Cheyenne, Chickasaw, Creek, Delaware, Hesquiat, Illinois-Miami, Iroquois, Malecite, Menominee, Micmac, Mohawk, Paiute, Potawatomi, Tete-de-Boule, Ute, Winnebago and Zuni.

Similar entries exist for ca. 700 plants. We revisit Bloodroot, May apple, Blue cohosh, Spikenard, Jack-in-the Pulpit, Horsetail, Joe-Pye weed, St. John's wort, Elm, Ash and numerous other plants we already talked about.

Native American Ethnobotany by Moerman [15] is another superb book. It also contains sections on comparative use of medicinal plants by different tribes, in addition to a wealth of other information.

Hartwell, who worked at the National Cancer Institute in Bethesda, Maryland, was inspired by the use of May apple for treatment of tumors by the Penobscot Indians of Maine. In the 1950s he was personally involved in the isolation and identification of the anti-cancer chemical agents from podophyllin resin from May apple [43], which led to the development of useful anti-cancer drugs [12, 44]. Hartwell then produced a magnificent series of papers in the period of 1967–1971, under the title *Plants Used Against Cancer, A Survey* [45–55]. He surveyed several thousand references "embracing the whole history of medicine, pharmacology, materia medica, medical botany, ethnobotany and folklore..." [45]. The history covered was from 2838 B.C.! In this gold mine of Hartwell's papers one finds also the uses of various plants against cancer by the Native American tribes. We were not able to find a systematic and comprehensive follow-up of Hartwell's work, a situation similar to Smith's work; this would consist of chemical analyses and pharmacological assessments by modern methods.

5 Conclusions and perspective

We have shown a wealth of information about the use of medicinal plants by the Wisconsin Indians. The information is from the 1920s and 1930s, and no systematic and comprehensive follow-up has been reported since. The Wisconsin Indians' knowledge of the medicinal plants was remarkable. The use of mixtures of medicinal plants by these Indians reveals their deep understanding of drug interactions.

We have provided readers with a selected number of the information science tools which are appropriate for searching the literature and various databases for new results on chemical analyses of plants and pharmacology of their active ingredients. These new results in some cases can be matched with the plants that Indians used as medicinal, and in such a way that the old information from Smith can be somewhat updated. In the limited number of plants that we have studied in such a manner, it was revealed that they indeed contain biologically active ingredients consistent with the reported medicinal use of the plant.

It is our hope that the subject of the herbal medicine of the Wisconsin Indians will be further studied in the future, and that pharmacological tests will be done with the plant mixtures. The latter tests may lead to a better understanding of drug interactions.

6 References

1   M.R. Reddy and A.L. Parrill, in: A.L. Parrill and M.R. Reddy (eds): Rational Drug Design, Novel Methodology and Practical Applications. American Chemical Society, Washington, D.C. 1999, 1–11.

2   D.B. Boyd, in: A.L. Parrill and M.R. Reddy (eds): Rational Drug Design, Novel Method-

ology and Practical Applications, American Chemical Society, Washington, D.C. 1999, 346–356.

3   J. Josephson: Modern Drug Discovery *5*, 45–46, 49–50 (2000).

4   S. Bank: The Scientist, July 10, 8–9 (2000)

5   M.J. Plotkin: Tales of a Shaman's Apprentice, Penguin Books, New York 1994.

6   M.J. Plotkin: Medicine Quest, Viking, New York 2000.

7   D.J. Chadwick and J. Marsh (eds): Bioactive Compounds from Plants, CIBA Foundation Symp. 154, J. Wiley, New York 1990.

8   V.E. Tyler: J. Nat. Prod. *62*, 1589–1592 (1999).

9   P. J. Houghton: J. Chem. Ed. *78*, 175–184 (2001).

10   D.M. Hosler and M.A. Mikita: J. Chem. Ed. *64*, 328–332 (1987).

11   Y-Z. Shu: J. Nat. Prod. *61*, 1053–1071 (1998).

12   M. Hamburger, A. Marston and K. Hostettmann: Adv. Drug. Res. *20*, 167–215 (1991).

13   J.M. Douglas: The Indians in Wisconsin History, The Milwaukee Public Museum, Milwaukee, Wisconsin 1954.

14   H.H. Smith: Ethnobotany of the Ojibwe Indians, Bull. of the Public Museum of the City of Milwaukee 4 (3), 327–525 (plates 46–77) (1932).

15   D.E. Moerman: Native American Ethnobotany, Timber Press, Portland, Oregon, 1998.

16   H.H. Smith: Ethnobotany of the Forest Potawatomi Indians, Bull. of the Public Museum of the City of Milwaukee 7 (1), 1–230 (plates 1–38), (1933).

17   H.H. Smith: Ethnobotany of the Meskwaki Indians, Bull. of the Public Museum of the City of Milwaukee 4 (2), 175–326 (plates 37–46), (1928).

18   H.H. Smith: Ethnobotany of the Menomini Indians, Greenwood Press Publ., Westport, Conn. 1970 (republication of 1923 edn.).

19   T. Johnson: CRC Ethnobotany Desk Reference, CRC Press, Boca Raton, Fla. 1999.

20   A.R. Torkelson: The Cross Name Index to Medicinal Plants, CRC Press, Boca Raton, Fla. 1996.

21   S.N. Hooper and R.F. Chandler: J. Ethnopharmacol. *10*, 181–194 (1984).

22   R.F. Chandler, S.N. Hooper, D.L. Hooper, W.D. Jamieson, C.G. Flinn and L.M. Safe: J. Pharm. Sci. *71*, 690–693 (1982).

23   R.F. Chandler, S.N. Hooper, D.L. Hooper, W.D. Jamieson and E. Lewis: Lipids *17*, 102–106 (1982).

24   R.F. Chandler and S.N. Hooper: J. Ethnopharmac. *6*, 275–285 (1982).

25   S.N. Hooper and R.F. Chandler: Canad. J. Pharm. Sci. *16*, 56–59 (1981).

26   R.F. Chandler and S.N. Hooper: Canad. J. Pharm. Sci. *14*, 103–106 (1979).

27   R.F. Chandler, L. Freeman and S.N. Hooper: J. Ethnopharmacol. *1*, 49–68 (1979).

28   Native Wisconsin, Special Sesquicentennial Edition, Official Guide to Native American Communities in Wisconsin, Great Lakes Inter-Tribal Council, Inc., Lac du Flambeau, Wisconsin 1998.

29   C. Waldman: Encyclopedia of Native American Tribes, Facts on File Publications, New York 1988.

30   J.M. Dunn: The Relocation of the North American Indian, Lucent Books, World History Series, San Diego, California 1995.

31   L.J. Hauptman and L.G. McLester III (eds.): The Oneida Indian Journey, From New York to Wisconsin 1784–1860, The University of Wisconsin Press, Madison, WI 1999.

32   R.D. Edmunds: The Potawatomis, Keepers of the Fire, University of Oklahoma Press, Norman, OK 1978.

33 R. Landes: The Prairie Potawatomi, Tradition and Ritual in the Twentieth Century, The University of Wisconsin Press, Madison, WI 1970.

34 Indian Tribes of Wisconsin, Wisconsin Division of Tourism, Madison, WI 2001.

35 W.W. Warren: History of the Ojibway People, Minnesota Historical Society Press, St. Paul, MN 1984 (first published in 1885).

36 J.G. Kohl: Kitchi-Gami, Life Among The Lake Superior Ojibway, Minnesota Historical Society Press, St. Paul, MN 1985 (first published in 1859 in German).

37 F. Densmore: How Indians Use Wild Plants for Food, Medicine & Crafts (formerly entitled "Uses of Plants by the Chippewa Indians"), Dover Publications, Inc., New York 1974 (first published in 1928).

38 V.J. Vogel: American Indian Medicine, University of Oklahoma Press, Norman, OK 1970.

39 C. Erichsen-Brown: Medicinal and Other Uses of North American Plants, A Historical Survey with Special Reference to the Eastern Indian Tribes, Dover Publications, Inc., New York 1989.

40 A.R. Hutchens: Indian Herbalogy of North America, Shambhala, Boston, Mass. 1991.

41 A.R. Hutchens: A Handbook of Native American Herbs, Shambhala, Boston, Mass. 1992.

42 J.A. Duke: Handbook of Northeastern Indian Medicinal Plants, Quarterman Publications, Inc., Lincoln, Mass 1986.

43 M.G. Kelly and J.L. Hartwell: J. Natl. Cancer Inst. *14*, 967–1010 (1954).

44 J. Bruneton (ed.): Pharmacognosy, Phytochemistry, Medicinal Plants; Intercept Limited, Andover, England 1995, 247–249.

45 J.L. Hartwell: Lloydia *30*, 379–436 (1967).

46 J.L. Hartwell: Lloydia *31*, 71–170 (1968).

47 J.L. Hartwell: Lloydia *32*, 70–107 (1969).

48 J.L. Hartwell: Lloydia *32*, 153–205 (1969).

49 J.L. Hartwell: Lloydia *32*, 247–296 (1969).

50 J.L. Hartwell: Lloydia *33*, 97–194 (1970).

51 J.L. Hartwell: Lloydia *33*, 288–392 (1970).

52 J.L. Hartwell: Lloydia *34*, 103–160 (1971).

53 J.L. Hartwell: Lloydia *34*, 204–255 (1971)

54 J.L. Hartwell: Lloydia *34*, 310–361 (1971).

55 J.L. Hartwell: Lloydia *34*, 386–437 (1971).

Progress in Drug Research, Vol. 58 (E. Jucker, Ed.)
© 2002 Birkhäuser Verlag, Basel (Switzerland)

The impact of multiple drug resistance (MDR) proteins on chemotherapy and drug discovery

By Paul L. Skatrud

Elanco Animal Health Science
A Division of Eli Lilly and Company
2001 West Main Street, DC GL52
Greenfield, Indiana 46140, USA

<Skatrud_Paul_L@Lilly.com>

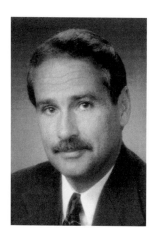

Paul L. Skatrud

*Ph.D., 1986, Pharm. & Toxicol., Indiana U. School of Medicine;
M.S., 1977, Microbiol., U. of Wisconsin; B.A., 1974, Biology,
Luther College
Eli Lilly and Company: Research Scientist – Elanco Animal Health
Research (current); Infectious Diseases Research (1992–2000);
Senior Molecular Biologist – Molecular Genetics Research
(1988–92); Assistant Senior Microbiologist – Antibiotic Culture
Development (1986–87); Microbiologist – Antibiotic Culture Devel-
opment (1983-86); Associate Microbiologist – Antibiotic Culture
Development (1982–83)
Miller Brewing Co.: Microbiologist (1980–82); Associate Microbiol-
ogist (1977–80);
Scientific Contributions: More than 100 publications (including
journal articles, book chapters, books edited, published abstracts,
and posters); 38 issued US Patents
Awards: Fellow, Industrial Society for Microbiol. 2000; Outstanding
Alumnus, Indiana U. School of Medicine, Pharm. & Tox. Dept.
1999; Powell Award, Indiana Branch of ASM 1992*

Summary

Transportation of molecules across the cell membrane in living organisms is a critical aspect of life. Transportation includes importation of nutrients from the environment and exportation of toxic compounds. When export includes therapeutic compounds, then the practice of clinical medicine may become compromised. Often efflux of therapeutic compounds is mediated by a large superfamily of proteins referred to as multidrug resistance (MDR) proteins. The initial sections of this chapter are focused on MDR proteins and their negative impact on clinical medicine in cancer chemotherapy as well as infectious diseases mediated by bacteria, fungi and parasites. A brief description of major classes of MDR proteins found in microbes is followed by a more exhaustive treatment of ABC transporters in lower eukaryotes and parasites as well as cancerous mammalian cells. Later sections deal with potential and real positive aspects and applications brought about by a growing knowledge of MDR proteins. Examples described include improved antibiotic production, leveraging MDR proteins in drug discovery, new therapeutic options, dual therapy in treatment of cancer and infectious diseases, and finally MDR proteins as targets for new classes of therapeutic compounds.

Contents

Key words

Multidrug resistance, ABC transporter, cancer chemotherapy, antibacterial, antifungal, parasites, drug discovery, antibiotic production, ATP-binding cassette, transport, efflux pumps, combination therapy, potentiation.

Glossary of abbreviations

ABC, ATP-binding cassette; hu MDR1, human multiple drug resistant protein; *hu mdr1*, gene encoding hu MDR1; MATE, multidrug and toxic compound extrusion; MDR, multiple or multidrug resistance; MFP, membrane fusion protein; MFS, major facilitator superfamily; MRP, multidrug resistance associated protein; MSR, membrane spanning region; OMP, outer membrane protein; RNP, resistance-nodulation-cell division transporters; SAR, structure activity relationship; SMR, small multidrug resistance; TM, transmembrane

1   Introduction

Generally the words "multiple drug resistance" or the corresponding acronym "MDR" carry a negative connotation in the medical community and research environment. Certainly, resistance to antibiotics, antifungals, antiseptics and parasiticides is a major problem world-wide in the clinical setting. It is even more problematic when a particular organism responsible for an infection is resistant to more than one traditionally used therapeutic compound, as is the case for MDR. Cancer chemotherapy has also been compromised by drug efflux *via* MDR proteins. However, like many situations in life, there is more than one side to this situation and thus the importance of being open to new ideas is emphasized. MDR proteins achieved their negative status because of their ability to eject therapeutic compounds from many different disease-causing organisms and in life-threatening diseases, resulting in clinical treatment failures. This ability is to some extent due to the relatively wide variety of compounds transported by many MDR proteins. The "natural" physiological roles of MDR-like proteins are clearly not fully appreciated. A great deal of information has been published concerning MDR proteins in the last decade. During that time it has become evident that the MDR phenomenon presents several positive opportunities when carefully considered from different perspectives. It is hoped that during the course of reading this manuscript you will once again heighten your awareness to the threat MDR poses and become convinced that there are positive aspects/uses for the genes and proteins involved in some forms of MDR.

1.1   Transport, an essential life process

Environmental interactions probably present the single most challenging set of obstacles that living organisms must contend with. A cell depends upon its environment for life-sustaining nutrients, whether it is a microbe, a single cell in a highly differentiated organism, or a relatively simple parasite living inside another cell or drawing life-sustaining nutrients from another cell. However, that same environment is also the source of numerous dangers in the form of toxic substances and wildly varying osmotic pressures. Thus it is necessary to be able to transport molecules into the cell that will provide that all-important nutrition and, at the same time, selectively exclude toxic molecules and remove toxic metabolic products from the cell. In addition, a critical balance of solutes must be maintained in a cell, as compared to its external environment, in order for it to thrive. A number of mechanical (i.e., cell walls, cell membranes) and functional barriers (passive or active import and/or export, toxin modification) are employed by different types of organisms/cells to achieve harmony with their environment. Figure 1 illustrates four mechanisms cells commonly employ to deal specifically with toxic molecules and, more specifically for the sake of this discussion, therapeutic drugs. Descriptions of mechanisms in this figure are not intended to be all-inclusive but rather illustrative. The cell membrane and cell wall (if present) present a formidable mechanical barrier protecting the cell from its external environment at least to some extent. Drug metabolism or, as illustrated, enzymatic modification which renders a therapeutic inactive, can occur inside (i.e., transferases that modify aminoglycoside antibiotics) as well as outside of the cell (i.e., β-lactamase inactivation of β-lactam antibiotics). Genetic plasticity permits organisms to modify therapeutic targets by mutations that directly interfere with the interaction of a therapeutic compound and its target. Finally, active efflux or removal of toxins/therapeutics from the interior of the cell or the cell membrane is an effective means of avoiding their negative effect. In the case of an intracellular target, an efficacious concentration of compound is thus avoided at the target site. For the purpose of this discussion, a focus will be placed on microbial disease-causing organisms and resistance mediated by efflux pumps. However, efflux of oncolytic drugs in human cells must also be addressed at least to some extent for a proper historical perspective and to illustrate its impact on chemotherapy and drug discovery. The process of toxin efflux *via* ABC transporters and other efflux mechanisms is usually not limited to a single substrate for a particular transporter. Thus the term "multiple drug resistance" (MDR) has become popular. The author recognizes that there are many other important types of transporters using alternative mechanisms of transport and those that transport only a single substance. For a more comprehensive review of microbial efflux pumps the reader is referred to the recent work of Saier [1].

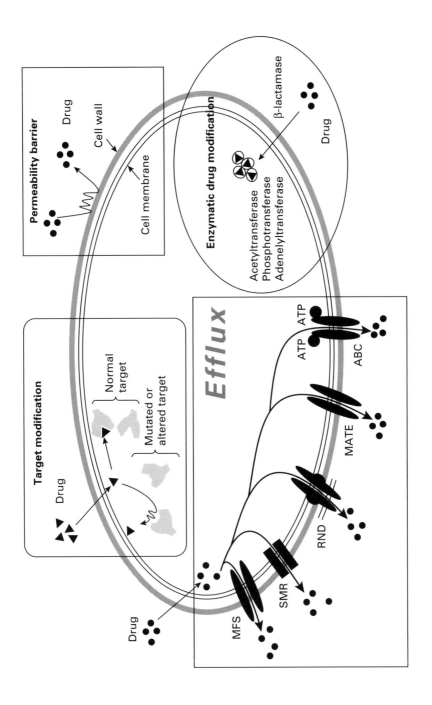

Fig. 1
Cartoon of a hypothetical cell illustrating various means to avoid the toxic effects of therapeutic, metabolic and environmental compounds.

1.2   Multidrug resistance in cancer chemotherapy

Historically, perhaps the most widely studied MDR phenomenon is the human P-glycoprotein, also referred to as human MDR1 (hu MDR1). Over half a century ago, Burchenal and colleagues observed the phenomenon of tumor MDR [2]. In 1973, Dana described the "drug pump" model to explain the MDR phenotype [3]. Since then an enormous amount of scientific literature has been devoted to elucidating the precise mechanism of action of hu MDR1 as well as the clinical relevance of hu MDR1. Recent studies have questioned the pump model. These studies resulted in a new model called "altered partitioning" that attempts to explain the drug efflux mechanism [4–7]. At this point, neither the precise mechanism nor its clinical relevance is completely understood; however, as Roepe [4] has pointed out, "hu MDR1 protein remains an extremely important window in on the complex pathways that lead to induced chemotherapeutic drug resistance". This importance was recently re-highlighted by the work of Chan and colleagues [8]. They observed reversal of drug resistance when a *hu mdr1* antisense RNA was expressed in cultures of human HepG2 cells. Chen et al. [9] demonstrated that also in cell culture (sarcoma cell line MES-SA), the predominant resistance mechanism selected by exposure to vinblastine was *hu mdr1* activation. With regard to the clinical aspect, Plaat et al. [10] compared two different clinical manifestations of cancer in patient populations. They concluded that patients had a better survival rate if their malignancies collectively expressed MDR proteins to a lesser extent. One approach for treatment of tumors with elevated levels of MDR expression would be co-administration of a pharmacokinetically similar compound that would block efflux of the therapeutic compound. This type of approach is actively being pursued within the pharmaceutical industry as well as in the academic setting. For example, Tiberghien et al. [11] demonstrated that aureobasidin A inhibits the activity of hu MDR1. Interestingly, aureobasidin A was initially described as an antifungal agent. Furthermore, hu MDR1 inhibitory activity does not correlate with antifungal activity during structure activity relationship (SAR) studies. Calcium antagonists, such as verapamil and related compounds, also inhibit the function of hu MDR1, rendering treated cells more susceptible to the action of oncolytic drugs [12]. More details and examples of co-therapy stimulated by the MDR phenomenon will be presented in a subsequent section describing therapeutic options in cancer chemotherapy (section 6.3.1).

2 Microbial efflux pumps

Drug/toxin efflux *via* MDR-like proteins and other pumps is by no means limited to the mammalian world. Very similar types of transporters exist in both eukaryotic and prokaryotic cells. Bambeke and colleagues have recently produced a summation of transporters in eukaryotes [13]. In the microbial world there are at least five distinct families of drug efflux pumps currently recognized and split between two classes or types. These drug transporter families have been extensively reviewed by Jenkinson [14] and Putman et al. [15]. The Type I transporters include the ATP-dependent multidrug transporters, also referred to as the ATP-binding cassette (ABC) multidrug transporters. The secondary or Type II multidrug transporters are those driven by the proton motive force. The secondary transporters include the major facilitator superfamily (MSF), the small multidrug resistance family (SMR), the resistance-nodulation-cell division family (RND), and the multidrug and toxic compound extrusion family (MATE). A short description of each family follows along with brief comments on how their presence has had an impact with regard to chemotherapy.

2.1 Major facilitator superfamily of transporters (MFS)

The expulsion of compounds from bacterial cells *via* members of the MSF drug pumps utilize the proton motive force as an energy source in uniport, antiport, or symport (i.e., for each molecule transported, one proton goes in the opposite direction). In a general sense, the structure of these transporters, which is highly conserved within the MFS, is reminiscent of the ABC-type transporters in that they possess twelve or fourteen transmembrane (TM) domains. However, nucleotide-binding sites, a defining characteristic of ABC transporters, are not found in the MFS super family. Amino acid motifs highly conserved within the MFS transporters are typically not found in ABC transporters. Members of the MFS family of transporters are generally comprised of about 400 amino acids [14] and are divided into subgroups based on the number of TM domains (i.e., twelve or fourteen). MFS proteins with twelve TM domains contain five conserved amino acid sequence motifs. Three of these motifs are also found in MFS proteins with fourteen TM domains. MFS proteins with fourteen TM domains have four additional highly conserved motifs [15].

A wide variety of compounds can be moved by members of the MFS family including sugars, Krebs cycle intermediates, phosphate esters, oligosaccharides and various antibiotics [16]. Examples of MFS-type efflux pumps with twelve TM domains include TetA from *Escherichia coli* (Gram negative) which confers resistance to tetracycline [17] and NorA which provides protection from quinolones and chloramphenicol in *Staphylococcus aureus* (Gram positive) [16, 18]. In *Streptococcus pneumoniae*, a reserpine-sensitive multidrug transporter, PmrA [19], imparts resistance to the fluoroquinolone antibiotics ciprofloxacin and norfloxacin [20–23]. Treatment of tuberculosis, the single most devastating microbial disease on earth, is complicated by intrinsic resistance of *Mycobacterium tuberculosis* to aminoglycosides and tetracycline, which is mediated by the Tap multidrug efflux pump [24]. Until recently (i.e., after the mid to late 1990s), the degree of involvement of MDR proteins in intrinsic antimicrobial resistance to numerous antibacterials, as well as antifungals, was probably not fully appreciated.

MFS transporters with fourteen membrane spanning (MS) domains are also found in both Gram positive and Gram negative organisms (i.e., QacA and B in *S. aureus* and its homologue ErmB in *E. coli*, respectively) [15]. Efflux mediated by QacA in the hospital setting has caused emergence of resistance to bacteriostatic antiseptic and disinfectant agents such as chlorhexidine [25, 26]. Expression of the efflux pump VceAB in the Gram negative enteric pathogen *Vibrio cholera* protects this organism from nalidixic acid and chloramphenicol [27]. In addition to the above-mentioned antibiotic resistances mediated by efflux in *M. tuberculosis*, it has been suggested that fluoroquinolone resistance is mediated in this organism by an efflux pump encoded by *lfrA* that belongs to the MSF family with 14 MS domains [28, 29]. In the world of fungal opportunistic pathogens, MDR, a representative of this transporter family from *Candida albicans*, is responsible for efflux and intrinsic resistance to the antifungals benomyl and methotrexate [30]. Both intrinsic and acquired resistance through up-regulation of the MFS transporters has caused problems in the clinical setting in the treatment and control of bacterial and fungal infections.

2.2 Small multidrug resistance transporter family (SMR)

The SMR family of transporters, also members of the Type II class of transporters, was so named because proteins in this family are the smallest known multidrug transporters (roughly 100 amino acids) [16, 31, 32]. QakC from *S. aureus* [33] and YkkC/YkkD from *Bacillus subtilis* [34] are two distinctive representatives of this family in Gram positive species. This distinction is based on evidence that transport activity is acquired only after formation of multi-subunit enzymes which is typical for this family. It has been suggested that most SMR proteins form homo-oligomers, as is the case for QacC [35,36]. However, both YkkC and YkkD are required to express drug resistance in *B. subtilis* apparently through the formation of a heterodimer or multimers of heterodimers [34].

QakE, a protein which confers resistance to antiseptics, is a representative of SMR transporters in Gram negative bacteria [35]. This transporter is present in *E. coli* on what appears to be a mobile genetic element. The presence of QakE in many Gram negative bacteria suggests that the mobile genetic element may have played a role in the spread of this gene to other Gram negative bacteria [37]. SMR transporters rely on proton motive force for movement of substances across the cell membrane. Compounds transported by the SMR family of transporters are usually lipophilic and cationic, for example, tetracyclines, erythromycin and sulfadiazine [38]. Topologically, members of the SMR family of transporters possess four TM regions; in comparison, other families of transporters described herein (i.e., MSF, RND, MATE, and ABC transporters) have 12–14 membrane spanning regions (MSRs). Chung and Saier recently published a comprehensive review containing a phylogenetic analysis of the SMR-type MDR pumps [39].

2.3   Resistance-nodulation-cell division (RND) transporter family

The RND family of multidrug transporters is found in Gram negative bacteria [15]. RND transporters are unique with respect to structure compared to other transporters. Their presence in Gram negative bacteria demands that they physically traverse the cell membrane, the periplasmic space, the cell wall and the outer membrane in order to deliver molecules to the external environment. This process in some cases requires an interaction with a membrane fusion protein (MFP) and an outer membrane protein (OMP). Consequently, transporters of the RND family are larger than the MFS and SMR family members. Class II RND transporters are typically composed of roughly 900 amino acids [14]. Structurally, RND proteins consist of twelve MSRs with two large loops, one after the first MSR and the second occurring after the seventh MSR [40, 41]. RND transporters are unrelated to the MFS or SMR families of transporters at the primary structure level. However, similar to the MFS family of transporters, the RND transporters are capable of extruding a rather broad variety of compounds, including amphiphilic and charged substrates such as tetracycline, quinolones, chloramphenicol and β-lactams [42–44].

2.4 Multidrug and toxic compound extrusion family (MATE)

Members of the MATE family of transporters resemble the MFS family in that they possess twelve TM domains. However, like all other members of the Type II family of transporters, they rely on proton motive force, not ATP. Amino acid comparisons of the MATE family reveal no conserved motifs or general sequence similarity to the MFS proteins. Representatives of this family, the NorM transporter from *Vibrio parahaemolyticus* and its homologue in *E. coli*, YdhE, impart resistance to aminoglycosides, dyes and fluoroquinolones [45].

2.5 ATP-binding cassette (ABC) transporters

ABC transporters, also referred to as ABC traffic ATPases, are responsible for transport of a wide range of substrates in a variety of organisms including mammals, yeast, bacteria, insects, protozoa, nematodes and fungi. As their name implies, these proteins utilize energy imparted by ATP and possess at least one region that binds ATP (i.e,. the ATP-binding cassette domain or the ABC domain). The ATP-binding domains are typically 200 amino acids in length and reside on the cytoplasmic side of the cell membrane. Specific characteristics of the ABC domains include the presence of the Walker A and B motifs and a unique ATP-binding cassette signature sequence (LSGGQ) that is present in all family members of ABC proteins [46–48]. The ATP-binding domains are associated with two hydrophobic integral membrane domains. Each hydrophobic domain is comprised of six alpha helical MSRs. ABC multidrug transporters will typically be arranged in the following combination: two cytoplasmic ABC domains plus two MS domains (i.e., twelve alpha helical regions). The members of the functional unit can be encoded in separate genes or in some cases all components are present on a single transcript [49–52].

It is important to understand the distinction between an ABC protein and an ABC multidrug transporter. An ABC protein contains a domain that binds and hydrolyzes ATP. The energy released from this hydrolysis may be used in quite divergent physiological processes, including transport. The cytoplasmic ATP-binding domain of an ABC multidrug transporter is associated with or fused to a domain which transverses the cell membrane several times as indicated above.

In section 1.2 above, the role of MDRs and, more specifically, ABC transporters, was discussed in relationship to human cancer chemotherapy. That subject in itself is the focus of a voluminous amount of literature that will not be dealt with here. It was presented at that point in this discussion for the historical perspective of discovering and laying the foundation for understanding the MDR phenomenon.

3 ABC transporters in bacteria

A great deal of work has focused on determining the "normal" physiological function of ABC transporters in bacteria and other organisms. This super family of transporters has been implicated in functions as diverse as cell division, translation elongation, and maintenance of cell volume [53, 54], in addition to efflux of natural metabolites and drug resistance. ABC transporters are also involved in the importation of a wide range of small molecular weight molecules [55]. For this discussion a focus will be placed on efflux. The importance of ABC transporters in the life style or livelihood of organisms can be highlighted by considering how many are present in bacteria, where they are the largest single superfamily of proteins. For example, the ABC transporter superfamily in bacteria represents the largest set of paralogous genes; five per cent of all genes encode ABC transporter systems in *E. coli* and *Bacillus subtilis*. Tomii and Kanehisa performed a comparative analysis of ABC transporters found in seven completed microbial genomes and in the process established 25 orthologous groups of ABC transporters correlated with their function [56]. Predictions were then made for the function of ABC transporters found in other bacteria.

3.1   Non-MDR related functions of ABC transporters in bacteria

Before examining efflux of therapeutic compounds, the involvement of ABC transporters in movement of other types of molecules will be mentioned briefly. Once again, this is not intended to be all-inclusive, but rather illustrative of other roles for these proteins. For example, ABC transporters are involved in providing materials for the surface structure of bacteria and perhaps for other organisms as well. MsbA is an ABC transporter in *E. coli* involved in moving lipids through the inner membrane to the inner surface of the outer membrane [57]. The "ABC-2 transporters" or "ABC-A2 transporters" in Gram negative and Gram positive bacteria mobilize glycosylated compounds to the cell surface. These hydrophilic compounds include small glycosylated molecules as well as much more complex carbohydrates (lipopolysaccharides, teichoic acids and capsular polysaccharides) [58, 59]. An ABC transporter was identified within a cluster of genes devoted to antigenic capsular biosynthesis in the human pathogen *Enterococcus faecalis*. This transporter was similar to other ABC transporters involved in export of sugar polymers from Gram positive and Gram negative bacteria [60]. Synthesis of capsular polysaccharide occurs near the cytoplasmic membrane, perhaps in association with transport proteins [61]. Capsular polysaccharides play a pivotal role in the virulence of many human and animal pathogens. For example, capsule-deficient mutants of the Gram positive human pathogen *Streptococcus pneumoniae* are rendered avirulent [62]. In this case, ABC transporters functionally help create the pathogenic capacity of a bacterium and enable the disease process. The movement of polysaccharide capsular material to the cell surface of bacteria and fungi will be addressed later as a potential therapeutic arena.

Bacteria are able to sense population density through extracellular communication molecules. ABC transporter proteins are utilized to export communication molecules to the external environment. In Gram positive bacteria these molecules are peptides, in contrast to Gram negative bacteria where N-acyl homoserine lactones are used. The ABC transporter responsible for export of communication molecules in Gram positive bacteria has been identified and homologues have been found in Gram negative bacteria as well [63]. In this case the ABC transporters are actively participating in cell-to-cell communication.

Microbes are provided with an arsenal of offensive weapons and, in some cases, a self-defensive weapon *via* ABC-mediated transport. In this case exogenously added antibacterial compounds are not being considered, but rather compounds produced by the bacterium itself are at the center of attention. On the offensive weapons side, at least in some instances, they may take the form of antibiotics. For example, many divergent classes of antibiotic molecules are produced by Gram positive bacteria, especially by species of *Streptomyces*. To gain an offensive advantage from such molecules, they must be moved to the external environment. In the external environment, antibiotics may have a positive impact on the organism's ability to compete for nutrients by elimination of competing species. For the sake of argument, one could just as well have characterized the effect of externalized antibiotics as a defensive weapon. In any case, the same potential advantage is afforded to the producing organism. ABC transporters have been shown to be responsible for the export of class I and II bacteriocins in Gram positive organisms [64]. Complex macrolide antibiotics such as tylosin and carbomycin in the streptomycetes [65, 66], as well as peptide antibiotics, such as bacitracin in *B. licheniformis*, are expelled by ABC peptide transporters [67]. In tylosin-producing *Streptomyces fradiae*, an ABC transporter is located immediately upstream of the polyketide synthetase responsible for tylosin production [68]. It should be noted that some of these antibiotics produced by bacteria are toxic not only to other organisms, but also to the producing organism. In the case of *S. fradiae*, efflux mediated by the ABC transporter adjacent to the polyketide synthetase plays a key role in self-resistance to the antibiotic produced by this organism.

Another example of self-defense and deployment of an offensive weapon is evident in the biosynthetic production of the antibacterial compound bacitracin. Recently, Neumuller and colleagues dissected the bacitracin biosynthetic pathway in *Bacillus licheniformis* [69]. They identified ABC transporters (bcrABC genes) involved in export of bacitracin. Bacitracin is active against most Gram positive bacteria, but the producing organism is insensitive during antibiotic production. The amount of the ABC transporters present that is utilized for bacitracin transport was increased during idiophase, consistent with induction of transport in response to bacitracin biosynthesis and accumulation. Thus, from a defensive standpoint, externalization of antibiotic compounds is at least sometimes essential for self-survival of the antibiotic producer. The ABC transporters that serve in self-protection have the same domain organization as other ABC transporters that provide resistance to therapeutic agents in other microbes.

3.2 ABC transporters and drug resistance in bacteria

Thus far evidence accumulated indicates that Type II MDR proteins play the most important role in the resistance of bacteria to antibacterial compounds. The role of ABC transporters in drug resistance in Gram negative bacteria appears even somewhat less important than the role they play in Gram positive bacteria. This situation may stem from the fact that they contain many more representatives of the Type II MDR transporters or it may be due to the external physical architecture of Gram negative bacteria (i.e., in particular the presence of the external membrane outside of the peptidoglycan layer). In Gram positive bacteria an example of an ABC transporter playing a role in drug resistance may occur in *Staphylococcus epidermidis*. An ABC transporter was identified which interacted with MsrA, contributing to significantly high levels of erythromycin resistance in this human pathogen [70]. Another ABC transporter associated with drug efflux was identified in *Lactobacillus lactis* [71, 72]. The LmrA protein confers multidrug resistance on this organism. As more completed genomic DNA sequences become available for disease-causing bacteria, a more comprehensive understanding will emerge for the role of ABC transporters in drug resistance.

4 Multidrug resistance transporters in fungi

Human antifungal therapy has recently been complicated by an increased incidence of resistance to clinically utilized compounds. Unfortunately front-line antifungals have been affected the most. In particular, azole-resistant strains of the yeast-like organism *Candida albicans* have appeared, especially during prolonged treatment of oral candidiasis in immunocompromised patients [73]. At the same time the immunocompromised patient population is generally on the increase due to AIDS and the increasing prevalence of major invasive surgical procedures that either require or cause a reduction in immuno-efficiency. Two major classes of transporter proteins have been found in fungi, the MFS family and the ABC transporters. Del

Sorbo and colleagues have recently provided a concise and informative review of efflux in well-studied fungal species [74].

4.1 Multidrug resistance transporters in *Candida albicans*

C. albicans causes more fungal infections in humans than all other fungal opportunistic pathogens combined. Efflux has been implicated as the mechanism of resistance in fluconazole-resistant and multiazole-resistant strains of *C. albicans* and *C. glabrata* [75, 76]. In *C. albicans*, evidence for increased mRNA production for two transporters (CDR1 and MDR1) in the presence of fluconazole provided early evidence for the inducible nature of these genes in fungi [14,76]. Fluconazole and miconazol resistance in *C. albicans* is to a large degree due to the ABC transporter CDR1 [76, 77]. Three additional highly related ABC transporters (CDR2, CDR3 and CDR4) in *C. albicans* have been reported [78–80]. CDR2 and CDR4 have been implicated in drug resistance. CDR3 is expressed only during the opaque phase of the life cycle and its function remains unknown [81]. In contrast to the ATP-dependent CDR transporters, MDR1 is a member of the MFS family of transporters in *C. albicans* and confers resistance to benomyl and methotrexate [82]. FLU1, another member of the MFS family of transporters, was recently isolated and characterized by Calabrese and colleagues [83]. When this *C. albicans* gene was expressed in *S. cerevisiae*, FLU1 mediated resistance to fluconazole. When FLU1 was deleted from *C. albicans*, the mutant only became slightly more susceptible to fluconazole, suggesting that other drug transporters, perhaps with an overlap in substrate specificity, or other mechanisms of resistance were also involved in fluconazole resistance. Interestingly, the FLU1-deleted *C. albicans* mutant did become markedly sensitive to mycophenolic acid. Such observations point out the overlapping specificity of transport for various types of compounds by different MDR proteins and helps us to recall that other mechanisms of drug resistance are also operative in the fungi.

Clinically problematic infections due to other species of *Candida* have recently been on the increase due to intrinsic resistance factors. Two MDR-related ABC transporter proteins (ABC1 and ABC2) have been identified in *Candida krusei*. This yeast-like fungus is naturally resistant to fluconazole. Investigation revealed an up-regulation ABC1 in response to azole antifungal compounds, as well as other unrelated antifungals [84], leading to the speculation that ABC1 was involved in antifungal resistance in *C. krusei*.

4.2 ABC transporters in *Cryptococcus neoformans*

Another human opportunistic fungal pathogen is the encapsulated yeast *Cryptococcus neoformans*. This organism is a particular threat in immuno-compromised patients such as those with full-blown AIDS. *C. neoformans* meningeal and systemic infections have been noted as the fourth leading cause of death in AIDS patients [85]. Thornewell and colleagues [86] reported the complete sequence of *Cne*MDR1, a gene encoding an ABC transporter. A second ABC transporter was also detected in this clinical isolate of *C. neoformans* during the course of that study by reverse transcriptase-PCR (*Cne*MDR2). A clear-cut role for *Cne*MDR1 and *Cne*MDR2 in drug efflux or resistance was not established in the above-mentioned study. However, some interesting parallels and potential functions in addition to drug resistance were highlighted. In *C. neoformans*, four factors have been associated with virulence: ability to grow at 37 °C, production of melanin, polysaccharide capsule, and mating type [87–90]. ABC transporters are clearly associated with two of these processes in other organisms. For example, in the bacterium *Haemophilus influenzae* type b, an ATP-driven efflux mechanism is responsible for transport of capsular polysaccharide to the cell surface. Disruption of this efflux system renders *H. influenzae* avirulent [91]. It is conceivable that *Cne*MDR1 and/or *Cne*MDR2 might be involved in capsule transport. An alternative route for these proteins to have an impact on virulence might be that these transporters have a role in mating-type factor export. *C. neoformans* has two mating types. The α mating type is 30–40 times more virulent than the a mating type [89]. In the budding yeast *Saccharomyces cerevisiae*, STE6, an ABC transporter protein related to human MDR1, is responsible for export of mating-type factors [92]. Perhaps one or both of the *C. neoformans* ABC transporters play a role in mating factor export. This is an opportune juncture to once again stress the fact that we certainly do not understand the physiological role for all ABC transporters. However, this brief discussion of *C. neoformans* ABC transporters has highlighted three potential ways for these proteins to have an impact in the clinical setting: drug resistance *via* export of therapeutic compounds, or virulence manifested either through movement of capsular material to the cell surface or *via* mating factor transport.

4.3 Multidrug resistance in filamentous fungal human opportunistic pathogens

Of the filamentous fungi, *Aspergillus flavus* and *A. fumigatus* are the most frequently encountered human opportunistic pathogens. Like *C. albicans* and *C. neoformans*, they are particularly problematic in immunocompromised individuals. In such patients, systemic infections with these organisms are uniformly fatal if not treated. Invasive pulmonary aspergillosis is most commonly caused by *A. fumigatus* [93]. The "gold standard" treatment, Amphotericin B, either alone or in combination with another antifungal, is fraught with toxicity problems, in particular nephrotoxicity [94]. Unfortunately, only a few antifungal compounds have presented themselves as alternatives to Amphotericin B for the treatment of aspergillosis. The first observation of the MDR phenomenon in an *Aspergillus* species was in a laboratory mutant of *Aspergillus nidulans* selected for resistance to a range of azole antifungals and related compounds. Resistance to these compounds was due to the inability of the organism to accumulate a toxic concentration in the cytoplasm [95]. A detailed genetic explanation for this observation became available nearly two decades later.

Although, in general, *C. albicans* does not produce the most life-threatening fungal infections, it does represent by far the most frequently encountered fungal opportunistic pathogen in human medicine. In the search for new antifungal compounds using whole-cell screens, *C. albicans* is usually the organism of choice. Compounds identified in such screens as active against *C. albicans* will frequently lack activity against some or all of the key *Aspergillus* species. Such observations led Tobin and colleagues [96] to suggest that the ability of *Aspergillus* species to withstand antifungal therapy was due at least in part to the presence of effective efflux systems. With this in mind they mounted a search to find MDR-like genes in the human opportunistic pathogens *A. fumigatus* and *A. flavus*. Degenerate PCR primers were used to amplify regions of genomic DNA from these fungi. The primers were based on the conserved regions of the ATP-binding domain of several MDR genes, including fungal and human sources. This effort very quickly revealed two

MDR-like genes in *A. fumigatus* (*AfuMDR1* and *AfuMDR2*) and one in *A. flavus* (*AflMDR1*). When *AfuMDR1* was expressed in *S. cerevisiae*, the transformed yeast cells became resistant to the antifungal compound cilofungin. Thus, the experimental results were consistent with the suggested role of efflux being a factor in resistance and suggested a role for *AfuMDR1* in drug resistance. The encoded proteins, AfuMDR1 and AflMDR1, possessed the typical structure of MDR proteins – two hydrophobic domains with six TM regions and two nucleotide-binding domains. In contrast, analysis of AfuMDR2 revealed only one hydrophobic region with four TM regions and one nucleotide-binding domain (i.e., a half MDR protein). Recently Robey and colleagues reported a half MDR protein (ABCG2) associated with flavopiridol resistance in human breast cancer cells [97]. The role of AfuMDR2 in drug transport in *A. fumigatus* has not been elucidated [96]. The search for MDR proteins in these fungi was by no means exhaustive. It was anticipated that many more ABC transporters are present in these *Aspergillus* species. This anticipation was probably reasonable in light of the fact that in the yeast *S. cerevisiae*, which has a smaller genome, at least 29 ABC transporter proteins have been identified [98]. As the genomic sequences of these *Aspergillus* species become available, many more ABC transporters will undoubtedly be identified and at least some will have a role in drug resistance.

4.4 Multidrug resistant ABC transporters in *Aspergillus nidulans*

As indicated above, the original biochemical observation of energy-dependent efflux of drugs in filamentous fungi was observed in *A. nidulans* during the 1970s. Then, in the late 1990s, some of the individuals in that original group of investigators began to clarify the genetics surrounding efflux in *A. nidulans*. This organism is not a common direct human opportunistic pathogen. However, it and closely related *Aspergillus* species are problematic in the agricultural setting from the standpoint of aflatoxin production which is a potent toxic and carcinogenic agent [99, 100]. De Waard and colleagues reported the cloning and characterization of *atrA* and *atrB* from *A. nidulans* in 1997 [101]. A clear role for the ABC transporter encoded by *atrB* in MDR, as well as efflux of other toxic compounds, was established [102]. Shortly thereafter they, along with collaborators from Eli Lilly and Company, reported the cloning and characterization of *atrC* and *atrD*; these genes also

117

encoded ABC transporters. Gene disruption of *atrD* in *A. nidulans* revealed that the MDR-like protein encoded by this gene provided protection to a variety of toxic compounds including cycloheximide [103].

5   ABC transporters in human and animal parasitic diseases

Humans are parasitized by a large number of different types of organisms. Of the diseases caused by parasites, malaria is the most recognized. It has gained its notoriety because of the immense toll it takes on the human population in terms of morbidity and mortality. Malaria is second only to tuberculosis in the number of human lives it claims annually. Three to five hundred million clinical cases resulting in roughly a million deaths are recorded each year (World Health Organization Fact Sheet 94, revised 1998, available at http://www.who.ch/). Malaria is caused by four different species of the single-celled protozoan parasite, *Plasmodium*: *P .falciparum*, *P. vivax*, *P. ovale* and *P. malariae*. Of these, *P. falciparum* accounts for the majority of infections and produces the most lethal infections.

If diagnosed early, malaria is relatively responsive to treatment. However, resistance to clinically used agents has been reported in several regions with endemic malaria. Malarial parasites carrying resistance mutations in the dehydrofolate reductase and dehydropteroate synthase genes and, notably, pfmdr1, have been reported [104]. High-level chloroquine resistance is associated with mutations of the MDR encoded by pfmdr1 in *P. falciparum* [105]. Polymorphisms in pfmdr1 were also found to be responsible for resistance to some of the newer antimalarial drugs such as mefloquine and halofantrine [106]. On the one hand, changes in amino acid sequence of the transporter encoded by pfmdr1 has led to resistance, however, laboratory studies have demonstrated that enhanced sensitivity to the antimalarials mefloquine and artemisinin can be induced by other mutations in this gene [107]. In the clinical setting, treatment with antimalarial compounds selects for increased resistance, not enhanced susceptibility. However, the concept of enhancing susceptibility by altering transport points to the potential utility of combination therapy involving common antimalarial compounds plus an efflux pump blocker. Other investigators, focused on a different human parasite, *Leishmania tropica*, came to the same conclusion. This conclusion was based on their ability to identify a compound which blocked ABC-transporter-mediated resistance in *L. tropica* [108].

Over two billion people are infected with parasitic worms. For the most part these are soil-transmitted helminths such as *Ascaris lumbricoides* (hookworms) and schistosomes. The burden on human health is enormous, with over 300 million people suffering from severe infections resulting in developmental problems and loss of cognitive function [109]. Recently the World Health Assembly approved a resolution to initiate mass drug treatment of school-age children in areas with endemic infections caused by helminths and schistosomes. At this point in time there are no major indications of the MDR phenomenon being involved in drug resistance in these organisms. However, as discussed below, resistance *via* ABC transporters is present in the animal health sector dealing with parasitic nematodes. With prolonged use of therapeutic agents against these organisms, it is predictable that resistance will be selected for and become problematic.

In addition to rising concerns in the human health arena, the animal health sector has also realized a negative impact on therapeutic options due to MDR activity in parasitic organisms. The most widely used group of anthelmentic compounds in the animal health arena are the macrocyclic lactones represented by ivermectin and related compounds. *Haemonchus contortus* is a sheep nematode parasite that causes significant economic loss. Xu and colleagues reported the presence of a P-glycoprotein/MDR in *H. contortus* that was related to MDR proteins from humans, mice, and *Caenorhabditis elegans,* a frequently studied nematode. Changing the level of expression of this MDR resulted in altered levels of resistance to ivermectin and furthermore, addition of the MDR blocking agent, verapamil, increased susceptibility to ivermectin and moxidectin [110].

The life style of obligate parasitic worms presents numerous practical barriers for studying the effects of MDR proteins on drug resistance. In contrast, *C. elegans*, a free-living nematode that is highly related to parasitic nematodes such as *H. contortus*, provides a convenient vehicle for such studies, as its life cycle can be completed in three days on a laboratory medium. Studies have demonstrated, in parallel with the parasitic worms, the role of MDR and MRP proteins in protection of *C. elegans* from naturally occurring toxins such as heavy metals and the antinematode compound produced by *P. aeruginosa* (pyocyanin) [111, 112]. More than 50 ABC transporters (potential MDR proteins) have been identified in *C. elegans* through genomic sequencing. It is likely that parasitic nematodes have a similar number of ABC transporters. Interestingly, the pgp-3 encoded MDR in C. *elegans* confers resistance to colchicine and the antimalarial chloroquine [113]. Thus C. *elegans* may be a useful model organism to study the MDR phenomenon and how it affects drug resistance of parasites in the human health as well as the animal health sectors.

6 Potential beneficial aspects of the MDR phenomenon

In the preceding sections the focus has been to a large extent on the negative impact of the MDR phenomenon on clinical medicine. It is clear that all living organisms have the capacity to move materials in and out of their cells, whether they are complex multicellular organisms or simple single-celled organisms. Unfortunately, the ability to export therapeutic compounds does get in the way of human and veterinarian medical practice. However, because of the impact on human health, the MDR phenomenon has caused scientists to study the process very closely and from many different angles. As a result, a new appreciation for the MDR process is evolving and novel ideas are gaining momentum with regard to applications involving various aspects of toxin efflux. The next sections will highlight some of these recent observations and draw attention to potential benefits.

6.1 Enhancing the production of antibiotics

In addition to producing the toxic compound aflatoxin, A. *nidulans* strains also produce the β-lactam antibiotic penicillin, a life-saving compound. Andrade and colleagues made an interesting observation regarding the ABC transporter encoded by *atrD* in A. *nidulans*. When *atrD* was disrupted, the amount of extracellular penicillin produced was dramatically decreased, suggesting that this ABC transporter played a role in secretion of penicillin [103]. In this instance, the *atrD* encoded ABC transporter was not playing a role in self-protection *via* resistance, because A. *nidulans* is not susceptible to the action of penicillin. Rather, one might speculate that this ABC transporter is part of an offensive/defensive weapon system used to protect this organism's niche from invasion by bacteria. From a standpoint of human medicine and/or industrial efficiency, efflux of penicillin by an ABC transporter might be taken advantage of in a positive sense. Providing extra copies of *atrD* or by enhancing its expression in a penicillin-producing strain should, theoretically, enhance the amount of penicillin reaching the outside. Previous studies have demonstrated that extra copies of certain genes involved in β-lactam biosynthesis have yielded a beneficial effect on the total amount of antibiotic produced [114, 115]. By rapidly removing the final product of this biosynthetic pathway through efflux, any chance for feedback inhibition in earlier steps should be eliminated, thus perhaps increasing overall productivity. A similar strategy may be useful in bacterial species that produce antibiotics to which they are susceptible.

6.2   Discovery of novel drugs for treatment of infectious diseases

Clearly, intrinsic resistance to therapeutic compounds, as well as naturally occurring toxins, *via* efflux is a common strategy found in virtually every infectious disease category. Rapidly rising rates of resistance mediated by still other mechanisms have stimulated a great deal of research directed at new classes of therapeutic compounds for treatment of bacterial, fungal and parasitic infections. However, due to market constraints, researchers have to some extent been compromised in their ability to be successful. In the search for new antifungal compounds, for example, whole-cell high-throughput screens have been frequently designed to detect compounds effective in killing *C. albicans*. This organism was most commonly selected because it is the most frequently occurring fungal pathogen in human infections. Compounds with the capacity to kill *C. albicans* were subsequently tested against other fungal pathogens such as the aspergilli. These compounds frequently lacked the broader spectrum needed for marketability and were dropped from consideration early in the discovery process. As a consequence, the number of compounds to select for SAR studies became limited. Failure of anti-*Candida* compounds to exhibit the desired spectrum of activity was often due to intrinsic resistance mediated by drug efflux in the aspergilli. This failure could be interpreted as a lack of sensitivity in the design of the high-throughput screen.

In an effort to implement more sensitive screens, pharmaceutical company investigators over the last two decades have moved toward mechanism-based biochemical assays for high-throughput screens. Such endeavors have revealed compounds with exquisite capacity to inhibit a variety of key enzymatic targets *in vitro* from various infectious disease-causing organisms. All too frequently, these highly active enzyme inhibitors exhibited limited capacity to gain access to and hit the target in a live cell. A trend to return to whole-cell screens is now emerging. The obvious advantage of whole-cell screens is the fact that many pharmacological factors, as they pertain to the disease-causing organism, are resolved during the screening process. However, the issue of sensitivity still remains. To address this concern, several companies have gone to hypersensitive whole-cell high-throughput screens. One popular way to create such hypersensitive strains is to compromise the target organism's ability to expel toxic compounds. Examples of this strategy have emerged for both antifungal and antibacterial drug discovery.

Rogers and coworkers demonstrated that deletion of seven ABC transporter genes plus two transcriptional activators rendered *S. cerevisiae* roughly 2–200 times more sensitive to a collection of 349 toxic compounds [116]. Sulavik and colleagues examined the effect of disrupting many different *E. coli* genes and operons involved in efflux, including members of the MFS, RNP, SMR, ABC transporter families, and outer membrane proteins [117]. This work produced strains of *E. coli* hypersensitive to a broad range of compounds as compared to the wild type. Davis and colleagues took a similar approach with *Enterococcus faecalis* MDR transporters [118]. This organism is somewhat naturally resistant to antibiotic therapy and clinical isolates also frequently carry the liability of vancomycin resistance. These investigators identified 34 potential MDR transporter sequences from the unannotated *E. faecalis* DNA sequence database (TIGR). Gene disruptions in these genes helped identify which transporters were important for drug efflux and guided them in the construction of hypersensitive strains for high-throughput screening [118].

Intrinsic resistance caused by efflux of compounds prevents the discovery of marginally active compounds during the high-throughput screening process. Using hypersensitive fungal or bacterial strains will be beneficial in the detection of a broader range of active compounds. Although more compounds possessing the desired activity should be found, they will be less potent against the wild-type organism. However, by providing a broader range of chemicals for the medicinal chemists to examine, a higher probability exists to discover molecules that are amenable to chemical modification and establishment of SARs. If potency can be improved against the wild-type offending organism and spectrum expansion achieved, then lead compounds will emerge. It is also very important to note that this strategy also maximizes the utility of existing compound libraries within pharmaceutical companies. In a sense, utilization of hypersensitive strains will expand the effective chemical diversity found in chemical compound and natural product libraries.

6.3 Emerging therapeutic options engendered by multidrug resistance

Clearly, MDR is a major problem in many therapeutic areas. When a problem of this magnitude in human clinical medicine becomes apparent, it produces a dedicated response in scientists to find solutions to the problem. The resolve to solve the problem caused by MDR is portrayed to some extent in the following discussion in which examples of new therapeutic strategies are emerging. The use of dual therapy is the most advanced in the area of cancer chemotherapy (i.e., MDR blocker plus an oncolytic).

6.3.1 Cancer chemotherapy

Although this chapter is highly focused on infectious microbial organisms, it is fitting that consideration be given to the study of cancer chemotherapy. It is from these studies that a more clear understanding of the MDR phenotype has emerged and also some of the more progressive ideas in terms of therapeutic options as well. Multidrug resistance has been and continues to be a major obstacle in cancer chemotherapy. A great deal of work has been undertaken to overcome this problem. Two general approaches are readily obvious. First one can attempt to avoid efflux by treating with anticancer agents that are not included in the spectrum of compounds transported. Second, one could develop a compound or series of compounds that block the activity of key MDR proteins and add this compound to an existing or new oncolytic agent. This approach has been pursued extensively and is nearing clinical success. Szabo and colleagues examined the physical properties of chemosensitizers that block ABC transporter efflux of anticancer agents. These compounds are usually lipid-soluble at physiological pH, contain a basic nitrogen atom and two or more co-planar rings. Chirality of the compounds did not affect MDR blocking. They concluded that resistance modifiers that block efflux combined with cytostatics would be chemotherapeutically more effective for cancer patients [119].

Investigators at Eli Lilly and Company have extensively analyzed the MDR phenomenon as it affects cancer chemotherapy. These studies led to the development of molecules capable of interfering with resistance. Briefly, the MDR phenotype in resistant tumor cells is frequently associated with P-glycoprotein (Pgp) and/or MRP1/MRP2 expression. LY329146 is a compound that reverses the drug resistance phenotype in MRP1 overexpressing cells [120]. In comparison, LY335979 does not affect efflux by MRP1 or MRP2 but is an extremely potent Pgp inhibitor [121]. The pharmacological properties of LY335979 were consistent with a compound that might be effective *in vivo*. This cyclopropyl-dibenzosuberane modulator of Pgp-mediated drug resistance exhibited high affinity binding to Pgp, very strong potency for *in vitro* drug resistance reversal, a good therapeutic index, and no adverse interactions with coadministered oncolytic agents [122]. *In vivo* studies with LY335979 revealed effectiveness in blocking the MDR phenomenon, increasing life span, and enhancement of the antitumor activity of the oncolytic Taxol [123]. The favorable selectivity and potency properties of LY335979 have permitted this compound to enter human clinical trials. These trials are currently in progress [124].

Baekelandt and colleagues recently reported the results of phase I/II clinical studies for another MDR modulator (valspodar). Valspodar was coadministered with two clinically used oncolytic agents for the treatment of refractory ovarian cancer. Although results were encouraging, the value of valspodar in reversing resistance mediated by Pgp remains to be determined [125]. These examples of reversal of MDR in cancer therapy were not meant to be comprehensive – but rather, they were mentioned to illustrate that success in this approach may be realized very soon.

A third option for chemotherapeutic intervention in cancer may be targeting Pgp-mediated efflux itself. As mentioned earlier in this discussion, all physiological functions of ABC transporters are not fully appreciated. Toxic molecules are produced within a cell and, if not removed or detoxified, will manifest a negative effect on the producing cell – that is clear in antibiotic-producing bacteria. Thus it is plausible that blocking efflux in mammalian cancer cells may turn out to be a therapeutic option. For example, certain Pgp inhibitors slow cell proliferation and cause death by apoptosis in some MDR cancer cell lines [126].

6.3.2 Combination therapy for bacterial or fungal infections

Several companies have initiated programs to discover and develop inhibitors of efflux pumps (MDR blockers) for use in antimicrobial therapy [127]. Potentiation is another term frequently used when referring to dual therapy. This strategy is intended to extend the usefulness and improve the clinical performance of already existing antimicrobial therapies and for new therapeutics as well. Augmentin is a successful example of dual therapy in the antibacterial therapeutic arena. In this case, resistance was due to degradation of the β-lactam molecule by a β-lactamase – not efflux. Nonetheless, resistance was overcome by adding a potentiating compound, in this case a β-lactamase inhibitor.

Fluoroquinolone resistance in clinical isolates of *Pseudomonas aeruginosa* is at least partially an intrinsic characteristic of this organism. Investigators at Microcide Pharmaceuticals implemented a genetic study to determine which efflux pumps were important for resistance to fluoroquinolones in *P. aeruginosa* [128]. This study was followed by a search for and discovery of MDR blockers effective against the key efflux pumps. They determined that inhibition of efflux pumps reduced intrinsic resistance significantly, reversed acquired resistance, and decreased the frequency of emergence of *P. aeruginosa* highly resistant to fluoroquinolones [129]. This work was continued by Renau and colleagues who developed a series of compounds that function as efflux pump inhibitors in *P. aeruginosa* [130, 131]. They were able to demonstrate potentiation of levofloxacin antipseudomonal activity in an *in vivo* model of infection. Two general sets of problems exist with this type of approach to therapy. First an effective inhibitor must be found and, second, the inhibitor must have pharmacokinetic properties similar to the therapeutic compound in order to successfully treat an infected patient. The above studies demonstrate the potential utility of this approach.

The above strategy might be applied with equal efficacy in antifungal chemotherapy. Marchetti and coworkers demonstrated that the activity of fluconazole was potentiated by the MDR reversing agent cyclosporin [132].

6.3.3 MDR proteins as targets for new classes of antibacterials and antifungals

Previously in this discussion, two organisms were mentioned that utilized efflux as a mechanism to present virulence factors to the external environment (i.e., the bacterium *H. influenzae* and the fungus *C. neoformans* – this function was a speculation for this organism). It is plausible that an agent that would interfere with the formation of capsule, or with the movement of the polysaccharide material to the cell surface in the case of either of these organisms, would constitute a useful antibiotic. This type of antimicrobial agent would not directly cause death to the offending bacterium or fungus. Rather, the host organism would be required to remove the infection *via* its own immune system. As a consequence, there would be no or little selective pressure placed on the bacterium or fungus. In the presence of such a virulence-modifying compound, the offending organism would be safe in or on the host unless it entered a site of infection where it expressed its virulence factors (capsular polysaccharide in this example). It is conceivable that there would be a reduced incidence of antibiotic or antifungal resistance with such a treatment strategy, due to the lack of selective pressure. An added benefit may also manifest itself from the exposure of the host immune system to a pathogen. An effective immune response would be induced, thus in a sense indirectly providing the effect of a vaccine.

Perhaps the "Achilles Heel" in this strategy lies in the timing of treatment. It is unclear what would happen if you were to interfere with capsule export in an already well-established infection. Another issue would be the likely narrow spectrum of activity for such an antibacterial or antifungal compound. However, with diagnostic procedures becoming more rapid and accurate, narrow-spectrum antibiotics or antifungals may become the desired treatment modality. Another concern would be the ability to discover a small molecule that would be specific enough to avoid toxicity issues. MDR-like transport systems are ubiquitous and many can interact with multiple substrates as the name implies. There may be a liability of disrupting essential host transport processes; however, there are concerted efforts to find specific MDR blockers in a number of pharmaceutical companies. The example above in cancer chemotherapy suggests that this issue can be overcome.

7   Summary

The dark side of the MDR phenomenon is evident in the problems it has caused and continues to cause in the clinical treatment of cancer and infectious diseases caused by bacteria, fungi and parasites. However, through diligent study, it has also become quite apparent that there is a bright side of the MDR phenomenon to be considered as well. First of all, simply being aware of and understanding the MDR phenotype/problem in various organisms has armed scientists with critical knowledge needed to deal with a variety of disease states. A well-defined problem can usually be more readily solved. It is hoped that a clinical success in dual therapy for resistant cancer cells will strongly stimulate use of that concept in other therapeutic arenas. As the other physiological functions for MDR proteins are identified, they themselves may become the target for chemotherapy. For example, modulation of virulence by blocking efflux pumps required to display cell surface factors may provide a new avenue to treat infectious diseases with less risk of resistance development. Benefits made possible by knowledge of the MDR phenomenon may also arise in the arenas of drug discovery and natural product production. Hypersensitive fungal, bacterial and parasitic organisms used in high-throughput screens may reveal new classes of antimicrobial compounds for development. Finally, enhancing the effectiveness of efflux in the case of organisms producing antimicrobial compounds at the industrial scale may facilitate higher titer yields during production.

Acknowledgements

The author thanks Dr. Jesus Gutierrez for critical reading of the manuscript and helpful suggestions. The officers and managers of Elanco Animal Health and Eli Lilly and Company are also acknowledged for their continuing support.

References

1   M.H. Saier Jr.: Microbiol. Mol. Biology Reviews 64, 354 (2000).
2   J.H. Burchenal, E. Robinson, S.F. Johnston and M.M. Kushida: Science 111, 116 (1950).
3   K. Dano: Biochim. et Biophys. Acta 323, 466 (1973).
4   P.D. Roepe: Current Pharmaceutical Design 6, 241 (2000).
5   P.D. Roepe: Biochemistry 31, 12555 (1992).
6   P.D. Roepe: Biochim. et Biophys. Acta 1241, 385 (1995).
7   P.D. Roepe, L.-Y. Wei and D. Carlson: Biochemisty 32, 11042 (1993).
8   J.Y. Chan, A.C. Chu and K.P. Fung: Life Sci. 67 (17), 2117 (2000).
9   G.K. Chen, G.E. Duran, A. Mangili, L. Becketic-Oreskovic and B.I. Sikie. Br. J. Cancer 83, (7), 892 (2000).

10   B.E. Plaat, H. Hollema, W.M. Molenaar, G.H. Torn Broers, J. Pijpe, M.F. Mastik, H.J. Hoekstra, E. van den Berg, R.J. Scheper and W.T. van der Graaf: J. Clin. Oncol. *18*, (18), 3211 (2000).

11   F. Tiberghien, T. Kurome, K. Takesako, A. Didier, T. Wenandy and F. Loor: J. Med. Chem. 43, (13), 2547 (2000).

12   V. Hollt, M. Kouba, M. Dietel and G. Vogt: Biochem. Pharm. 43, (12), 2601 (1992).

13   F. Van Bambeke, E. Balzi and P.M Tulkens: Biochem. Pharmacol. 60, 457 (2000).

14   H.F. Jenkinson: J. Dent. Res. *75* (2), 736 (1996).

15   M. Putman, H. W. van Veen and W.N. Konings: Microbiol. and Mol. Biol. Reviews *64* (4), 672 (2000)

16   M.D. Marger and M.H. Saier, Jr.: Trends Biochem. Sci. *18*, 13 (1993)

17   S.B. Levy: Antimicrob. Agents Chemother. *36*, 695 (1992).

18   H. Yoshida, M. Bogaki, S. Nakamura, K. Ubukata and M. Konno: J. Bacteriol. *172*, 6942 (1990).

19   M.J. Gill, N.P. Brenwald and R. Wise: Antimicrob. Agents Chemother. *43*, 187 (1999).

20   N.N. Varanova and A.A. Neyfakh: Antimicrob. Agents Chemother. *41*, 1396 (1997).

21   N.P. Brenwald, M.J. Gill and R. Wise: Antimicrob. Agents Chemother. *40*, 458 (1997).

22   N.P. Brenwald, M.J. Gill and R. Wise: Antimicrob. Agents Chemother. *42*, 2032 (1998).

23   V. Zeller, C. Janoir, M. Kitzis, L. Gutmann and N.J. Moreau: Antimicrob. Agents Chemother. *41*, 1973 (1997).

24   J.A. Ainsa, M.C. Blokpoel, I. Otal, D.B. Young, K.A.L. De Smet and C. Martin: J Bacteriol *180*, 5836 (1998).

25   J.M. Tennent, B.R. Lyon, M. Midgley, G. Jones, A.S. Purewal and R.A. Skurray: J. Gen. Microbiol. 135, 1 (1989).

26   I.T. Paulsen, M.H. Brown and R.A. Skurray: J. Bacteriol. *180*, 3477 (1998).

27   B.J. Colmer, J.A. Fralick and A.N. Hamood: Mol. Microbiol. *27*, 63 (1998).

28   J. Liu, H.E. Takiff and H. Nicaido: J. Bacteriol. *178*, 3791 (1996).

29   H.E. Takiff, M. Cimino, M.C. Musso, T. Weisbrod, R. Martinez, M.B. Degado, L. Salazar, B.R. Bloom and W.R. Jacobs, Jr.: Proc. Natl. Acad. Sci. USA *93*, 362 (1996).

30   R. Ben-Yaacov, S. Knoller, G.A. Caldwell, J.M. Becker and Y. Koltkin: J Antimicrob. Agents Chemother. *38*, 648 (1994).

31   I.T. Paulsen, R.A. Skurray, R. Tam and M.H. Saier, Jr.: Mol. Microbiol. *19*, 1167 (1996).

32   C.F. Higgins: Ann. Rev. Cell Biol. *8*, 67 (1992).

33   T.G. Littlejohn, D. DiBerardino, L.J. Messerotte, S.J. Spiers and R.A. Skurray: Gene *101*, 59 (1991).

34   D.L. Jack, M.L. Storms, J.H. Tchieu, I.T. Paulsen and M. H. Saier, Jr.: J. Bacteriol. *182*, 2311 (2000).

35   I.T. Paulsen, T.G. Littlejohn, P. Radstrom, L. Sundstrom, O. Skold, G. Swedberg and R. A. Skurray: Antimicrob. Agents Chemother. *37*, 761 (1993).

36   I.T. Paulsen, M.H. Brown, S.J. Dunstan and R.A. Skurray: J. Bacteriol. *177*, 2827 (1995).

37   H. Kazama, H. Hamashima, M. Sasatsu and T. Arai: FEMS Microbiol. Lett. *159*, 173 (1998).

38   F. Van Bambeke, E. Balzi and P.M. Tulkens: Biochemical Pharmacology *60*, 457 (2000).

39   Y.J. Chung and M.H. Saier, Jr.: Curr. Opin. Drug Discov. Devel. *4*, 237 (2001).

40   M.H. Saier Jr., R. Tam, a. Reizer and J. Reizer: Mol. Microbiol. 11, 841 (1994).

41   L. Guan, M. Ehrmann, H. Yoneyama and T. Nakae: J. Biol. Chem. *274*, 10517 (1999).

42   K. Poole, K. Krebes, C. McNally and S. Neshat: J. Bacteriol. *175*, 7363 (1993).

43 X.Z. Li, D.M. Livermore and H. Nickaido: Antimicrob. Agents Chemother. *38*, 1732 (1994).

44 M.M. Hamzehpour, J.-C. Pechere, P. Plesiat and T. Kohler: Antimicrob. Agents Chemother. *39*, 2392 (1995).

45 Y. Morita, K. Kodama, S. Shiota, T. Mine, A. Kataoka, T. Mizushima and T. Tsuchiya: Antimicrob. Agents Chemother. *42*, 1778 (1998).

46 J.E. Walker, M. Saraste, M.J. Runswick and N.J. Gay: EMBO J. *1*, 945 (1982).

47 C.F. Higgins, I.D. Hiles, G.P. Salmond, D.R. Gill, J.A. Downie, I.J. Evans, I.B. Holland, L. Gray, S.D. Buckel, A.W. Bell et al.: Nature *323*, 448 (1986).

48 E. Schneider and S. Hunke: FEMS Microbiol. Rev. *22*, 1 (1998).

49 J. Young and I.B. Holland: Biochimica et Biophysica ACTA *1461*, 177 (1999).

50 M.J. Fath and R. Kolter: Microbiol. Rev. *57*, 995 (1993).

51 C.F. Higgins: Annu. Rev. Cell Biol. *8*, 67 (1992).

52 S.C. Hyde, P. Emsley, M.J. Hartshorn, M.M. Amimmack, U. Gileady, S.R. Pearce, M.P. Gallagher, D.R. Gill, R.E. Hubbard and C.F. Higgins: Nature *346*, 362 (1990).

53 C.F. Higgins and J. Bioenerg: Biomembr. *27*, 63 (1995).

54 S. Thiagalingham and L. Grossman: Nucleic Acids Res. *268*, 18382 (1993).

55 G. Kuan, E. Dassa, W. Saurin, M. Hofnung and M.H. Saier, Jr.: Res. Microbiol. *146*, 271 (1995).

56 K. Tomii and M. Kanehisa: Genome Res. *8*, 1048 (1998).

57 I.T. Paulsen, J.H. Park, P.S. Choi and M.H. Saier, Jr.: FEMS Microbiol. Lett. *156*, 1 (1997).

58 J. Reizer, A. Reizer and M.H. Saier, Jr.: Protein Sci. *1*, 1326 (1992).

59 W. Saurin, M. Hofnung and E. Dassa: J. Mol. Evol. *48*, 22 (1999).

60 Y. Xu, B.E. Murray and G.M. Weinstock: Infect. Immun. *66*, 4313 (1998).

61 G.P. Rigg, G.P., B. Barrett and I.S. Roberts: Microbiology 144, 2905 (1998).

62 Hoskins, J.A., W. E. Alborn, Jr., J. Arnold, L. C. Blaszczak, S. Burgett, B. S. DeHoff, S. T. Estrem, L. Fritz, D.-J. Fu, W. Fuller et al.: J. Bacteriol. *183*, 5709 (2001).

63 J. Michiels, G. Dirix, J. Vanderleyden and C. Xi: Trends Microbiol. *9*, 164 (2001).

64 I.F. Nes, D.B. Diep, L.S. Havarstein, M.B. Brurberg, V.G.H. Eijsink and H. Holo: Antonie von Leeuwenhoek *70*, 113 (1996).

65 P.R. Rosteck, P.A. Reynolds and C.L. Hershberger: Gene *102*, 27 (1991).

66 B. Schoner, M. Geistlich, P. Rosteck, R.N. Rao, E. Seno, P. Reynolds, K. Cox, S. Bergett and C. Hershberger: Gene *115*, 93 (1992).

67 Z. Podlesek, A. Comino, B. Herzog-Velikonja, D. Zgur-Bertok, R. Komel and M. Grabnar: Mol. Microbiol. *16*, 969 (1995).

68 E. Cundliffe, L.A. Merson-Davies and G.H. Kelemen: In: R.H. Baltz, G.E. Hegeman and P.L. Skatrud (eds): Industrial Microorganisms: Basic and Applied Molecular Genetics, ASM Press, Washington DC 1993, 235–243.

69 A.M. Neumuller, D. Konz and M.A. Marahiel: Eur. J. Biochem. *268*, 3180 (2001).

70 J.I. Ross, E.A. Eady, J.H. Cove and S. Baumberg: Gene *153*, 93 (1995).

71 H. Bolhuis, H.W. van Veen, D. Molenaar, B. Poolman, A.J.M. Driessen and W.N. Konings: EMBO J. *15*, 4239 (1996).

72 H.W. van Veen, R. Callaghan, L. Soceneantu, A. Sardini, W.N. Konings and C.F. Higgins: Nature *391*, 291 (1998).

73 L. Millon, A. Manteaux, RG. Reboux, C. Drobacheff, M. Monod, T. Barale and Y. Michel-Briand: J. Clin. Microbiol. *32*, 1115 (1994).

74   G. Del Sorbo, H. Schoonbeek and M.A. De Waard: Fungal Genetics and Biology *30*, 1 (2000).

75   T. Parkinson, D.J. Falconer and C.A. Hitchcock: Antimicrob. Agents Chemother. *39*, 1696 (1995).

76   D. Sanglard, K. Kuchler, F. Ischer, J.-L. Pagani, M. Monod and J. Bille: Antimicrob. Agents Chemother. *39*, 2378 (1995).

77   R. Prasad, P. Dewergifosse, A. Goffeau and E. Balzi: Curr. Genet. *27*, 320 (1995).

78   D. Sanglard, F. Ischer, M. Monod and J. Bille: J. Microbiol. *143*, 405 (1997).

79   I. Balan, A.M. Alarco and M. Raymond: J. Bacteriol. *179*, 7210 (1997).

80   R. Franz, S. Michel and J. Morschhauser: Gene *220*, 91 (1998)

81   I. Balan, A.M. Alarco and M. Raymond: J. Bacteriol. *179*, 7210 (1997).

82   M.E. Fling, J. Kopf, A. Tamarkin, J.A. Gorman, H.A. Smith and Y. Koltin: Mol. Gen. Genet. 227, 318 (1991).

83   D. Calabrese, J. Bille and D. Sanglard: Microbiol. *146*, 2743 (2000).

84   S.K. Katiyar and T.D. Edlind: Med. Mycol. *39*, 109 (2001).

85   W.G. Powderly: Clin. Infect. Dis. *14*, S54 (1992).

86   S.J. Thornewell, R.B. Peery and P.L. Skatrud: Gene *201*, 21 (1997).

87   K.J. Kwon-Chung, I. Polacheck and T.J. Popkin: J. Bacteriol. *150*, 1414 (1982).

88   K.J. Kwon-Chung and J.C. Rhodes: Infect. Immun. *51*, 218 (1986).

89   K.J. Kwon-Chung, J.C. Edman and B.L. Wickes: Infect. Immun. *60*, 602 (1992).

90   J.C. Rhodes, I. Polacheck and K.J. Kwon-Chung: Infect. Immun. *36*, 1175 (1982).

91   J.S. Kroll, B. Loynds, L.N. Brophy and E.R. Moxon: Mol. Microbiol. *4*, 1853 (1990).

92   K. Kuchler, R.R. Sterne and J. Thorner: EMBO J. *8*, 1853 (1989).

93   M.G. Rinaldi: Rev. Infect. Dis. *5*, 1061 (1983).

94   C.A. Lyman and T.J. Walsh: Drugs *44*, 9 (1992).

95   M.A. De Waard and J.G.M. Van Nistelrooy: Pestic. Biochem. Physiol. *10*, 219 (1979).

96   M.P. Tobin, R.B. Peery and P.L. Skatrud: Gene *200*, 11 (1997).

97   R.W. Robey, W.Y. Medina-Perez, K. Nishiyama, T. Lahusen, K. Miyake, T. Litman, A.M. Senderowicz, D.D. Ross and S.E. Bates: Clin. Cancer Res. *7*, 145 (2001).

98   A. Decottignies and A. Goffeau: Nature Genet. *15*, 137 (1997).

99   T.E. Cleveland, A.R. Lax, L.S. Lee and D. Bhatnagar: Appl. Environ. Microbiol. *53*, 1711 (1987).

100 C. Stora and I. Dvorackova: J. Med. *18*, 23 (1987).

101 G. Del Sorbo, A.C. Andrade, J.G.M. Van Nistelrooy, J.A.L. Van Kan, E. Balzi and M.S. De Waard: Mol. Gen. Genet. *254*, 417 (1997).

102 A.C. Andrade, G. Del Sorbo, J.G.M. Van Nistelrooy and M.A. De Waard: Microbiol. *146*, 1987 (2000).

103 A.C. Andrade, J.G.M. Van Nistelrooy, R.B. Peery, P.L. Skatrud and M.A. De Waard: Mol. Gen. Genet. *263*, 966 (2000).

104 H.S. Nagesha, Din-Syafruddein, G.J. Casey, A.I. Susanti, D.J. Fryauff, J.C. Reeder and A.F. Cowman: Trans. R. Soc. Trop. Med. Hyg. *95*, 43 (2001).

105 H.A. Babiker, S.J. Pringle, A. Abdel-Muhsin, M. Mackinnon, P. Hunt and D. Walliker: Infect. Dis. *183*, 1535 (2001).

106 M.B. Reed, K.J. Saliba, S.R. Caruana, K. Kirk and A.F. Cowman: Nature *403*, 906 (2000).

107 M.T. Duraisingh, C. Roper, D. Walliker and D.C. Warhurst: Mol. Microbiol. *36*, 955 (2000).

108 J.M. Perez-Victoria, F.J. Perez-Victoria, A. Parodi-Talice, I.A. Jimenez, A.G. Ravelo, S. Castanys and F. Gamarro: Antimicrob. Agents Chemother. *45*, 2468 (2001).

109 D.G. Colley, P.T. LoVerde and L. Savioli: Science *293*, 1437 (2001).

110 M. Xu, M. Molento, W. Blackhall, P. Ribeiro, R. Beech and R. Prichard: Mol. Biochem. Parasitol. *91*, 327 (1998).

111 A. Broeks, B. Gerrard, R. Allikmets, M. Dean and R.H. Plasterk: EMBO J. *15*, 6132 (1996).

112 T.H. Lindblom, G.J. Pierce and A.E. Sluder: Curr. Biol. *11*, 864 (2001).

113 A. Broeks, H.W. Janssen, J. Calafat and R.H. Plasterk: EMBO J. *14*, 1858 (1995).

114 P.L. Skatrud, A.J. Tietz, T.D. Ingolia, C.A. Cantwell, D.L. Fisher, J.L. Chapman and S.W. Queener: Bio/Technol *7*, 477 (1989).

115 P.L. Skatrud: Trends in Biotechnol. *10*, 324 (1992).

116 B. Rogers, A. Decottignies, M. Kolaczkowski, E. Carvajal, E. Balzi and A. Goffeau: J. Mol. Microbiol. Biotechnol. *3*, 207 (2001).

117 M.C. Sulavik, C. Houseweart, C. Cramer, N. Jiwani, N. Murgolo, J. Greene, B. DiDomenico, K.J. Shaw, G.H. Miller, R. Hare et al.: Antimicrob. Agents Chemother. *45*, 1126 (2001).

118 D.R. Davis, J.B. McAlpine, C.J. Pazoles, M.K. Talbot, E.A. Alder, C. White, B.M. Jonas, B.E. Murray, G.M. Weinstock and B.L. Rogers: J. Mol. Microbiol. Biotechnol. *3*, 179 (2001).

119 D. Szabo, H. Keyzer, H.E. Kaiser and J. Molnar: Anticancer Res. *20*, 4261 (2000).

120 B.H. Norman, A.H. Dantzig, J.S. Kronin, K.L. Law, L.B. Tabas, R.L. Shepard, A.D. Palkowitz, K.L. Hauser, M.A. Winter, J.P. Sluka et al.: Bioorg. Med. Chem. Lett. *9*, 3381 (1999).

121 A.H. Dantzig, R.L. Shepard, K.L. Law, L. Tabas, S. Pratt, J.S. Gillespie, S.N. Binkley, M.T. Kuhfeld, J.J. Starling and S.A. Wrighton: J. Pharmacol. Exp. Ther. *290*, 854 (1999).

122 J.J. Starling, R.L. Shepard, J. Cao, K.L. Law, B.H. Norman, J.S. Kroin, W.J. Ehlhardt, T.M. Baughman, M.A. Winter, M.G. Bell et al.: Adv. Enzyme Regul. *37*, 335 (1997).

123 A.H. Dantzig, R.L. Shepard, J. Cao, K.L. Law, W.J. Ehlhardt, T.M. Baughman, T.F. Bumol and J.J. Starling: Cancer Res. *56*, 4171 (1996).

124 A.H. Dantzig, K.L. Law, J. Cao and J.J. Starling: Curr. Med. Chem. *8*, 39 (2001).

125 M. Baekelandt, G. Lehne, C.G. Trope, I. Szanto, P. Pfeiffer, B. Gustavsson and G.B. Kristensen: J. Clin. Oncol. *19*, 2983 (2001).

126 G. Lehne: Curr. Drug Targets *1*, 85 (2000).

127 O. Lomovskaya and W. Watkins: J. Mol. Microbiol. Biotechnol. *3*, 225 (2001).

128 O. Lomovskaya, A. Lee, K. Hoshino, H. Ishida, A. Mistry, M.S. Warren, E. Boyer, S. Chamberland and V.J. Lee: Antimicrob. Agents Chemother. *43*, 1340 (1999).

129 O. Lomovskaya, M.S. Warren, A. Lee, J. Galazzo, R. Fronko, M. Lee, J. Blais, D. Cho, S. Chamberland, R. Renau, et.al.: Antimicrob. Agents Chemother. *45*, 105 (2001).

130 T.E. Renau, R. Leger, E.M. Flamme, M.W. She, C.L. Gannon, K.M Mathias, O. Lomovskaya, S. Chamberland, V.J. Lee, T. Ohta et al.: Bioorg. Med. Chem. Lett. *12*, 663 (2001).

131 T.E. Renau, R. Leger, E.M. Flamme, J. Sangalang, M.W. She, R. Yen, C. L. Gannon, D. Griffith, S. Chamberland, O. Lomovskaya et al.: J. Med. Chem. *42*, 4928 (1999).

132 O. Marchetti, P. Moreillon, M.P. Glauser, J. Bille and D. Sanglard: Antimicrob. Agents Chemother. *44*, 2373 (2000).

Progress in Drug Research, Vol. 58 (E. Jucker, Ed.)
©2002 Birkhäuser Verlag, Basel (Switzerland)

Potassium channels: Gene family, therapeutic relevance, high-throughput screening technologies and drug discovery

By John W. Ford,
Edward B. Stevens,
J. Mark Treherne,
Jeremy Packer, and
Mark Bushfield

BioFocus PLC
Cambridge Science Park
Milton Road
Cambridge CB4 0FG, UK

<jford@biofocus.co.uk>
<estevens@biofocus.co.uk>

John W. Ford

is currently Team Leader of Receptors and Channel Hit Discovery at BioFocus PLC, Cambridge. His interests include potassium channel drug discovery, specialising in high-throughput screening and assay technology. Prior to joining BioFocus PLC, he completed his Ph.D. at the University of Leeds on the Structure/Function of Trp channels.

Edward B. Stevens

is Team Leader of Ion Channel Assay Development and Hit-to-Lead Discovery at BioFocus PLC, Cambridge. He obtained a Ph.D. in electrophysiology of epithelial K^+ channels from Imperial College, London University. His post-doctoral experience was in structure-function studies of G-protein-coupled K^+ channels at Cambridge University, and the involvement of voltage-gated Na^+ channel auxiliary subunits in pain processing at Parke-Davis Neuroscience Research Centre, Cambridge.

J. Mark Treherne

obtained his Ph.D. in receptor neuropharmacology from Cambridge University, where he subsequently worked on neuronal ion channel biophysics. He then moved on to hold a Senior Faculty position in Switzerland at the Biozentrum in Basel, before returning to the UK to initiate a neuroscience research programme targeting ion channels at Pfizer's research facility at Sandwich. Mark co-founded Cambridge Drug Discovery (CDD) as Chief Executive in 1997 and is now Commercial Director of BioFocus PLC, which acquired CDD in 2001. Mark is a Visiting Senior Lecturer in Neuroscience at the University of Kent at Canterbury and Chairman of the Eastern Region Biotechnology Initiative, which has over 190 members and represents the Biotechnology Sector in the east of England.

Jeremy Packer

is Head of the Bioinformatics group at BioFocus PLC. His interests include elucidating patterns in sequence data that are relevant to drug discovery and exploring the diversity and evolution of target-rich gene families.

Mark Bushfield

After completing his Ph.D. on calcium signalling, Mark worked for five years in Stony Brook, New York and Glasgow, Scotland, studying the regulation of cyclic nucleotide metabolism. He joined Pfizer Central Research in 1991 and led several successful drug discovery teams in the areas of lead discovery, urogenitals, and gastrointestinal diseases. Mark co-founded CDD in 1997 and is now Director of Biology at BioFocus PLC.

Summary

Existing drugs that modulate ion channels represent a key class of pharmaceutical agents across many therapeutic areas and there is considerable further potential for potassium channel drug discovery. Potassium channels represent the largest and most diverse sub-group of ion channels and they play a central role in regulating the membrane potential of cells. Recent advances in genomics have greatly added to the number of these potential drug targets, but selecting a suitable potassium channel for drug discovery research is a key step. In particular, the potential therapeutic relevance of a potassium channel should be taken into account when selecting a target for screening. Potassium channel drug discovery is being driven by a need to identify lead compounds that can provide tractable starting points for medicinal chemistry. Furthermore, advances in laboratory automation have brought significant opportunities to increase screening throughput for potassium channel assays, but careful assay configuration to model drug-target interactions in a physiological manner is an essential consideration. Several potassium channel screening platforms are described in this review in order to provide some insight into the variety of formats available for screening, together with some of their inherent advantages and limitations. Particular emphasis is placed on the mechanistic basis of drug-target interaction and those aspects of structure/function that are of prime importance in potassium channel drug discovery.

Contents

Key words

Potassium channels, drug discovery, high-throughput screening, genomics, drug target selection, ligand binding assays, ion flux assays, fluorescent dyes, electrophysiology, selectivity assays, laboratory automation.

Glossary of abbreviations

ABC, ATP-binding cassette; ADP, adenosine diphosphate; ATP, adenosine triphosphate; BK, large conductance calcium-activated potassium channel; CRAC, Ca^{2+}-release-activated-Ca^{2+}; CNS, central nervous system; G, GTP-binding protein; GIRK, G-protein-coupled inwardly rectifying potassium channel (GIRK); HTS, high-throughput screening; IP_3, inositol triphosphate; IK, intermediate conductance calcium-activated potassium channel; KCO, K^+ channel openers; $Kv_{(ur)}$, cardiac ultrarapid delayed rectifier; $Kv_{(r)}$, cardiac rapid delayed rectifier; $Kv_{(s)}$, cardiac slow delayed rectifier; SK, small conductance calcium-activated potassium channel; NMDA, N-methyl-D-aspartate; NMDA channel, non-selective cation channel; MEQ, 6-methoxy-N-ethyl-quinolinium iodide; PIP_2, phosphatidylinositol-4,5-bis-phosphate; TEA, tetra-ethylamine; FRET, fluorescence resonance energy transfer; $DiBAC_4(3)$, dis-(1,2-dibutylbarbituric acid) trimethine oxonol; FLIPR, fluorometric imaging plate reader; VIPR, voltage ion probe reader; CCD, charge coupled device; WCPC, whole-cell patch clamp; TEVC, two-electrode voltage clamp; PDMS, polydimethylsiloxilane; UBSM, urinary bladder smooth muscle.

1   Introduction

An in-depth analysis of the molecular nature of drug targets found that all known drugs bind to about 500 distinct molecular targets [1]. Only 5% of these molecular targets, however, were classed as ion channels (Fig. 1). This relatively low percentage (compared with G-protein-coupled receptors, for example) may have resulted from a lack of suitable starting points for medicinal chemistry and difficulties in configuring relevant screens to identify novel chemical series. Nevertheless, existing drugs that modulate ion channels represent a key class of pharmaceutical agents with a total market value

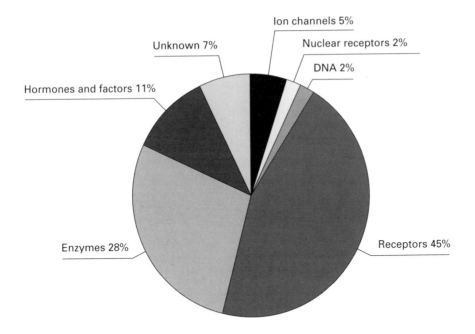

Fig. 1
Biochemical classes of drug targets of corrent therapies. Data taken and redrawn from [1], illustrates the classes of drug targets defined by their molecular nature and the relative percentages of those classes out of the 483 targets identified.

in excess of $ 6,000 million in 1995 [2] and which has now grown to approximately $ 10,000 million. The uses of these drugs span many therapeutic areas including cardiovascular diseases, disorders of the central and peripheral nervous systems, as well as metabolic dysfunction. These observations suggest that there is considerable further potential for ion channel drug discovery. Ion channels are proteins that span the lipid bilayer of the cell membrane and provide an aqueous pathway through which specific ions, such as Na^+, K^+, Ca^{2+} and Cl^-, can pass [3]. The ability of channels to distinguish between different ionic species is a fundamental aspect of their function and is achieved by specific amino acid residues within the pore of the channel [4–6]. The selective permeability and gating of ion channels are responsible for maintaining cell membrane potential and controlling cellular excitability [7]. Given their key role in cell functioning, it is not surprising that ion channels are such important drug targets [8].

Table 1
Diversity of mammalian potassium channel subunits. The number of genes indicated is based on a non-redundant set of sequences collated from (a) the Human and Rodent sections of the EMBL database and (b) human and rodent entries in the Geneseq database of sequences from patent applications (Derwent Ltd).

Channel type	Membrane topology	Number of genes
Voltage gated, Kv		27
Voltage gated, Klqt		5
Voltage gated, ether-a-go-go-like		8
Calcium activated, small conductance, SK and IK		4
Calcium activated, large conductance, BK, slo		3
Inward rectifying, Kir		15
Two-pore domain, TASK, TREK, TWIK, etc.		15

Table 1 (continued)

Subunit type	Associated with	Number of genes
Kvβ	Kv1.x	3
MinK/MiRP	Kvlqt, HERG	5
Sloβ	BK	4
SUR	Kir6.1, Kir6.2	2
KCHAP	Kv2.1	1
KChIPS	Kv4.2, Kv4.3	3

It is estimated that approximately 300 pore-forming ion channel subunits are encoded in the human genome, giving rise to many more functional channels by combination with various auxiliary subunits. Ion channels are classified into distinct sub-groups by their selective permeability to different ions. Potassium channels, which selectively pass potassium ions, represent the largest and most diverse sub-group of ion channels and play a central role in regulating the membrane potential of cells [9, 10]. It is this central role that has resulted in the realisation that potassium channel inhibitors and openers offer significant therapeutic opportunities in cardiac, smooth muscle, neuronal, immune and secretory systems [11]. A simplified summary of known potassium channel subunits is given in Table 1. Potassium channel nomenclature and structure are discussed in more detail elsewhere [10, 12–14]. The general structure of potassium channels is shown in Figure 2. Key features of the pore-forming subunits of potassium channels (α-subunits) are: a pore region that allows flow of potassium ions across the plasma membrane; a selectivity filter that allows K^+ but not other ions to pass through; and a gating mechanism that allows the channel to switch between open and closed states in response to changes in membrane potential or ligand presence. In most, if not all cases, the alpha-subunit co-assembles with an auxiliary protein (e.g., β-subunit) that regulates channel expression, ligand- and voltage-sensitivity and kinetics of activation and inactivation.

Potassium channel drug discovery is being driven by a need to identify lead compounds that can provide tractable starting points for medicinal chemistry. Furthermore, the chemistry must be directed at novel, therapeutically relevant drug targets and guided by functionally relevant screens. The search for new lead compounds that modulate potassium channels has been

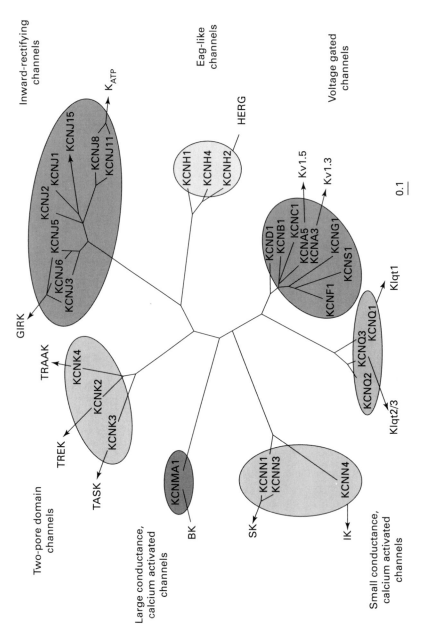

stimulated by the discovery of an ever-larger number of interesting potassium channels with no known pharmacology. In particular, recent advances in genomics and proteomics have greatly added to the number of these potential drug targets. This review summarises the scope of the potassium channel gene family and then goes on to identify potassium channels of known, or potential, therapeutic relevance.

The introduction of parallel synthesis techniques in chemistry has further highlighted the need for novel assay formats and screening systems capable of dealing with compound collections of 100,000 molecules or more. Advances in laboratory automation, instrumentation and assay miniaturisation have brought significant increases in the potential for screening throughput. For potassium channel assays, however, careful assay configuration, together with the ability of a high-throughput screen (HTS) to model drug-target interactions in a physiological manner, remains a fundamental consideration for assay design. A number of potassium channel screening platforms are described in this review to provide some insight into the variety of formats available for HTS, together with some of their inherent advantages and limitations. Particular emphasis is placed on the mechanistic basis of drug-target interaction and those aspects of structure/function that are of prime importance in the design of HTS approaches. For example, an important aspect of the development of potassium channels as drug targets is their ability to exist in multiple conformational states (e.g., open, closed and inactivated) and show "state-dependent" drug sensitivity (e.g., see [11]). This property of "state-dependent" blockade can be exploited therapeutically to discover drugs that selectively target the form of the channel present under pathological conditions, whilst sparing normal channel functioning. The benefits of being able to select "state-dependent" potassium channel modulators from screens can be of key importance in the discovery of potassium channel modulators.

Fig. 2
Phylogenetic tree of mammalian potassium channels. The tree is based on a multiple sequence alignment of the pore-forming domain and flanking transmembranes (with the N-terminal domain being used for the 2-pore domain containing sequences) and was constructed using a distance matrix method (the programs Protdist and Fitch from the Phylip package). HUGO gene symbols (http://www.gene.ucl.ac.uk/nomenclature/genefamily/KCN.shtml) are used to identify the sequences.

2 Potassium channel gene family

The efforts of gene cloning programmes in academic and industrial laboratories have led to the discovery of a large number of genes encoding potassium channel subunits. A significant challenge facing drug discovery scientists is to establish the molecular identity of the channel responsible for a physiological current. This is a complex task as a physiological channel may be formed from an oligomer of several gene products and a simple one gene – one target model need not necessarily apply. Furthermore, certain channel subunits are subject to extensive splice variation. Simple reconstitution experiments often do not produce a functional channel whose properties are identical to those of a physiological current, suggesting that the physiological channel is indeed more complex than the reconstituted channel.

2.1 Genes encoding α-subunits

Full-length mammalian sequences are currently available for a total of 77 potassium channel α-subunits, based on an exhaustive mining of the EMBL database (including finished genomic sequences) and the GeneSeq database of sequences from published patent applications (Derwent Ltd). Table 1 shows how these sequences are distributed between the seven families of potassium channels.

Figure 2 is a phylogenetic tree that shows the relationships between the seven families of potassium channels and illustrates the relative positions of therapeutically interesting targets within the superfamily. A comprehensive phylogenetic analysis of potassium channel subunits was published recently [15]. This publication analysed 67 sequences. Since then, 7 two-pore-domain channel subunits and three voltage-gated channel homologues have been identified. An updated set of phylogenetic trees is maintained and made available on the World-Wide Web at http://www.biofocus.com/TargetBASE. The HUGO Gene Nomenclature Committee (HGNC) also maintains a catalogue of known potassium channel-encoding genes (http://www.gene.ucl. ac.uk/nomenclature/genefamily/KCN.html). Sixty-nine α-subunit genes are currently annotated there.

Splice variation occurs in some α-subunits. Multiple splice variants have been identified in the extended C-terminal domain of the large conductance calcium-activated potassium channel (BK) [16]. These variants are differentially expressed in specific brain regions. The C-terminal domain is responsible for calcium sensing, and the splice variants differ in calcium sensitivity. C-terminal splice variants that differ in calcium sensitivity have also been reported recently for the small conductance calcium-activated potassium channel (SK1) [17, 18]. Splice variants in the C-terminal domain are also known in Kir3.1 [19], and the voltage-gated potassium channels, HERG [20], Klqt2 [21, 22], Klqt5 [23], Kv3.4 [24] and Kv4.3 [25]. An N-terminal variant of Kv3.4 lacks the inactivation ball that confers fast inactivation on Shaw-type channels [24]. Two N-terminal variants of Klqt1 co-assemble in different ratios to generate currents in endo- and mid-myocardium [26].

2.2   Pore-forming heterotetramers

The crystal structure of the bacterial KcsA potassium channel illustrates how a functional potassium channel is formed from the interaction of four pore-forming domains. With the likely exception of the rather poorly characterised family of two-pore domain containing subunits, each α-subunit contributes a single pore domain to a tetrameric pore-forming complex. Whilst the majority of physiological channels are likely to be homotetramers of a single class of α-subunit, increasing evidence points to some native potassium channels being formed from heterotetramers of at least two distinct α-subunits.

The majority of heterotetramers are formed from subunits with closely related sequences. For example, the very closely related Klqt2 and Klqt3 co-assemble to give rise to the neuronal M-current [27]. Kv1.1/1.2, Kv1.1/1.4 and Kv1.1/1.2/1.3/1.4 heteromultimers have been identified in the human central nervous system (CNS) [28] and Kv1.1/1.2/1.6 has been shown in rat brain [29].

A number of mammalian Kv homologues (belonging to the Kv5, 6, 8 and 9 subfamilies) do not form functional channels at all when expressed alone. Rather, subunits of these subfamilies co-assemble with Kv2 and Kv3 subunits to produce functional channels [30]. The effect of the co-assembly of Kv2 with Kv5, 6 or 9 subunits is to shift the inactivation curve to more negative potentials.

Outside the voltage-gated channel family, Slo2, a divergent member of the large-conductance, calcium-dependent potassium channel family, co-assembles with BK to form channels with intermediate gating properties [31]. These intermediate-conductance channels may be important in the CNS.

2.3   Genes encoding auxiliary subunits

A number of membrane-spanning and peripheral proteins associate with the pore-forming α-subunits of potassium channels. The known members of each class of auxiliary subunits are summarised in Table 1.

Voltage-gated channels of the Kv1 (shaker) subfamily consist of α4βn oligomers, where n is 0–4 [32]. The β-subunits are associated with the cytoplasmic face of the membrane. The inactivation properties of the channel are determined by the precise nature of the β-subunit. Kvβ1 and Kvβ3 have inactivation domains at the N-terminal domain. Kvβ2 (which always assembles in an α4β4 complex) lacks the inactivation domain. N-terminal splice variants of Kvβ1 differ in their channel blocking properties [33].

MinK and the related MiRP subunits are encoded by the KCNE gene family. These proteins have single transmembrane domains. MinK associates with Klqt1 and the resulting channel gives rise to the $K_{v(s)}$ cardiac current [34, 35]. MiRP1 is also expressed in the heart, but associates with HERG α-subunits and forms the $K_{v(r)}$ current [36]. MiRP2 associates with Kv3.4 in skeletal muscle [37] and with Klqt1 in the intestine [38]. Thus, members of the KCNE family of β-subunits are found in association with members of three different families of pore-forming subunits.

Four genes, KCNMB1-4, have been identified as encoding auxiliary subunits of the BK channel. The proteins have two transmembrane domains. BK channels lacking β-subunits do not inactivate. In contrast, channels with β-subunits do inactivate and show enhanced calcium sensitivity. β-subunits affect the pharmacology of the channels and have been shown to be involved in charybdotoxin binding [39].

The adenosine triphosphate (ATP)-sensitive potassium channel (K_{ATP}) consists of pore-forming subunits Kir6.1 or Kir6.2 co-assembled with auxiliary subunits belonging to the ATP-binding cassette (ABC) transporter superfamily. The channels are blocked by sulphonylureas that bind to the auxiliary subunits, designated the sulfonylurea receptor (SUR1 and SUR2). Multiple splice variants of SUR1 and SUR2 confer different ATP-sensitivity on the channel.

KChIPS are cytosolic proteins that interact with the N-terminal domain of Kv4 subunits [40]. They are thought to confer calcium sensitivity on the channel complex.

3   Potassium channels of therapeutic relevance

Given the large number of potassium channel α-subunits and auxiliary sub-units, and the ability of different α-subunits to form heteromultimeric channels in combination with other α-subunits within the same family, there is a potentially vast array of physiologically distinct potassium channels. This channel diversity should potentially allow very selective potassium channel modulators to be discovered as therapeutic agents.

3.1 K_{ATP} channels

K_{ATP} channels are weak inwardly rectifying potassium channels, which are regulated by intracellular ATP and, therefore, couple cellular metabolism to membrane excitability.

K_{ATP} channels are heteromeric complexes of Kir6 pore-forming subunits and SUR regulatory subunits. The Kir6 subunit confers sensitivity to ATP. The SUR subunit belongs to the ABC superfamily and determines channel sensitivity to ADP, sulfonylureas and channel openers such as diazoxide [41]. K_{ATP} channels are predominantly expressed in the pancreas and brain (SUR1-Kir6.2), cardiac and skeletal muscle (SUR2A-Kir6.2) and smooth muscle (SUR2B-Kir6.1) [42].

K^+ channel openers (KCOs) acting on K_{ATP} channels cause hyperpolarization of the membrane potential and reduction in cellular excitability and muscle relaxation. Due to tissue-specific distribution of hetermultimeric channel isoforms, selective K_{ATP} channel openers can potentially target different diseases. K_{ATP} openers have been shown to be useful in treatment of asthma, hypertension, urinary incontinence, angina and myocardial ischaemia.

The bladder detrusor muscle (smooth muscle) normally contracts to empty the bladder after filling from the kidneys. During urge incontinence, the bladder contractions become unstable, leading to spontaneous bladder emptying. K_{ATP} channels are expressed in human urinary bladder smooth muscle (UBSM) and are thought to be an attractive target for urge incontinence [43]. The tertiary carbinol, ZD-6169, and the arylsquarates, WAY-133537 and WAY-151616, are claimed to have bladder selective properties over cardiovascular parameters in animal models [44–46]. Studying *in vivo* rat models, these different classes of compounds have been shown to reduce bladder overactivity [45–48]. ZD-0947, a variant of ZD-6169, is now in clinical trials for bladder instability.

3.2   GIRK

The GTP-binding (G) protein-coupled inwardly rectifying potassium channel (GIRK) is a receptor-coupled potassium channel that opens in response to binding of G-protein $\beta\gamma$-subunits. $G\beta\gamma$ binding is dependent on the presence of phosphatidylinositol-bis-phosphate (PIP_2) [49] and is synergized by binding of Na^+ and Mg^{2+} [50].

The GIRK channel is predominantly expressed in the brain and heart. The channels consist of heteromultimers of Kir3.1 with Kir3.2, Kir3.3 and Kir3.4 within the brain and heart [51]. In the brain, GIRK channels have been shown to be important in post-synaptic inhibition. The weaver mouse mutation results in degeneration of cerebellar granule cells and dopaminergic neurons in the substantia nigra and is associated with spontaneous seizures. The weaver mutation is a single residue in the pore region of Kir3.2, implicating GIRK channels in seizure-related disorders [52].

GIRK has been suggested to be an important pain target. Both ethanol and the non-opioid analgesic, flupirtine, have been shown to directly activate GIRK channels [53–55]. Also, there is an absence of analgesia in the presence of ethanol and opioid agonists (morphine and U-50488) in the weaver mouse [56]. The use of flupirtine as an anti-convulsant and for neuroprotection suggests that GIRK channels may be a target for other CNS disorders [57]. Recent clinical trials have used flupirtine for treatment of variant Creutzfeldt-Jakob disease [58].

3.3   Kv1.3

During T-cell activation, binding of mitogens to the T-cell receptor causes activation of phospholipase C, production of inositol triphosphate (IP_3) and a transient release of Ca^{2+} from intracellular stores due to activation of the IP_3 receptor. Depletion of Ca^{2+} from the endoplasmic reticulum activates the Ca^{2+}-release-activated-Ca^{2+} (CRAC) channel allowing influx of extracellular Ca^{2+}. The voltage-gated K^+ channel, Kv1.3, which is upregulated during T-cell activation, sets the resting membrane potential of human peripheral T cells and determines the driving force for Ca^{2+} entry [59].

Blockers of Kv1.3 have been shown to prevent T-cell activation and proliferation *in vitro*, e.g., the Kv1.1/Kv1.3 selective toxins margatoxin and kaliotoxin [60], the nortriterpene correolide (purified from the tree *Spachea correae*) [61], the piperidine UK-78,282 [62] and the nonpeptide agent CP-339,818 [63]. *In vivo*, margatoxin and correolide have been shown to inhibit delayed-type hypersensitivity reaction in miniswine [61, 64]. Therefore, Kv1.3 is a useful target for immuno-suppression.

3.4   Kv1.5

Kv1.5 is thought to underlie the cardiac ultra-rapid delayed rectifier ($Kv_{(ur)}$) in humans. Kv1.5 shares biophysical and pharmacological properties similar to $Kv_{(ur)}$ [65], while antisense oligonucleotides to Kv1.5 reduce $Kv_{(ur)}$ amplitude in human atrial myocytes [66]. Electrophysiological recordings have demonstrated that $Kv_{(ur)}$ is selectively expressed in atrial, but not ventricular myocytes [67]. As $Kv_{(ur)}$ has an important role in repolarization of atrial myocytes, Kv1.5 blockers could prolong action potentials and prevent atrial fibrillation and atrial flutter.

The benzopyran compound NIP-142 has been shown to block Kv1.5 channels, prolong atrial refractory period and to terminate atrial fibrillation and flutter in *in vivo* canine models [68].

3.5   Klqt channels

The M-current is a subthreshold voltage-gated K^+ channel which inhibits neuronal excitability. The channel is coupled to various receptors, including M1 muscarinic receptors which inhibit the current. Native M-currents in neurones are thought to consist of heteromultimers of Klqt3 associated with Klqt2 or Klqt5, due to similar biophysical and pharmacological properties.

Klqt2, Klqt3 and Klqt5 show overlapping distributions throughout the brain and sympathetic neurones, due to similar biophysical and pharmacological properties [69, 70]. The Klqt4 gene is expressed in outer hair cells and nuclei of the central auditory pathway [71].

Homomeric and heteromeric combinations of Klqt2, Klqt3, Klqt4 and Klqt5 subunits (but not Klqt1) show high sensitivity to the novel anticonvulsant retigabine [72–75]. Retigabine enhances current amplitudes by hyperpolarizing the conductance-voltage relationship of the channel. Retigabine also activates M-currents in rat sympathetic neurones causing hyperpolarization of the membrane potential [73]. Retigabine is currently in phase II clinical trials as an anti-epileptic agent. Selective drugs to M-current subtypes could provide useful anti-convulsant therapies.

M-current blockers have been developed as cognition enhancers for neurodegenerative diseases such as Alzheimer's disease, as the block of the M-current is associated with enhanced acetylcholine release. Both linopirdine and its analogue XE-991 have been shown to block M-currents [76, 77]. Linopirdine and the analogues XE-991 and DMP-543 increase acetylcholine release in rat brain, while, in addition, linopirdine has been shown to improve learning and memory in rat models [78, 79].

Klqt1 is associated with the regulatory subunit MinK and forms the slowly activating component of the delayed rectifier in the heart. The Klqt1/MinK channel is a target for class-III anti-arrhythmic compounds. For example, the benzodiazepine L-735,821 is a Klqt1/MinK blocker which has been shown to increase the action potential duration of guinea pig ventricular myocytes [80].

3.6 BK channels

The BK channel consists of 4 α-subunits encoded by the *KCNMA1* gene. Extensive splice variation of the α-subunit is observed. The α-subunit forms a heteromultimer and associates with 1 of 4 β-subunits (β1–4). The smooth muscle/cardiac β1-subunit increases Ca^{2+}-sensitivity of the channel and alters BK pharmacology [81].

BK channels are potential targets for muscle relaxation during urinary incontinence, because they are expressed in human UBSM and control repolarization of the action potential and the resting membrane potential [82,

83]. The BK openers, NS004 and NS008, caused relaxation of guinea pig bladder strips [84], while the BK opener, NS1608, hyperpolarizes rat UBSM resting membrane potential [82]. *In vivo*, NS008 has been reported to increase bladder volume and inhibit bladder contractions in the rat, while introduction of recombinant *KCNMA1* DNA into rat bladder *in vivo* has been shown to reduce bladder hyperactivity [85].

Erectile dysfunction is due to altered tone of smooth muscle in the *corpus cavernosum* (the two expandable sacs that become engorged with blood). Promotion of smooth muscle relaxation (e.g., by elevating cGMP levels by phosphodiesterase 5 inhibition) is an effective therapeutic strategy for treating erectile dysfunction. BK channels that are expressed in human corporal smooth muscle also have a role in relaxation and are a potential target for erectile dysfunction [86]. Block of BK with 1 mM tetra-ethylamine (TEA) attenuates nitroglycerin (a nitrate donor)-stimulated relaxation [87], while PGE1-induced relaxation activates BK channels and reduces Ca^{2+} influx [88]. Injection of *KCNMA1* cDNA into the rat *corpus cavernosum* resulted in increased intra-cavernous pressure and altered nerve-stimulated erection [89].

BK openers have been developed as neuroprotective compounds during ischemic stroke [90]. BK openers hyperpolarize neurones reducing the influx of extracellular Ca^{2+}, which is associated with cell death. The fluoro-oxindole BMS-204352, a selective BK opener, is an effective neuroprotective agent in rat models of permanent large-vessel stroke [91]. BMS-204352 has now progressed to clinical trials for acute stroke.

3.7 IK channels

Intermediate conductance Ca^{2+}-activated K^+ channels (IK) channels are up-regulated during T-cell activation and set the membrane potential of lymphocytes. Therefore, similar to Kv1.3, the IK1 channel is considered an immunosuppression target. The triarylmethanes, clotrimazole and TRAM-34, have been shown to reduce T-cell proliferation in mitogen-stimulated lymphocytes [92, 93].

The erythrocyte Gardos channel, now identified as IK1, promotes erythrocyte dehydration, concentration and polymerization of abnormal haemoglobin and sickling of erythrocytes in sickle cell anaemia. Block of the

Gardos channel using clotrimazole has been shown to reduce erythrocyte dehydration in humans [94]. Therefore, the Gardos channel is a potential target for sickle cell anaemia. ICA-17043 has been shown to prevent red blood cell dehydration *in vitro* and in a mouse model of sickle cell anaemia [95]. ICA-17043 has progressed to phase I clinical trials.

3.8 SK channels

Small conductance Ca^{2+}-activated K^+ channels (SK) are found in a variety of cells, including neurones and smooth muscle. In neurones, SK channels underlie the after-hyperpolarization following an action potential [96]. The SK family consists of three genes, SK1, SK2 and SK3. SK2 and SK3, are blocked by apamin, whereas SK1 is apamin-insensitive [97]. In human tissue, SK1 is restricted to CNS, while SK2 and SK3 are more widespread [98]. The Ca^{2+}-sensitivity of the SK channel is bestowed by association of calmodulin with the SK α-subunit [99]. Using apamin block, SK channels have been shown to be involved in smooth muscle relaxation in gastro-intestinal and genito-urinary tracts [83], while regulation of SK channels in CNS are thought to be important in synaptic plasticity [100, 101]. SK channels are thought to be targets for memory disorders, epilepsy and gastro-intestinal dismobility. However, drugs specific for SK subtypes need to be developed; e.g., the bis-quinolone UCL-1530 can discriminate between neuronal and peripheral SK channels [102].

3.9 Two-pore domain potassium channels

Specific members of the recently identified diverse family of two-pore domain K^+ channels have been shown to be activated by volatile anaesthetics. TREK1, TREK2, TASK1 and TASK2 are activated to different extents by chloroform, diethylether, halothane and isoflurane [103]. Clinically relevant concentrations of inhalation anaesthetics activate TASK-1 currents in rat somatic motor neurones and locus coeruleus cells, causing membrane hyperpolarization and decrease in cell excitability [104]. Therefore these channels are important anaesthetic targets.

TREK and TRAAK are activated by cell swelling, intracellular acidosis and polyunsaturated fatty acids, as occurs during brain ischaemia. Activation of

TRAAK or TREK would cause hyperpolarization of neurones and reduce Ca^{2+} influx through voltage-gated Ca^{2+} channels and N-methyl-D-aspartate (NMDA) channels. Therefore TRAAK and TREK are potential neuroprotective targets. The neuroprotective compound, riluzole, has been shown to directly activate both TRAAK and TREK [105].

4 Potassium channel high-throughput screening technologies

High-throughput, homogeneity, low false-positive hit rate, no false negatives, reliability, reproducibility, detection of fast channel activation and inactivation, good correlation with electrophysiology, generic, low cost, and amenable to miniaturisation, are characteristics which would make the ideal ion channel assay platform. Although there have been some very exciting developments over the last decade, there are still no high-throughput ion channel assay platforms available which meet all these criteria.

Ion channel assay platforms can be separated into several categories: ligand binding, ionic flux, fluorescence, electrophysiology and novel technologies. These different areas will be reviewed, focusing on potassium channels and recent technological advances reported in the literature or developed in-house.

4.1 Ligand binding assays

Many ligands have been identified which bind to potassium channels and activate or modulate their function (Tab. 2). Typically, the ligand is radiolabelled, and compounds are identified which competitively displaced or allosterically affected ligand binding to the ion channel. This approach often resulted in "me too" drug discoveries, as only compounds which behaved mechanistically similarly to the labelled ligand were identified.

Ligand binding assays have been used for discovering and validating some of the first- (tolbutamide, chlorpropamide, acetohexamide and tolazamide) and second- (glibenclamide, glipizide, glibornuride) generation sulfonylureas. Sulfonylureas stimulate insulin secretion by binding to sulfonylureas receptors leading to the closure of the K_{ATP} channel. Many of the "me too" sulfonylureas, which were used in the treatment of Type-2 diabetes, suffered from several side-effects. Poor selectivity and long half-life of sulfonylureas often resulted in cardiac complications and excessive lowering of the plasma glucose levels, respectively. The ligand binding approach had limited success, as compounds which modulated ion channel activity independently of sulfonylurea binding went undetected. New improved classes of compound, unrelated to sulfonylureas, have now been discovered using functional assays rather than the traditional ligand binding assays [106].

Ligand binding assays have also been used for identifying compounds with undesirable pharmacological properties. For example, compounds displaying toxicity towards HERG may prolong the QT phase of a typical cardiac electrocardiogram [107]. Long QT can result in the onset of ventricular arrhythmia and occasional sudden death. Dofetilide is a drug used to treat cardiac arrhythmias which functions by blocking HERG. Due to its HERG blocking capabilities, radiolabelled dofetilide is routinely used to identify other compounds that modulate HERG activity by performing radioligand-binding assays. Radiolabelled dofetilide is incubated with whole cell or membrane preparations containing HERG; compounds are then added and assessed for their ability to displace bound dofetilide. Compounds that modulate HERG activity via an alternative mechanism to dofetilide are not identified. This is a serious disadvantage, considering the structural diversity of known compounds that modulate HERG activity [108]. Accordingly, for HERG safety pharmacology profiling, functional assays are often performed to complement radioligand binding data.

Following the advances in fluorescent-dye chemistry and screening technology for fluorescence assays, a rapid transition from radiolabelled to fluorescent-based binding assays in the ion channel field would have been expected. However, after reviewing the literature, it appears that the application and number of fluorescent ion channel ligands commercially available are limited. Green-fluorescent-glibenclamide and red-fluorescent-glibenclamide have been used to identify sulphonylurea receptors associated with K_{ATP} channels [109, 110]. Elsewhere, green fluorescent apamin derivatives have been developed for localising small-conductance calcium-activated potassium channels (Molecular Probes). Generally, the application of modified fluorescent ligands to ion channel pharmacology was restricted as a result of reduced binding affinity for the modified ligand compared to unlabelled ligand.

Table 2
Summary of some potassium channel ligands that have been used in potassium channel drug discovery as toxicological, pharmacological, or assay tools. Prefix "r" denotes recombinant expression of ligand.

Ligand	Potassium ion channel
rAgitoxin-2 / *Leiurus quinquestriatus hebraeus*	Kv1.1, Kv1.3, Kv1.6
rAgitoxin-3 / *Leiurus quinquestriatus hebraeus*	Kv1.1, Kv1.3, Kv1.6
Apamin / *Apis mellifera*	SK-type
BDS-I / *Anemonia sulcata*	Kv3.4
BDS-II / *Anemonia sulcata*	Kv3.4
rCharybdotoxin / *Leiurus quinquestriatus hebraeus*	BK, IK1, Kv1. 3
α-Dendrotoxin / *Dendroaspis angusticeps*	Kv1.1, Kv1.2, Kv1.6
β-Dendrotoxin / *Dendroaspis angusticeps*	Some Kv
γ-Dendrotoxin / *Dendroaspis angusticeps*	Some Kv
δ-Dendrotoxin / *Dendroaspis angusticeps*	Some Kv
Dendrotoxin K / *Dendroaspis p. polylepis*	Kv1.1
Dendrotoxin-I / *Dendroaspis p. polylepis*	Some Kv
Dofetilide	HERG
E- 4031	HERG
Glibenclamide	KATP
rIberiotoxin / *Buthus tamulus*	BK
Kaliotoxin / *Androctonus m. mauritanicus*	Some Ca^{2+}-activated and Kv channels
rMargatoxin / *Centruroides margaritatus*	Kv1.3
MCD-Peptide / *Apis mellifera*	Some Kv
rNoxiustoxin / *Centruroides noxius*	Some Ca^{2+}-activated and Kv channels
Paxilline / *Penicillium paxilli*	BK
Penitrem A / *Penicillium palitans*	BK
Stichodactyla toxin / *Stichodactyla heliantus*	Some Kv
Tertiapin / *Apis mellifera*	Kir1.1, Kir3.1, Kir 3.2, KAch
rTityustoxin Kα / *Tityus serrulatus*	Some Kv
Verruculogen / *Penicillium verruculosum*	BK

In summary, the application of ligand binding assays to ion channel pharmacology is unattractive because of the limited information content and the inability to identify compounds which modulate ion channel activity independently of the mechanism of the labelled ligand. Further disadvantages include difficulties in modifying or synthesising the ligand of interest and the influence of numerous parameters known to affect ligand binding. These include state-dependent ligand binding, voltage-dependent ligand binding, and the binding of the ligand to multiple binding sites. Additionally, potassium channels such as Kv1.5 are not amenable to ligand binding assays as there are no known selective high-affinity ligands available. Applications of labelled ligands outside of ion channel pharmacology include ion channel localisation studies, isolation and identification of the ligand-binding partner, and a drug discovery platform for the identification of compounds which up/down modulate ion channel surface expression (see Section 4.5).

4.2   Ion flux assays

The pore of a potassium channel is permeable to other monovalent cations such as Rb^+ and Tl^+. By looking at the cellular efflux of potassium channel permeable ions, which are radioisotopic, one can monitor potassium channel activity. For potassium channels, $[^{86}Rb^+]$ is the preferred isotope, due to its high-energy β and γ emission characteristics which allow its quantification by Cerenkov counting without the requirement of liquid scintillation fluid addition. This radiometric flux assay principle has also been used to look at other ion channel types: $[^{14}C]$-guanidinium or $[^{22}Na^+]$ for sodium channels, $[^{45}Ca^{2+}]$ for calcium channels, and $[^{125}I^-]$ for chloride channels.

The assay principle for voltage gated potassium channels is summarised in Figure 3. Calcium-activated potassium channels and ligand-gated potassium channels are activated by the addition of calcium under depolarising conditions or ligand addition, respectively.

Use of radioisotopes, requirement of cell washing to remove unloaded isotope, production of cell lines with high-level functional expression of the target channel, requirement of assay conditions which delay ion channel inactivation, and confinement to the 96-well microplate format are features/requirements which have hindered the development of HTS ionic flux assays.

Several of these disadvantages have been overcome, making ion channel flux assays attractive and extremely valuable to ion channel drug discovery. Amersham Pharmacia have developed homogenous ion channel flux assays. Their proprietary Cytostar-T scintillating microplate technology coats the base of the microplate with a scintillation material that will only detect radioisotopes in close proximity to it. Thus, growing a mono-layer of cells on the scintillant bed and adding radioisotope allows radioisotope that has entered the cell through target ion channels to be quantified without the requirement of cell washing. BioFocus has miniaturised the conventional

154

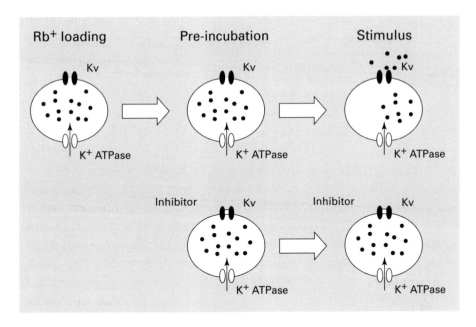

Fig. 3
Ionic flux assays. Cells are loaded with [^{86}Rb$^+$] *via* K$^+$ATPase. Unloaded [^{86}Rb$^+$] is removed by cell washing and cells are preincubated in the presence or absence of test compound. Voltage gated-potassium channels (Kv) are activated by the addition of a high content potassium buffer. Flux is allowed to occur over a pre-determined time course. The reaction supernatant is separated from the cell monolayer, and the percentage [^{86}Rb$^+$] efflux is determined by analysing both samples by Cerenkov counting. Compounds that inhibit the channel result in reduced [^{86}Rb$^+$] efflux.

potassium channel efflux protocol to 384-well microplate format and integrated it with their Robocon HTS system. This has provided HTS capabilities in excess of 30,000 compounds/week.

The use of high-energy radioisotopes is probably the strongest reason for not performing flux assays to study ion channel activity. Radioactive [^{86}Rb$^+$] has been substituted with non-radioactive [^{85}Rb$^+$], and the amount of [^{85}Rb$^+$] present in a given solution is accurately quantified by atomic absorption spectroscopy [111]. The integration of atomic absorption spectroscopy with HTS has taken place at BioFocus by modifying conventional atomic absorption spectrometers to accommodate microtitre plates. The correlation between radiometric and non-radiometric flux for a cell-based HERG assay is given in Figure 4, which shows IC$_{50}$ determinations for the known HERG blocker, E4031. There was no shift in E4031 potency, and atomic absorption spectroscopy gave better sensitivity (increased signal:background) compared to conventional radiometric detection methods.

4.3 Fluorescent dye assays

For ion channels, fluorescent dyes function in one of two ways. First, dyes may be directly affected by the ion of interest, e.g., Ca^{2+} chelating to Fluo-3 results in fluorescence, and halide ions colliding with 6-methoxy-N-ethyl-quinolinium iodide (MEQ) quenches fluorescence. Second, dyes may indirectly monitor ion channel activity, e.g. dyes which are sensitive to changes in the cell resting membrane potential which is dictated by the ion channel of interest. These conventional single dye systems are susceptible to variation in dye loading, cell density, and cell volume. The use of a second dye during the assay allows ratiometric analysis and will account for any artefacts such as dye loading and cell density variation.

Fluorescent cell-based assays that monitor potassium channel activity often rely on membrane potential-sensitive dyes such as dis-(1,2-dibutylbarbituric acid) trimethine oxonol ($DiBAC_4(3)$). Membrane potential-sensitive dyes are charged molecules, which migrate across a lipid bilayer depending on the cell membrane potential. For example, a stable cell line expressing a voltage-gated potassium channel will be hyperpolarized, and the negatively charged bis-oxonol dye $DiBAC_4(3)$ will be unable to migrate across the cell membrane into the cell. Blocking the voltage-gated potassium channel will set the resting membrane potential to a less hyperpolarized state, allowing $DiBAC_4(3)$ to migrate into the cell. Fluorescence produced from dye present in the cell can be quantified by bottom plate reading on a conventional fluorescent plate reader in the presence of a cell impermeable dye quencher. Open potassium channels give low fluorescent counts and blocked potassium channels give high fluorescent counts. An alternative approach to monitor changes in the cell resting membrane potential involves coupling membrane potential changes to intracellular calcium concentrations through the co-expression of voltage-gated calcium channels. Complications can arise when compounds directly modulate calcium store depletion or the co-expressed voltage-gated calcium channel.

Membrane potential-sensitive dyes, such as $DiBAC_4(3)$, suffer from slow-response times, small dynamic range (< 1% change in fluorescence/mV),

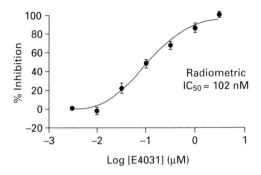

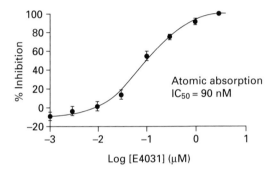

Fig. 4

Correlation between cell-based radiometric and non-radiemetric flux assays. Comparison IC_{50} determinations were carried out for E4031, a potent compound known to block HERG. Recombinant cell lines expressing HERG were loaded with [^{86}Rb$^+$] or [^{85}Rb$^+$] and subjected to the protocol summarised in Figure 3. IC_{50} determinations were 102 nM and 90 nM for radiometric and non-radiometric platforms, respectively. This demonstrates that changing from radiometric to non-radiometric flux assays does not affect the pharmacology of the assay.

compound interference (fluorescent compounds and dye quenching), temperature sensitivity, and the sequestering of some dyes into sub-cellular compartments. Improved membrane potential-sensitive dye systems have recently been reported. Molecular Devices Corporation has recently introduced a faster responding (2 min) membrane potential-sensitive dye that is much less sensitive to temperature changes than DiBAC$_4$(3). Aurora Biosciences Corporation (recently acquired by Vertex Pharmaceuticals) has developed a fluorescence resonance energy transfer (FRET)-based dye system for looking at changes in membrane potential [112]. Briefly, an external voltage-insensitive donor dye (coumarin-linked phospholipid) is FRET-coupled to a fast voltage-sensitive acceptor dye, e.g., $DiSBAC_2(3)$. When cells are in a hyperpolarized state, $DiSBAC_2(3)$ migrates out of the cell and FRET couples with the coumarin-linked phospholipid. Blocking potassium channels dictating the resting membrane potential causes the cells to become less hyperpolarized. $DiSBAC_2(3)$ migrates back into the cell, and FRET, between donor and acceptor dyes, is unable to occur across the cell membrane. These FRET-coupled dye systems offer sub-second responses, ratiometric analysis, and reduced background fluorescence (since measurements are confined to the cell membrane).

BioFocus is developing an alternative cell-based dye assay for looking at potassium channels [113]. The assay platform uses halide reporters such as, but not limited to, halide-sensitive fluorescence dyes to report the flow of Tl^+ through potassium channels. This invention is based on the phenomenon that Tl^+ will form an insoluble precipitate upon interaction with halide ions such as iodide. By precipitating iodide from aqueous media, quenching of halide-sensitive fluorescent reporters can be reduced, resulting in an increase in fluorescence. Thus, it is possible to quantitatively correlate flow of Tl^+ through potassium channels by monitoring increases in fluorescence that accompanies unquenching of halide-sensitive dyes.

Instrumentation for performing fluorescent cell-based assays is widely available. Traditional fluorescent plate readers come with single well detection systems (long plate read times), multiple wavelength read capabilities, and limited liquid handling for reagent and compound addition. Modified cell-based fluorescent plate readers such as Fluorometric Imaging Plate Reader (FLIPR) (Molecular Devices Corporation) and Voltage Ion Probe Reader (VIPR) (Aurora Biosciences Corporation) have been specifically developed for ion channel drug discovery. The FLIPR uses a charge-coupled device (CCD) imaging system for simultaneous optical measurement on all wells of a 384- or 96-well microtitre plate and a simultaneous dispensing device for compound addition. Increased sensitivity (signal:background) is achieved by high-energy dye excitation from a water-cooled argon-ion laser and the use of an optical detection system that focuses on the cell monolayer. The VIPR is capable of simultaneous column measurements in 384- or 96-well microtitre plates and has liquid handling capabilities for reagent and compound addition. Additionally, its proprietary optical imaging system allows simultaneous dual emission fluorescence measurements, making VIPR compatible with its proprietary FRET technology. Next generation plate readers may introduce field stimulation capabilities for studying ion channels.

4.4 Automated electrophysiology

Electrophysiology is considered the "gold standard" for measuring modulatory effects of drugs on ion channels. The electrophysiological techniques used most commonly for drug discovery are either the whole-cell patch-clamp (WCPC) technique of mammalian cell lines transiently or stably expressing recombinant ion channels [114] or the two-electrode voltage clamp (TEVC) of the *Xenopus* oocyte heterologous expression system [115]. For both techniques, under voltage-clamp conditions, channel activity is monitored by measuring currents associated with flow of charged ions. The voltage-clamp technique is rapid and precise, allowing channel activity to be recorded over a millisecond time-scale at different voltages. During the discovery process, electrophysiology has traditionally been used to validate HTS data and generate accurate IC_{50} values. Also, electrophysiology has been essential for determining the mechanism of action of channel blockers by examining voltage dependence, state dependence and frequency dependence. However, recently electrophysiology has been considered a potential platform for HTS.

All of the HTS approaches mentioned in the preceding sections are indirect measurements of ion channel activity. Additionally, with the exception of the Aurora FRET technology, the temporal response for most of these assays is greater than a second. In contrast to HTS assays, voltage-clamp recordings are direct measurements of channel activity and have a rapid temporal response (in milliseconds). Also, voltage-clamp recordings are independent of the cell resting membrane potential, do not require modified external K^+ concentrations to alter membrane potential and have exceptional signal to noise characteristics. Therefore, when using electrophysiology to study the action of compounds on ion channels, analysis is performed under physiologically relevant timescales, voltages and ionic conditions. Although the quality and reproducibility of electrophysiological data are substantially higher than HTS data, throughput by electrophysiology is markedly lower. Therefore, considerable attention has been directed towards developing high-throughput electrophysiological assays.

4.4.1 Automated whole-cell patch-clamp systems

There are two commercially available automated patch-clamp systems using a modification of conventional patch-clamp techniques, Sophion's ApatchI and CeNeS's Autopatch1. The ApatchI system automatically loads pipettes from a rack containing up to 18 prefilled pipettes and selects cells from 8 microperfused chambers on a rotating carousel. The pipette and cell are located and positioned relative to each other using an automatic focusing and imaging analysis. The CeNeS system uses "interface technology", where the entire patch-clamp system is inverted and miniaturized by removing the need for cell visualisation (base of the unit is 800 mm^2). Cells are loaded into a glass capillary and allowed to sediment to the air-solution interface, while a patch pipette is positioned beneath the capillary. The capillary is lowered onto the patch electrode and contact with a cell is indicated by a reduction in pipette resistance. Both systems show significant improvement in throughput compared to conventional whole-cell patch clamp by an experienced user. Additionally, automation allows inexperienced users to run several machines in parallel.

4.4.2 Automated two electrode voltage-clamp systems

Both Multi Channel Systems and Axon have developed automated oocyte screening systems. Roboocyte (Multi Channel Systems) allows cDNA or cRNA injection and TEVC recording from *Xenopus* oocytes in a 96-well plate. TEVC of oocytes uses a plug-and-play measuring head containing glass electrodes, reference electrodes and perfusion ports. In collaboration with Roche and AstraZeneca, Axon is currently developing an automated oocyte TEVC system using eight oocytes in parallel based around their current electrophysiological amplifiers. Such systems have the potential of generating hundreds of data points per day and are suitable for hit validation and hit-to-lead development.

4.4.3 Planar patch-clamp techniques

Chip-based planar patch-clamp systems dispense with the need for borosilicate patch pipettes and instead use a substrate which has both optimal electrical insulation and membrane sealing behaviour (giving rise to gigaohm patches) with machined apertures into which individual cells are positioned. Membrane currents are recorded across the aperture containing the cell using a current-to-voltage converter. Axon is developing a planar patch-clamp system, "patch-on-a-chip", using surface treated polydimethylsiloxilane (PDMS or Sylgard), Nanion developed a glass chip based device, while Cytion used a Si_3N_4 aperture coated in SiO_2 [116]. Individual cells are automatically positioned into the aperture resulting in gigaohm seals, using either suction (Axon) or electrophoretic focusing exploiting electric fields surrounding the aperture (Cytion) [116]. Although the technology is still at the developmental stage and gigaohm seal failure rate high, planar patch-clamp systems are highly adaptable to parallel recording and therefore suitable for HTS. Essen Instruments is developing a high-throughput platch-clamp system capable of generating 10,000 data points/day, while demonstrating excellent background recordings (< 10 pA) and temporal resolution.

4.5   Novel ion channel assay platforms

Historically, compounds associated with ion channels modulate ion channel activity by directly binding to the target ion channel or one of its accessory subunits. For example, small molecule potassium channel blockers often function by binding to the inner vestibule pore region of the ion channel. Compounds with this mechanism may demonstrate poor selectivity over subfamily related ion channels. Alternative mechanisms are beginning to emerge for ion channel modulators which function independent of ion channel binding.

Modulators, which selectively regulate target ion channel expression, may be an alternative to the traditional ion channel blockers and openers. Additionally, compounds that are capable of up-modulating surface expression of defective ion channel trafficking mutants linked to channelopathies such as cystic fibrosis, may be valuable therapeutic agents. BioFocus is currently developing an assay for detecting compounds that down-regulate a voltage-gated potassium channel using its proprietary retroviral-displaying platform (Fig. 5). "Retroviral display" entails the fusion of polypeptides to the outer portion (N-terminus) of retroviral envelope proteins. For ion channel assays an ion channel-selective toxin or single chain antibody is displayed.

A retroviral display assay applied to ion channels would have a number of significant advantages over alternative methodologies available for quantifying ion channel surface expression. Since it is a cell-based assay, the compounds are tested in a relatively physiological environment. In addition, the assay produces a "positive read-out"; i.e., "hit" compounds that reduce the availability or number of cell-surface ion channels produce an increased signal. Compounds that are toxic, or that induce non-specific detrimental effects on the target cells, will, therefore, not be read as "false positives". This advantage overcomes a key problem in cell-based HTS. The assay format is convenient, since all components are encoded genetically.

Disrupting a protein:protein interaction that affects ion channel activity could also be another therapeutic approach for modulating ion channel activity. Many ion channel α-subunits have been shown to interact with accessory subunits which modulate their function. For example, the interaction between KChIPs and α-subunits of the Kv4 subfamily has been shown to be important for modulating ion channel density, inactivation kinetics, and the rate of recovery from inactivation [40]. Hence, disrupting this interaction may be an alternative approach for modulating the excitability of neurones and cardiac myocytes where this complex exists. Alternative protein:protein interaction targets in the ion channel field could include ion channel-cytoskeletal anchoring complexes and specific heteromultimeric ion channel complexes. There is a plethora of HTS technologies available for screening against protein:protein interactions *in vivo* and *in vitro*. ICAST™ is a new technology developed by Applied Biosystems that allows one to monitor specific functional protein:protein interactions *in vivo*. Two mutant forms of β-galactosidase proteins are fused to proteins of interest (A and B). If proteins A and B do not interact, or are prevented from interacting, the β-galactosidase mutants remain inactive. When A and B do interact, the β-galactosidase mutants will complement each other and form an active enzyme.

5 Concluding remarks

Potassium channel drug discovery is clearly an area of research with great therapeutic relevance to a number of important diseases. Historically, discovery of novel inhibitors and modulators of ion channels has been hampered by the lack of functionally relevant HTS. Electrophysiology, although

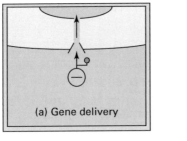 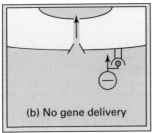

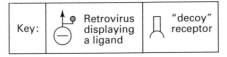

Fig. 5a
Receptor-mediated sequestration. The displayed polypeptide (ion channel selective toxin or single chain antibody) can bind to a "decoy" receptor (target ion channel) on the target cell surface. (a) In the absence of the decoy receptor, gene delivery proceeds. (b) When the decoy receptor is present, binding of the retrovirus to the virus receptor is impaired, and gene delivery is prevented.

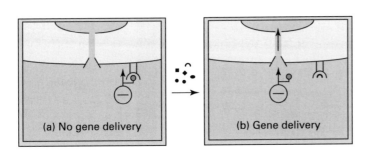

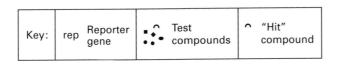

Fig. 5b
Assay for loss of free decoy receptor binding sites at the cell surface. (a) Virus is sequestered onto decoy receptors on the cell surface, preventing gene delivery. (b) "Hit" compounds reduce the cell-surface number or availability of the decoy receptors. This allows the virus to deliver the reporter gene (rep) to the target cell.

an excellent technique, is relatively slow in comparison to biochemical assays. Consequently, a number of novel assay platforms have recently been developed that will allow the discovery of novel drugs acting at potassium channels. Many of these drugs will have been optimised from novel hits discovered in HTS, where these hit compounds have opened up whole new avenues of research for medicinal chemistry to exploit. As long as medicinal chemistry can develop adequately selective molecules for the primary potassium channel target over other ion channels, then the pipeline of ion channel drugs entering the clinic will increase.

Acknowledgements

We would like to thank Sue Scott for help in preparing this manuscript, the Biofocus Retroviral Group (Mark Chadwick, Helen Sheldon, Bela Chopra and Andrew Cook) and Annik Panicker for their input on retroviral display and HERG assay development, respectively. We would like to acknowledge Thermo Elemental for help in modifying their Atomic Absorption Spectrometer for drug discovery purposes.

References

1   J. Drews: Science 287, 1960–1964 (2000).
2   K.K. Jain: Scrip Report, P.J. Publications Ltd., London 1995.
3   S.C. Herbert: Am. J. Med. 104, 87 (1998).
4   W.A. Catterall: Curr. Opinion Cell Biol. 6, 607–615 (1994).
5   W.A. Sather, J. Yang J and R.W. Tsien: Curr. Opinion Neurobiol. 4, 313–323 (1994).
6   C.I. Bargmann: Science 282, 2028–2033 (1998).
7   C.M. Armstrong and B. Hille: Neuron 20, 371–380 (1998).
8   F.M. Ashcroft and J. Roper: Curr. Opinion Cell Biol. 5, 677–683 (1993).
9   M.J. Coghlan, W.A. Carroll and M. Gopalakrishnan: J. Med. Chem. 44, 1627–1653 (2001).
10   G.J. Kaczorowski and M.L. Garcia: Curr. Opinion Cell Biol. 3, 448–458 (1999).
11   Q.Y. Liu: Can. J. Physiol. 14, 275 (1998).
12   K.G. Chandy and G.A. Gutman, in: A. North (ed.): Ligand and Voltage-Gated Ion Channels, CRC Press, Florida 1995, 1–71.
13   L.Y. Jan and Y.N. Jan: Ann. Rev. Neurosci. 20, 91–123 (1997).
14   C.C. Shieh, M. Coghlan, J.P. Sullivan and M. Gopalakrishnan: Pharmacol. Rev. 52, 557–594 (2000).

15 J. Packer, E. Conley, N. Castle, D. Wray, C. January and L. Patmore: Trends Pharmacol. Sci. *21*, 327–329 (2000).

16 J. Tseng-Crank, C.D. Foster, J.D. Krause, R. Mertz, R. Godinot, T.J. DiChiara and P.H. Reinhart: Neuron *13*, 1315–1330 (1994).

17 B.E. Shmukler, C.T. Bond, S. Wilhelm, A. Bruening-Wright, J. Maylie, J.P. Adelman and S.L. Alper: Biochim. Biophys. Acta *1518*, 36–46 (2001).

18 B.M. Zhang, V. Kohli, R. Adachi, J.A. Lopez, M.M. Udden and R. Sullivan: Biochemistry *40*, 3189–3195 (2001).

19 C.S. Nelson, J.L. Marino and C.N. Allen: Brain Res. Mol. Brain Res. *46*, 185–196 (1997).

20 I. Splawski, J. Shen, K.W. Timothy, G.M. Vincent, M.H. Lehmann and M.T. Keating: Genomics *51*, 86–97 (1998).

21 Z. Pan, A.A. Selyanko, J.K. Hadley, D.A. Brown, J.E. Dixon and D. McKinnon: J. Physiol. *531*, 347–358 (2001).

22 J.S. Smith, C.A. Iannotti, P. Dargis, E.P. Christian and J. Aiyar: J. Neurosci. *21*, 1096–1103 (2001).

23 B.C. Schroeder, M. Hechenberger, F. Weinreich, C. Kubisch and T.J. Jentsch: J. Biol. Chem. *275*, 24089–24095 (2000).

24 D. Vullhorst, H. Jockusch and J.W. Bartsch: Gene *264*, 29–35 (2001).

25 S. Ohya, M. Tanaka, T. Oku, T. Furuyama, N. Mori, W.R. Giles, M. Watanabe and Y. Imaizumi: Life Sci. *68*, 1703–1716 (2001).

26 Y. Pereon, S. Demolombe, I. Baro, F. Charpentier and D. Escande: Am. J. Physiol. Heart Circ. Physiol. *278*, H1908–H1915 (2000).

27 H.S. Wang, Z. Pan, W. Shi, B.S. Brown, R.S. Wymore, I.S. Cohen, J.E. Dixon and D. McKinnon: Science *282*, 1890–1893 (1998).

28 S.K. Coleman, J. Newcombe, J. Pryke and J.O. Dolly: J. Neurochem. *73*, 849–858 (1999).

29 F.C. Wang, D.N. Parcej and J.O. Dolly: Eur. J. Biochem. *263*, 230–237 (1999).

30 M. Salinas, F. Duprat, C. Heurteaux, J.P. Hugnot and M. Lazdunski: J. Biol. Chem. *272*, 24371–24379 (1997).

31 W.J. Joiner, M.D. Tang, L.Y. Wang, S.I. Dworetsky, C.G. Boissard, L. Gan, V.K. Gribkoff and L.K. Kaczmarek: Nat. Neurosci. *1*, 462–469 (1998).

32 J. Xu, W. Yu, J.M. Wright, R.W.Raab and M. Li: Proc. Natl. Acad. Sci. USA *95*, 1846–1851 (1998).

33 Z. Wang, J. Kiehn, Q. Yang, A.M. Brown and B.A. Wible: J. Biol. Chem. *271*, 28311–28317 (1996).

34 J. Barhanin, F. Lesage, E. Guillemare, M. Fink, M. Lazdunski and G. Romey: Nature *384*, 24–25 (1996).

35 M.C. Sanguinetti, M.E. Curran, A. Zou, J. Shen, P.S. Spector, D.L. Atkinson and M.T. Keating: Nature *384*, 80–83 (1996).

36 G.W. Abbott, F. Sesti, I. Splawski, M.E. Buck, M.H. Lehmann, K.W. Timothy, M.T. Keating and S.A. Goldstein: Cell *97*, 175–187 (1999).

37 G.W Abbott, M.H. Butler, S. Bendahhou, M.C. Dalakas, L.J. Ptacek and S.A. Goldstein: Cell *104*, 217–231 (2001).

38 B.C. Schroeder, S. Waldegger, S. Fehr, M. Bleich, R. Warth, R. Greger and T.J. Jensch: Nature *403*, 196–199 (2000).

39 H.G. Knaus, K. Folander, M. Garcia-Calvo, M.L. Garcia, G.J. Kaczarowski, M. Smith and R. Swanson: J. Biol. Chem. *269*, 17274–17278 (1994).

40   W.F. An, M.R. Bowlby, M. Betty, J. Cao, H.P. Ling, G. Mendoza, J.W. Hinson, K.I. Matts-son, B.W. Strassle, J.S. Trimmer et al.: Nature *403*, 553–556 (2000).

41   H. Yokoshiki, M. Sunagawa, T. Seki, N. Sperelakis: Am. J. Physiol. *274*, C25–37 (1998).

42   N. Inagaki and S. Seino: Jpn. J. Physiol. *48*, 397–412 (1998).

43   S.A. Buckner, I. Milicic, A. Daza, R. Davis-Taber, V.E. Scott, J.P. Sullivan and J.D. Brioni: Eur. J. Pharmacol. *400*, 287–95 (2000).

44   B.B. Howe, T.J. Halterman, C.L. Yochim, M.L. Do, S.J. Pettinger, R.B. Stow, C.J. Ohn-macht, K. Russell, J.R. Empfield, D.A. Trainor et al.: J. Pharmacol. Exp. Ther. *274*, 884–890 (1995).

45   A.M. Gilbert, M.M. Antane, T.M. Argentieri, J.A. Butera, G.D. Francisco, C. Freeden, E.G. Gundersen, R.F. Graceffa, D. Herbst, B.H. Hirth et al.: J. Med. Chem. *43*, 1203–1214 (2000).

46   J.A. Butera, M.M. Antane, S.A. Antane, T.M.Argentieri, C. Freeden, R.F. Graceffa, B.H. Hirth, D. Jenkins, J.R. Lennox, E. Matelan, N.W. Norton, D. Quagliato, J.H. Sheldon et al.: J. Med. Chem. *43*, 1187–1202 (2000).

47   R.K. Pandita, K. Persson and K.E. Andersson: J. Urol. *58*, 2300–2304 (1997).

48   A. Wojdan, C. Freeden, M. Woods G. Oshiro, W. Spinelli, T.J. Colatsky, J.H. Sheldon, N.W. Norton, D. Warga, M.M. Antane, S.A. Antane et al.: J. Pharmacol. Exp. Ther. 289, 1410–1418 (1999).

49   C.L. Huang, S. Feng, D.W. Hilgemann: Nature 391, 803–806 (1998).

50   J. Petit-Jacques, J.L.Sui and D.E. Logothetis: J. Gen. Physiol. *114*, 673–684 (1999).

51   M.D. Mark and S.G. Herlitze: Eur. J. Biochem. *267*, 5830–6 (2000).

52   Y.J. Liao, Y.N. Jan and L.Y. Jan: J. Neurosci. *16*, 7137–7150 (1996).

53   T. Kobayashi., K. Ikeda, H. Kojima, H. Niki, R. Yano, T. Yoshioka and T. Kumanishi: Nat. Neurosci. *2*, 1091–1097 (1999).

54   J. Kornhuber, S. Bleich, J. Wiltfang, M. Maler and C.G. Parsons: J. Neural Transm. *106*, 857–867 (1999).

55   R. Jakob and J. Krieglstein: Br. J. Pharmacol. *122*, 1333–1338 (1997).

56   K. Ikeda, T. Kobayashi, T. Kumanishi, H. Niki and R. Yano: Neurosci. Res. *38*, 113–116 (2000).

57   S. Perovic, M. Bohm, E. Meesters, A. Meinhardt, G. Pergande and W.E. Muller: Mech. Age-ing Dev. *101*, 1–19 (1998).

58   W.E. Muller, J.L. Laplanche, H. Ushijima and H.C. Schroder: Mech. Ageing Dev. *116*, 193–218 (2000).

59   M.D. Cahalan and K.G. Chandy: Curr. Opin. Biotechnol. *8*, 749–756 (1997).

60   C. Beeton, J. Barbaria, P. Giraud, J. Devaux, A.M. Benoliel, M. Gola, J.M. Sabatier, D. Bernard, M. Crest and E. Beraud: Immunol. *166*, 936–944 (2001).

61   G.C. Koo, J.T. Blake, K., Shah M.J. Staruch, F. Dumont, D. Wunderler, M. Sanchez, O.B. McManus, A. Sirotina-Meisher, P. Fischer et al.: Cell Immunol. *197*, 99–107 (1999).

62   D.C. Hanson, A. Nguyen, R.J. Mather, H. Rauer, K. Koch, L.E. Burgess, J.P. Rizzi, C.B. Donovan, M.J. Bruns, P.C. Canniff et al.: Br. J. Pharmacol. *126*, 1707–1716 (1999).

63   A. Nguyen, J.C. Kath, D.C. Hanson, M.S. Biggers, P.C. Canniff, C.B. Donovan, R.J. Mather, M.J. Bruns, H. Rauer, J. Aiyar et al.: Mol. Pharmacol. *50*, 1672–1679 (1996).

64   G.C. Koo, J.T. Blake, K. A. Talento, M. Nguyen, S. Lin, A. Sirotina, K. Shah, K. Mulvany, D. Hora Jr., P. Cunningham et al.: J. Immunol. *158*, 5120–5128 (1997).

65   Z. Wang, B. Fermini and S. Nattel: Circ. Res. *73*, 1061–1076 (1993).

66   J. Feng, B. Wible, G.R. Li, Z. Wang and S. Nattel: Circ. Res. *80*, 572–579 (1997).

67   G.R. Li, J. Feng, L. Yue, M. Carrier and S. Nattel: Circ. Res. *78*, 689–696 (1996).

68   T. Matsuda, H. Masumiya, N. Tanaka, T. Yamashita, N. Tsuruzoe, Y. Tanaka, H. Tanaka H and K. Shigenoba: Life Sci. *68*, 2017–24 (2001).

69   H.-S. Wang, Z Pan, B.S. Brown, R.S. Wymore, I.S. Cohen, J.E. Dixon and D. McKinnon: Science *282*, 1890–1893 (1998).

70   B.C. Schroeder, M. Hechenberger, F. Weinreich, C. Kubisch and T.J. Jentsch: J. Biol. Chem. *275*, 24089–24095 (2000).

71   T. Kharkovets, J.P. Hardelin, S. Safieddine, M. Schweizer, A. El-Amraoui, C. Petit and T.J. Jentsch: Proc. Natl. Acad. Sci. USA *97*, 4333–4338 (2000).

72   M.J. Main, J.E. Cryan, J.R. Dupere, B. Cox, J.J. Clare and S.A. and Burbidge SA.: Mol. Pharmacol. *58*, 253–262 (2000).

73   L. Tatulian, P. Delmas, F.C. Abogadie and D.A. Brown: J Neurosci 21, 5535–5545 (2001).

74   A.D. Wickenden, W. Yu, A. Zou, T. Jegla and P.K. Wagoner: Mol. Pharmacol. *58*, 591–600 (2000).

75   A.D. Wickenden, A. Zou, P.K. Wagoner and T. Jegla: Br. J. Pharmacol. *132*, 381–384 (2001).

76   M. Noda, M. Obana and N. Akaike: Brain Res. *794*, 274–280 (1998).

77   H.S. Wang, B.S. Brown, D. McKinnon and I.S. Cohen: Mol. Pharmacol. *57*, 1218–1223 (2000).

78   R. Zaczek, R.J. Chorvat and B.S. Brown: CNS Drug Rev. *3*, 103–119 (1997).

79   R. Zaczek, R.J. Chorvat, J.A. Saye, M.E. Pierdomenico, C.M. Maciag, A.R. Logue, B.N. Fisher, D.H. Rominger and R.A. Earl: J. Pharmacol. Exp. Ther. *285*, 724–730 (1998).

80   H.G. Selnick, N.J. Liverton, J.J. Baldwin, J.W. Butcher, D.A. Claremon, J.M. Elliott, R.M. Freidinger, S.A. King, B.E. Libby, C.J. McIntyre et al.: J. Med. Chem. *40*, 3865–3868 (1997).

81   S.I. Dworetzky, C.G. Boissard, J.T. Lum-Ragan, M.C. McKay, D.J. Post-Munson, J.T. Trojnacki, C.P. Chang and V.K Gribkoff : J. Neurosci. *16*, 4543–4550 (1996).

82   C. Siemer, M. Bushfield, D. Newgreen and S. Grissmer: J. Membr. Biol. *173*, 57–66 (2000).

83   G.M. Herrera, T.J. Heppner, M.T. Nelson: Am. J. Physiol. *279*, R60–R68 (2000).

84   S. Trivedi, L. Potter-Lee, J.H. Li, G.D. Yasay, K. Russell, C.J. Ohnmacht, J.R. Empfield, D.A. Trainor and S.T. Kau: Biochem. Biophys. Res. Commun. *213*, 404–409 (1995).

85   G.J. Christ, N.S. Day, C. Santizo, W. Zhao, T. Sclafani, V. Karicheti, M. Valcic and A. Melman: Urology *57*, 111 (2001).

86   S.F. Fan, P.R. Brink, A. Melman and G.J. Christ: J. Urol. *153*, 818–25 (1995).

87   J. Geliebter, A. Melman, G.J. Christ and J. Rehman: Patent Number US 6150338 (2000).

88   S.W. Lee, H.Z. Wang, W. Zhao, P. Ney, P.R. Brink and G.J. Christ: Int. J. Impot. Res. *11*, 189–99 (1999).

89   G.J. Christ, J. Rehman, N. Day, L. Salkoff, M. Valcic, A. Melman and J. Geliebter: Am. J. Physiol. *275*, H600–8 (1998).

90   V.K. Gribkoff, J.E. Starrett Jr. and S.I. Dworetzky: Neuroscientist *7*, 166–177 (2001).

91   V.K. Gribkoff, J.E. Starrett Jr, S.I. Dworetzky, P. Hewawasam, C.G. Boissard, D.A. Cook, S.W. Frantz, K. Heman, J.R. Hibbard, K. Huston et al.: Nat. Med. *7*, 471–7 (2001).

92   B.S. Jensen, N. Odum, N.K. Jorgensen, P. Christophersen and S.P. Olesen: Proc. Natl. Acad. Sci. USA *96*, 10917–10921 (1999).

93   H. Wulff, M.J. Miller, W. Hansel, S.Grissmer, M.D. Cahalan and K.G.Chandy: Proc. Natl. Acad. Sci. USA *97*, 8151–8156 (2000).

94   C. Brugnara, B. Gee, C.C. Armsby, S. Kurth, M. Sakamoto, N. Rifai, S.L. Alper and O.S. Platt: J. Clin. Invest. *97*, 1227–1234 (1996).

95   J. Stocker, L. de Franceschi, G. McNaughton-Smith and C. Brugnara: American Society of Hematology Annual Meeting (2000).

96   P. Pedarzani, J. Mosbacher, A. Rivard, L.A. Cingolani, D. Oliver, M. Stocker, J.P. Adelman and B. Fakler: J. Biol. Chem. *276*, 9762–9 (2001).

97   T.M. Ishii, J. Maylie and J.P. Adelman: J. Biol. Chem. *272*, 23195–23200 (1997).

98   R. Rimini, J.M. Rimland and G.C. Terstappen: Brain Res. Mol. Brain Res. *85*, 218–220 (2000).

99   M.A. Schumacher, A.F. Rivard, H.P. Bachinger and J.P. Adelman: Nature *410*, 1120–1124 (2001).

100   C. Messier, C. Mourre, B. Bontempi, J. Sif, M. Lazdunski and C. Destrade: Brain Res. *551*, 322–6 (1991).

101   M. Stocker, M. Krause and P. Pedarzani: Proc. Natl. Acad. Sci. USA *96*, 4662–4667 (1999).

102   P.M. Dunn, D.C. Benton, J. Campos Rosa, C.R. Ganellin and D.H. Jenkinson: Br. J. Pharmacol. *117*, 35–42 (1996).

103   A.J. Patel, E. Honore, F. Lesage, M. Fink, G. Romey and M. Lazdunski: Nat. Neurosci. *2*, 422–426 (1999).

104   J.E. Sirois, Q. Lei, E.M. Talley, C. Lynch 3rd and D.A. Bayliss: J. Neurosci. *20*, 6347–6354 (2000).

105   F. Duprat, F. Lesage, A.J. Patel, M. Fink, G. Romey and M. Lazdunski: Mol. Pharmacol. *57*, 906–912 (2000).

106   G. Emilien, J.-M. Maloteaux and M. Ponchon: Pharmacol Therapeutics *81*, 37–51 (1999).

107   F. De Ponti, E. Poluzzi and N. Montanaro: Eur. J. Clin. Pharmacol. *56*, 1–18 (2000).

108   J.I. Vandenberg, B.D. Walker and T.J. Campbell: Trends Pharmacol. Sci. *22*, 240–246 (2001).

109   I. Quesada, A. Nadal and B. Soria: Diabetes *48*, 2390–2397 (1999).

110   B. Lohrke, M. Derno, B. Kruger, T. Viergutz, H. Matthes and W. Jentsch: Pflugers Arch. *434*, 712–720 (1997).

111   G.C. Terstappen: Anal. Biochem. *272*, 149–155 (1999).

112   Gonzalez, K. Oades, Y. Leychkis, A. Harootunian and P. Negulescu: Drug Discovery Today *4*, 431–439 (1999).

113   N. Castle and J. Ford: Patent Number GB 9925799, PCT/GB00/04185, WO01/33219 (1999).

114   O.P. Hamill, A. Marty, E. Neher, B. Sakmann and F.J. Sigworth: Pflugers Archiv *391*, 85–100 (1981).

115   T.M. Shih, R.D. Smith, L. Toro, and A.L. Goldin, in: P.M. Conn (ed.): Methods in Enzymology (Ion Channel Part B), Academic Press, New York 1998.

116   C. Schmidt, M. Mayer and H.A. Vogel: Angew. Chem. Int. Ed. Engl. *39*, 3137–3140 (2000).

Progress in Drug Research, Vol. 58 (E. Jucker, Ed.)
©2002 Birkhäuser Verlag, Basel (Switzerland)

Dual serotonin and noradrenaline uptake inhibitor class of anti-depressants – Potential for greater efficacy or just hype?

By David T. Wong[1] and
Frank P. Bymaster[2]

[1]Neurobiology Program
Department of Psychiatry
Indiana University Medical School
Indianapolis, IN 46202
USA

[2]Neuroscience Research
Lilly Research Laboratories
Eli Lilly and Company
Lilly Corporate Center
Indianapolis, IN 46285-0510
USA
<F.Bymaster@Lilly.com>

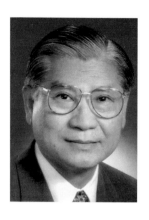

David T. Wong

received his Ph.D. in Biochemistry at the University of Oregon School of Medicine in 1966 following his M.S. in Biochemistry at Oregon State University, 1964 and B.S. in Chemistry at Seattle Pacific College, 1961. After spending post-doctoral years at the Department of Biophysics and Physical Biochemistry, Johnson Research Foundation, University of Pennsylvania, he joined the Lilly Research Laboratories, Eli Lilly and Company, as a Senior Biochemist, in the Division of Pharmacological Research in 1968. He and Mr. Bymaster belonged to the team involved in research on uptake inhibitors as potential antidepressant drugs, which led to the discovery and development of fluoxetine (Prozac), atomoxetine, duloxetine and daproxetine. They were also involved in the development and characterization of dopaminergic agents including the anti-Parkinson drug pergolide (Permax), an agonist of dopamine D_1 and D_2 receptors, other dopamine agonists, and the antipsychotic drug, olanzapine (Zyprexa), an antagonist at dopamine and serotonin receptors. After giving over 31 years of service in Eli Lilly and Company, Dr. Wong retired at the rank of Lilly Research Fellow in 1999. Dr. Wong is currently an adjunct professor in the Neurobiology Program, Department of Psychiatry, Indiana University Medical School, Indianapolis, IN.

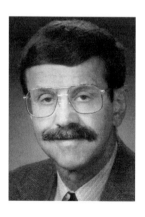

Frank P. Bymaster

received his B.S. in Pharmacy from Butler University in 1968 and a M.S. in pharmacology from Indiana University in 1975. He joined the Lilly Research Laboratories, Eli Lilly and Company, in 1970. His research interests have included development and characterization of antidepressant compounds including fluoxetine (Prozac) and duloxetine with Dr. Wong, characterization of the atypical antipsychotic olanzapine (Zyprexa) and investigation into muscarinic compounds for cognition and psychosis. He is currently a Senior Research Scientist in the Lilly Neuroscience Research Division and adjunct assistant professor at Butler University, Indianapolis, IN.

Summary

Preclinical and clinical studies support the rationale that development of single molecules, which would promote serotonergic and noradrenergic neurotransmission by inhibiting simultaneously the uptake of both monoamines, would potentially result in improved antidepressant drugs. Currently, the dual inhibitors of serotonin and noradrenaline uptake are venlafaxine, milnacipran and duloxetine. Based on the preclinical studies, the three drugs do show properties of inhibiting uptake of both monoamines *in vitro* and *in vivo* in the following order of decreasing potency: duloxetine, venlafaxine and milnacipran, and all exhibit low affinity at neuronal receptors of neurotransmitters, suggesting low side-effect potential. In double-blind, controlled studies, venlafaxine and milnacipran were repeatedly shown to be as efficacious as tricyclic antidepressant drugs in treating major depressive disorder, while one double-blind, placebo-controlled trial showed the antidepressant efficacy of duloxetine. Specifically designed comparative trials of dual uptake inhibitors against the other agents are needed to establish whether the dual uptake inhibitors show improvement in efficacy, rate of responders, antidepressive effects and/or remission.

Contents

Key words

Depression, antidepressants, tricyclic antidepressants, SSRI, serotonin selective reuptake inhibitors, dual uptake inhibitors, norepinephrine, serotonin, dopamine, duloxetine, venlafaxine, milnacipran, fluoxetine.

Glossary of abbreviations

AMPT, α-methylparatyrosine; cyclic AMP, cyclic adenosine monophosphate; CGI, Clinical Global Impression; DA, dopamine; L-DOPA, L-3,4-dihydroxyphenylalanine; ex, extracellular; ED_{50}, dose required to alter activity by 50%; NA, noradrenaline; 5-HT, 5-hydroxytryptamine, serotonin; HAM-D, Hamilton Rating Scale-Depression; L-5-HTP, L-5-hydroxytryptophan; IC_{50}, concentration required to inhibit activity by 50%; K_i, inhibition (dissociation) constant; Kd, dissociation constant; MADRS, Montgomery-Asberg Depression Rating Scale; MED, minimal effective dose; NMDA, N-methyl-D-aspartate; 8-OH-DPAT, 8-hydroxy-2-(di-n-propylamino)tetralin; PCPA, p-chlorphenylalanine; 1-PP, 1-(2-pyrimidinyl)piperazine; SSRI, selective serotonin reuptake inhibitor; TCA, tricyclic antidepressant; WAY 100635, N-[2-[4-(2-methoxyphenyl)-1-piperazinyl]ethyl]-N-(pyridinyl)cyclohexanecarboxamide.

1 Introduction and rationale for efficacy of dual uptake inhibitors

Current medications for treatment of depression have limited efficacy and delayed onset of therapeutic action. As a class of antidepressant drugs, selective serotonin (5-hydroxytryptamine, 5-HT) reuptake inhibitors (SSRI) have been considered to have comparable effectiveness to the earlier generation of tricyclic antidepressant (TCA) drugs [1–4]. The rates of response of the SSRIs and TCAs are similar and of 60–70% magnitude [3, 5] and the rate of remission is between 30–40% [6]. There is a controversy challenging the notion that the SSRIs are indeed as effective as the TCAs, especially for the treatment of severely depressed patients [4, 7–9]. However, the TCAs, because of undesirable side-effects, are not well tolerated [10, 11]. The SSRI class of antidepressant drugs has enjoyed patient acceptance due largely to their benign side-effect profile and the convenience of once-daily administration [3]. The onset of meaningful antidepressant effects of the SSRIs is also comparable to those reported for the TCAs and takes about 2 to 4 weeks to appear [3, 12–14]. In view of the limitations of the current antidepressant pharmaceuticals, tremendous research efforts are ongoing to search for a pharmacological treatment which may improve antidepressive efficacy, onset of action or even both therapeutic parameters [9, 15–17].

Effective treatment of depression with the SSRIs and the secondary amine containing TCA, desipramine, an inhibitor of noradrenaline (NA, also called norepinephrine) uptake, provides clinical research with the opportunity to test the dependence of efficacy on the availability of 5-HT and NA, respectively [18–20]. A dietary tryptophan depletion paradigm that transiently led to relapse of depressive symptoms more frequently occurred with patients remitted from treatment with the SSRI fluoxetine than those remitted from treatment with desipramine [18, 19]. These findings are consistent with the hypothesis that an intact 5-HT system is needed to maintain the antidepressive effect of a SSRI [19]. It was hypothesized that inhibition of 5-HT uptake with fluoxetine and in turn an enhancement of 5-HT neurotransmission could lead to a clinical antidepressive response [21–23]. The introduction of the SSRIs as a class of antidepressant drugs and the application of the dietary tryptophan depletion paradigm have strengthened the 5-HT hypothesis of antidepressant therapy [24, 25].

The long-held catecholamine hypothesis of antidepressant action [26, 27] has also recently been re-examined using a catecholamine-depleting paradigm. It is accomplished by treatment of patients with alpha-methyl-paratyrosine (AMPT), which inhibits tyrosine hydroxylase, an enzyme responsible for the conversion of tyrosine to L-DOPA (3,4-dihydroxyphenylalanine), the precursor of NA. Patients who remitted from treatment with the NA uptake-inhibiting antidepressant, desipramine, were more likely to experience transient relapse of depressive symptoms within hours upon AMPT treatment than those remitted from fluoxetine treatment [28, 29]. These recent findings have renewed interest in NA neurotransmission as an antidepressant pathway in development of new antidepressant drugs. Indeed, two small double-blind cross-over studies randomly treating in-patients with a SSRI, zimelidine, and desipramine suggested differential responses to the two classes of antidepressant drugs in some patients [30, 31].

Several small clinical studies have investigated the combination of SSRIs with TCAs. In one study, 30 depressed outpatients, with 90% meeting criteria for major depression, had fluoxetine (20–60 mg) added to their on-going and ineffective therapy, which included a tricyclic-like drug (56%) alone or in a combination of drugs (44%) including lithium, benzodiazepines or carbamazepine [32]. Positive response was reported for the combination in 26 of the 30 patients. The combination of fluoxetine and desipramine was evaluated in 14 patients with major depression [33]. The levels of desipramine were adjusted for the effects of fluoxetine on desipramine metabolism. The combination-treated group had a mean change of 42% in the Hamilton Depression Rating Scale in one week and eventually 71% achieved complete remission of symptoms, suggesting a rapid and robust therapeutic effect. Seth et al., 1992, used a combination of nortriptyline and either fluoxetine (63%) or sertraline to treat eight patients with resistant and recurrent depression [34]. Although many of these patients had failed on multiple drug regimes and electroconvulsive therapy, all improved on the combination of nortriptyline and SSRI. Overall, these studies suggest that the combination of a TCA that blocks NA uptake and a SSRI may have more rapid onset of action, overall greater efficacy or efficacy in treatment-resistant depression. However, these studies were small and open-label and need to be repeated in a double-blind, placebo-controlled trial.

A number of preclinical studies have indicated an interaction between the serotonergic and noradrenergic neuronal systems that may play a role in the therapy of depression. It has been proposed that antidepressant-induced β-adrenergic receptor down-regulation in the cortex and hippocampus and subsequent reduction in the formation of the second messenger cyclic AMP may play a key role in the action of antidepressants [35]. This was based on the finding that the down-regulation of β-adrenergic receptor and cyclic AMP formation took at least 2 weeks of treatment to occur with antidepressants of the TCA-class, consistent with the delayed onset of antidepressant effectiveness. However, not all antidepressants reduce β-adrenergic receptor and cyclic AMP formation, indicating that the down-regulation and desensitization of the β-adrenergic receptor is not required for antidepressant effectiveness [36, 37].

Several studies indicate a modulatory role of 5-HT neurons on NA neurotransmission. Specific lesions of 5-HT neurons to reduce 5-HT function abolished the reduction in β-adrenergic receptor density and cyclic AMP formation after chronic administration of the NA uptake inhibitor desipramine [38]. Moreover, selective lesions of 5-HT neurons increased β-adrenergic receptor density and cyclic AMP formation [39, 40]. In contrast, enhancement of serotonergic function by co-administration of fluoxetine to animals treated with desipramine accelerated the down-regulation of β-adrenergic receptor density and decreased cyclic AMP formation so that it was evident at 4 days, rather than 14 days as was found with repeated desipramine administration alone [41]. Fluoxetine alone had no effect on β-adrenergic receptor density. Thus, it appears that intact and functionally active 5-HT neurons play an obligatory role in the regulation of the desipramine-induced down-regulation and desensitization of β-adrenergic receptors.

In the dorsal raphe, 5-HT neurons are under stimulatory control mediated by the α-adrenergic receptor. Electrophysiological studies showed that dorsal raphe 5-HT neurons were excited by the administration of NA or the α_1-adrenergic agonist, phenylephrine, and the stimulatory effects could be blocked with prazosin, an antagonist at α_1-adrenergic receptors [42, 43]. Prazosin effectively lowered extracellular 5-HT levels in brain areas of conscious, freely moving rats [44, 45]. These pharmacologically manipulated studies indicate that 5-HT neurons in the dorsal raphe are dependent upon a tonically active adrenergic system [42, 46]. These findings of cross-talk between 5-HT and NA neuronal systems may indeed explain in part the aforementioned rapid onset of antidepressant activity or increased effectiveness when 5-HT uptake-inhibiting and NA uptake-inhibiting antidepressant drugs were combined to treat depressed patients. Areas of potential interaction of 5-HT and NA neuronal systems possibly resulting in synergistic effects are shown in Figure 1.

The finding that both 5-HT and NA neuronal pathways can serve in antidepressant mechanisms [18, 19, 28, 29], the encouraging clinical experience of combining SSRIs and TCAs [32–34], as well as inter-dependence between 5-HT and NA neuronal systems, suggest that the development of a single molecule that would increase availability of 5-HT and NA by blocking their respective transporter sites may result in pharmaceuticals with a broader profile in depression therapy [17, 20, 47]. Furthermore, patients who suffer from severe depressive disorders may particularly benefit from treatments that activate neurotransmission in both pathways [7]. In the present review, the pharmacological profile of three combined 5-HT and NA uptake inhibitors, venlafaxine, duloxetine and milnacipran, are compared. We will refer to compounds with similar affinity for 5-HT and NA uptake transporters as dual uptake inhibitors. It is of interest to search for clinical evidence that the dual 5-HT and NA uptake inhibitors as a class of antidepressant drugs are indeed an improvement over the SSRI and the TCA classes of antidepressant drugs [8–10].

2 Inhibition of *in vitro* uptake and transporter binding by antidepressant uptake inhibitors

Many antidepressants have high affinity for monoamine uptake processes and transporters. In Table 1, the antidepressants are divided into classes of

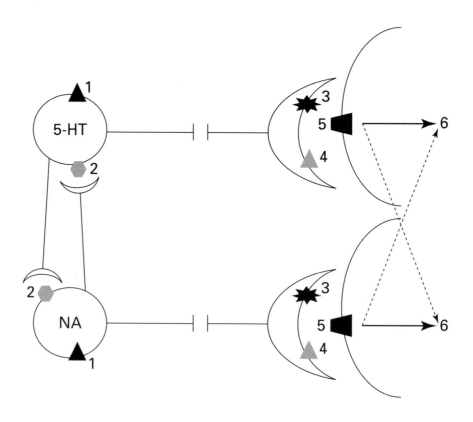

Fig. 1
Potential sites of interaction of dual uptake inhibitors.
There are a number of potential sites of interaction of 5-HT and NA neuronal systems that may have additive or synergistic effects on signal transduction and finally possibly enhanced or more rapid onset of antidepressant activity. Site 1 is the somatodendritic inhibitory autoreceptor (5-HT$_{1A}$ or α_2-adrenergic receptors). The dual uptake inhibitors do not have affinity for the autoreceptors, but activate them indirectly *via* increased monoamine levels due to uptake blockade at the cell bodies. Site 2 is potential cross-talk between respective raphe 5-HT cell bodies and locus coeruleus NA cell bodies. Evidence suggests that NA increases 5-HT cell body firing and this is a potential site of synergy. Site 3 is the transporter (uptake) site and the dual uptake inhibitors block both NA and 5-HT transporters and thereby enhance neurotransmission of each neuronal system which is a potential site of enhanced effectiveness. Site 4 is the presynaptic inhibitory autoreceptor (in some species 5-HT$_{1B/1D}$ and α_2-adrenergic receptors) and activation of these receptors decreases neurotransmitter release. Dual uptake inhibitors have no affinity for these receptors, but indirectly activate them by increased monoamine levels in the synapse due to uptake inhibition. Site 5 is the postsynaptic receptor which upon activation by the neurotransmitter presumably mediates the antidepressant action. Site 6 represents intracellular mechanisms including signal transduction, kinases, transcriptional factors and neurotrophic factors which presumably mediate the antidepressant effects. It is not known if there is interaction between the 5-HT and NA neuronal systems at this level.

Table 1.
In vitro inhibition of monoamine reuptake into rat synaptosomes by uptake inhibitors

Compound	Monoamine uptake		
	5-HT	NA	DA
		K_i, nM $\pm$ S.E.M.	
Dual uptake inhibitors			
Duloxetine[1]	4.6 $\pm$ 1.1	16 $\pm$ 2.9	369 $\pm$ 38
Venlafaxine[8]	77 $\pm$ 2	538 $\pm$ 43	6371 $\pm$ 1366
Milnacipran[3]	203 $\pm$ 50	100 $\pm$ 17	> 100000
Imipramine[2]	41 $\pm$ 3	14 $\pm$ 1	11000 $\pm$ 1000
Chlorimipramine[7]	1	16	3800
Amitriptyline[2]	84 $\pm$ 1	13.9 $\pm$ 0.8	8600 $\pm$ 600
SSRIs			
Fluoxetine[5]	20 $\pm$ 2	1230 $\pm$ 344	2884 $\pm$ 133
Citalopram[4]	1.8	6100	> 10000
Fluvoxamine[4]	3.8	620	42000
Paroxetine[2]	0.73 $\pm$ 0.04	33 $\pm$ 2	1700 $\pm$ 300
Sertraline[2]	3.4 $\pm$ 0.4	220 $\pm$ 40	260 $\pm$ 40
Indalpine[4]	3	2400	1300
Norepinephrine uptake inhibitors			
Desipramine[2]	180 $\pm$ 10	0.61 $\pm$ 0.07	11000 $\pm$ 2000
Nortriptyline[2]	154 $\pm$ 3	2.2 $\pm$ 0.1	3200 $\pm$ 200
Nisoxetine[7]	1000	1	360
Reboxetine[6]	1070	8	> 10000
Tomoxetine[2]	43 $\pm$ 2	0.7 $\pm$ 2	1400 $\pm$ 200

Subscripted numbers denote source of data: [1][47], [2][48], [3]=[49] (data are reported as IC_{50} values), [4][50], [5][51], [6][52], [7][53], [8][54]. Abbreviation: S.E.M., standard error of the mean.

compounds that *in vitro* are SSRIs, selective NA uptake inhibitors and dual uptake inhibitors of both NA and 5-HT. The diversity of chemical structures among the classes of antidepressant uptake inhibitors is shown in Figure 2. The SSRIs such as fluoxetine have high affinity for 5-HT uptake processes and much lower affinity for NA and DA uptake processes in rat brain regions. In contrast, the NA uptake inhibitors like reboxetine and tomoxetine have high affinity for NA and lower affinity for 5-HT and DA uptake processes.

Using membranes from cell lines transfected with human monoamine transporters, affinity for the uptake inhibitors was compared using the binding of selective transporter radioligands. Among inhibitors of uptake, there

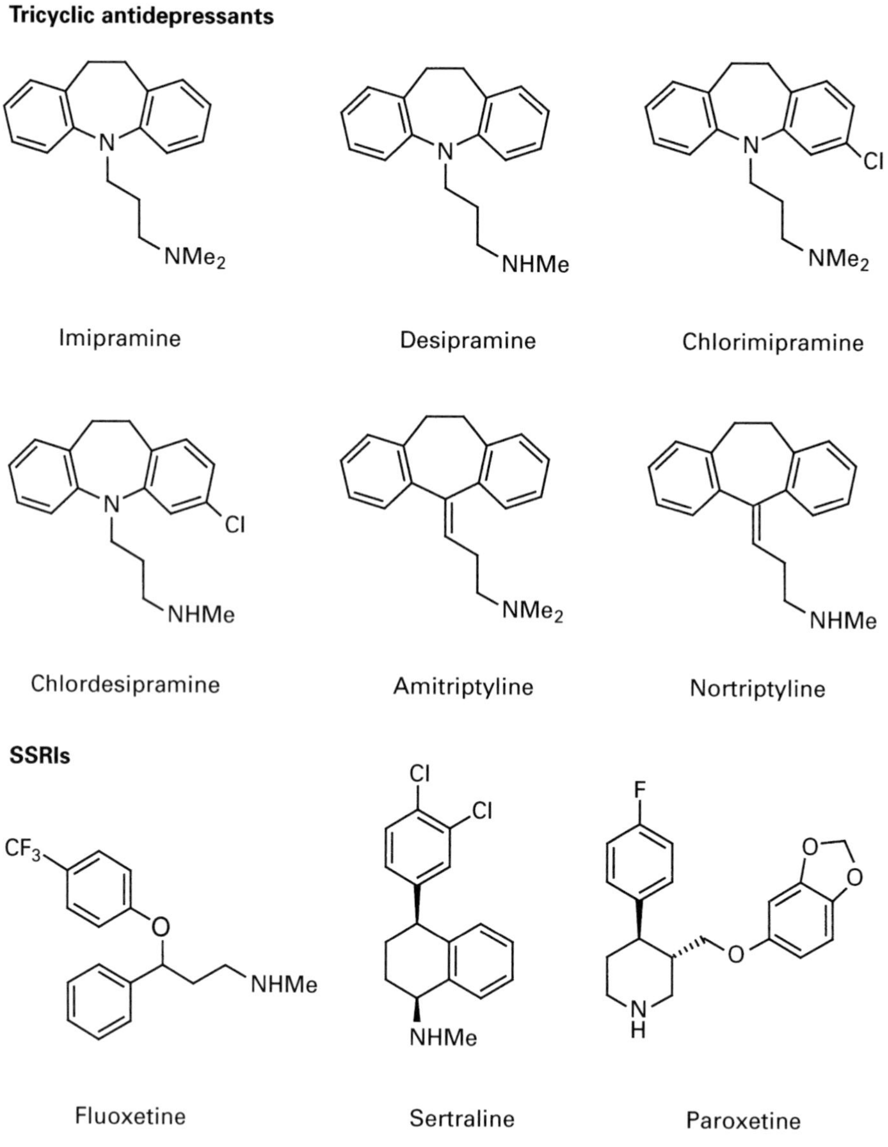
Tricyclic antidepressants
NMe2
NHMe
Cl
NMe2
Imipramine
Desipramine
Chlorimipramine
Cl
NHMe
NMe2
NHMe
Chlordesipramine
Amitriptyline
Nortriptyline
SSRIs
CF3
O
NHMe
Cl
Cl
NHMe
F
O
O
O
N
H
Fluoxetine
Sertraline
Paroxetine

Fig. 2
Structures of classes of antidepressants possessing uptake inhibitory properties

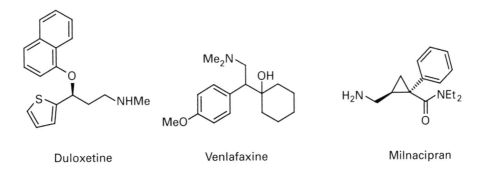

Fluvoxamine   **Citalopram**   **Indalpine**

Noradrenaline uptake inhibitors

Nisoxetine   **Tomoxetine**   **Reboxetine**

Dual uptake inhibitors

Duloxetine   **Venlafaxine**   **Milnacipran**

Fig. 2 continued

Table 2
Inhibition of radioligand binding to human monoamine transporters by uptake inhibitors

Compound	Transporter		
	5-HT	NA	DA
		K_i, nM ± S.E.M.	
Dual uptake inhibitors			
Duloxetine[1]	0.8 ± 0.04	7.5 ± 0.3	240 ± 23
Venlafaxine[1]	82 ± 3	2480 ± 43	7647 ± 793
Milnacipran[2]	43*	–	–
Imipramine[3]	1.4 ± 0.03	37 ± 2	8500 ± 100
Chlorimipramine[3]	0.28 ± 0.01	38 ± 1	2190 ± 40
Amitriptyline[3]	4.3 ± 0.1	35 ± 2	3250 ± 20
SSRIs			
Fluoxetine[3]	0.81 ± 0.02	240 ± 10	3600 ± 100
Citalopram[3]	1.16 ± 0.01	4070 ± 80	28100 ± 700
Fluvoxamine[3]	2.2 ± 0.2	1300 ± 30	9200 ± 200
Paroxetine[3]	0.13 ± 0.01	40 ± 2	490 ± 20
Sertraline[3]	0.29 ± 0.01	420 ± 20	25 ± 2
Norepinephrine uptake inhibitors			
Desipramine[3]	17.6 ± 0.7	0.83 ± 0.05	3190 ± 40
Nortriptyline[3]	18 ± 1	4.4 ± 0.07	1140 ± 30
Nisoxetine[5]	447 ± 23	9.7 ± 0.5	–
Reboxetine[4]	129 ± 13	1.1 ± 0.2	>10000
Tomoxetine[5]	77	5	1451

Subscripted numbers denote source of data: [1][54], [2][49] (IC$_{50}$ values), [3][55], [4][52], [5]Dr. David L. Nelson (unpublished observation); *denotes rat data. Abbreviation: S.E.M., standard error of the mean.

is good agreement between the relative affinity of compounds for rat monoamine transporters and affinity for human monoamine transporters. In general, the SSRIs have high affinity and selectivity for human 5-HT transporters, while the NA uptake inhibitors are selective for human NA transporters (Tab. 2).

The dual uptake inhibitors duloxetine, venlafaxine and milnacipran, as well as the secondary amine-containing TCAs imipramine, chlorimipramine and amitriptyline, are inhibitors of both 5-HT and NA uptake. Although the TCAs imipramine, chlorimipramine and amitriptyline have affinity for both the uptake transporters *in vitro*, rapid *in vivo* N-demethylation results in the formation of the corresponding desmethyl compounds desipramine, chlordesimipramine and nortriptyline, respectively, which are selective NA uptake inhibitors. For example, imipramine, chlorimipramine and amitriptyline were weak inhibitors of p-chloramphetamine-induced neurotoxicity, which is 5-HT transporter-dependent. However, they more potently blocked 6-hydroxydopamine-induced noradrenergic neurotoxicity, which is dependent on the NA transporter [56]. Furthermore, amitriptyline at doses up to 50 mg/kg p.o. increased extracellular levels of NA, but not 5-HT [57]. Thus, tertiary amine-containing TCAs are predominantly inhibitors of NA uptake and are not considered as dual uptake inhibitors *in vivo* in this review.

Amongst the non-tricyclic dual uptake inhibitors duloxetine, venlafaxine and milnacipran, duloxetine is the most potent of the compounds with K_i values of 4.6 ± 1.1, 16 ± 2.9 and 369 ± 38 nM, for 5-HT, NA and DA uptake processes, respectively (Tab. 1). Thus, duloxetine has 3.5-fold higher affinity for 5-HT uptake than NA uptake. Venlafaxine has K_i values of 77 ± 2, 538 ± 43 and 6371 ± 1366 nM for 5-HT, NA and DA uptake processes, respectively, and therefore has 7-fold higher affinity for 5-HT uptake than NA uptake processes. Milnacipran is a relatively weak uptake inhibitor of 5-HT and NA uptake in rat hypothalamus with IC_{50} values of 203 ± 50 and 100 ± 17 nM, respectively, and very low affinity for DA uptake (Tab. 1). However, although the IC_{50} values for milnacipran for 5-HT and NA are comparable, the comparative ratio of affinity for NA and 5-HT uptake processes for milnacipran cannot be appropriately compared without K_i values.

Duloxetine inhibited binding to the human 5-HT, NA and DA transporters with K_i values of 0.8 ± 0.04, 7.5 ± 0.3 and 240 ± 23, respectively, thus displaying 9.4-fold higher affinity for 5-HT transporters than NA transporters (Tab. 2). Venlafaxine inhibited binding of the human 5-HT, NA and DA transporters with K_i values 82 ± 3, 2483 ± 43 and 7647 ± 793, respectively, and 30-fold higher affinity for 5-HT transporters than NA transporters. Milnacipran has been reported to have 43 nM affinity for the rat 5-HT transporter and data have not been reported for human transporters.

Thus, duloxetine has moderately higher affinity for 5-HT transporters compared to NA transporters as measured either by inhibition of monoamine uptake in rat synaptosomes or by inhibition of radioligand binding to human transporters. The inhibition constant (K_i) ratios of NA/5-HT affinity from 3.5- to 9-fold suggest that *in vivo* duloxetine would be a balanced inhibitor and require slightly higher doses to inhibit NA uptake than 5-HT uptake. In contrast, venlafaxine has up to 30-fold higher affinity for 5-HT than NA uptake processes and transporters, consistent with markedly higher doses of venlafaxine being required to inhibit NA uptake than 5-HT uptake *in vivo*.

3 Neuronal receptor interactions of antidepressant drugs

The success of the TCAs for treatment of major depression resulted in investigation of the pharmacology of these drugs and the discovery that they not only interacted with monoamine uptake processes, but also had high affinity for a number of neuronal receptors. Blockade of certain neuronal receptors became associated with specific side-effects probably not related to efficacy. The development of effective antidepressants like fluoxetine without significant interaction with neuronal receptors indicated that blockade of these neuronal receptors was not required for antidepressant activity [53]. Although the side-effects of TCAs are quite bothersome early in the treatment, dose titration and compliance results generally in improved tolerability. As a class, TCAs have high affinity for α_1-adrenergic receptors, muscarinic receptors, histamine H_1 and 5-HT_2 receptors (Tabs. 3, 4) [58, 59].

Antagonism of α_1-adrenergic receptors has been associated with postural hypotension, sedation and possibly hypersalivation. Blockade of muscarinic receptors has been associated with a number of troublesome peripheral side-effects including dry mouth, blurred vision, constipation, urinary retention, tachycardia and exacerbation of glaucoma. The gastrointestinal and pupillary diameter effects are mediated largely by muscarinic M_3 receptors, whereas the chronotropic effects on the heart are mediated by muscarinic M_2 receptors [60]. Centrally, blockade of muscarinic receptors, probably of the M_1 subtype, results in inattention and memory impairment. Antagonism of histamine H_1 receptors causes sedation and weight gain. Dopamine (DA) D_2 receptor antagonism can result in extrapyramidal symptoms, tardive dyskinesias and dysphoria. Side-effects of TCAs produced by blockade of 5-HT_2 receptors, if any, are not clearly defined.

The development of high specific activity radioligands for neuronal receptors resulted in a ready tool to evaluate interaction of drugs with neuronal receptors. We developed a receptor binding battery of assays for neuronal receptors focused on receptors potentially responsible for adverse events [58]. The battery of receptor binding assays included α_1-, α_2- and β-adrener-

Table 3.
Inhibition of radioligand binding to neuronal receptors by uptake inhibitors

Compound	α_1-Adren.	α_2-Adren.	Hist. H_1	Musc. NS	Musc. M_3	Dop. D2
			K_i or K_d, nM ± S.E.M.			
Dual uptake inhibitors						
Duloxetine	8300	8600	2300	3000	–	14000
Venlafaxine	> 35000	> 35000	> 35000	> 35000	> 35000	> 35000
Milnacipran	> 10000	> 10000	> 10000	> 10000	–	> 10000
Imipramine	32 ± 5	3100 ± 100	37 ± 4	46 ± 2	60 ± 10	620 ± 90
Amitriptyline	24 ± 2	690 ± 20	0.95 ± 0.03	9.6* ± 0.3	12.8 ± 0.4	1460 ± 90
Chlorimipra-mine	80 ± 10	4500 ± 200	40 ± 10	230 ± 30	–	200
SSRIs						
Fluoxetine	3800 ± 300	13900 ± 200	5400 ± 500	590 ± 70	1000 ± 100	12000 ± 1000
Paroxetine	4600 ± 500	17000 ± 400	22000 ± 4000	108 ± 5	80 ± 10	32000 ± 4000
Sertraline	380 ± 50	4100 ± 200	24000 ± 5000	630 ± 30	1300 ± 100	10700 ± 800
Norepinephrine uptake inhibitors						
Desipramine	100 ± 10	5500 ± 200	60 ± 1	66 ± 2	210 ± 20	3500 ± 200
Nortriptyline	55 ± 2	2030 ± 30	6.3 ± 0.9	37 ± 1	50 ± 3	2570 ± 50
Reboxetine	10000 ± 2000	43000 ± 3000	1400 ± 200	3900 ± 200	2800 ± 100	9000 ± 5000
Tomoxetine	3800 ± 200	8800 ± 100	5500 ± 900	2060 ± 50	–	> 35000

Abbreviations: α_1-Adren., α_1-adrenergic; α_2-Adren., α_2-adrenergic; Hist. H_1, histamine H_1; Musc. NS, muscarinic non-selective; Musc. M_3, human muscarinic M_3 clonal; Dop. D_2, DA D_2; S.E.M., standard error of the mean. Values are K_i or K_d values. Milnacipran data in rat [49], duloxetine in rat [47], chlorimipramine in rat [58], musc. M_3 human [61], reboxetine in rat [52], remainder human tissue [59].

gic, histamine H_1, 5-HT_1, muscarinic non-selective, DA D_2, opiate, GABA and benzodiazepine receptors. Using this assay to profile antidepressant compounds, we found that the affinity of fluoxetine for these receptors was quite low, particularly compared to the TCAs. Based on these results, we correctly predicted the higher degree of tolerability of fluoxetine than TCAs.

Table 4
Inhibition of radioligand binding to serotonin receptor subtypes by uptake inhibitors

Compound	5-HT$_{1A}$	5-HT$_{2A}$	5-HT$_{2C}$
		K$_i$ or K$_d$, nM ± S.E.M.	
Dual uptake inhibitors			
Duloxetine	> 5000[3]	504 ± 87[3]	916 ± 190[3]
Venlafaxine	> 10000[3]	2230 ± 723[3]	2004 ± 808[3]
Milnacipran	> 10000[4]	> 10000[4]	–
Imipramine	5800 ± 500[1]	160 ± 7[2]	94 ± 26[2]
Amitriptyline	450 ± 20[1]	4.3 ± 2.4[2]	4.3 ± 0.8[2]
Chlorimipramine	–	15 ± 1[2]	22 ± 7[2]
SSRIs			
Fluoxetine	32400 ± 900[1]	708 ± 6[2]	42.6 ± 4.2[2]
Citalopram	>5000[6]	>1000[2]	269 ± 57[2]
Fluvoxamine	2935[6]	2592[6]	1563[6]
Paroxetine	> 35000[1]	3125[6]	3725[6]
Sertraline	> 35000[1]	> 1000[2]	> 1000[2]
Norepinephrine uptake inhibitors			
Desipramine	6400 ± 300[1]	121 ± 9[2]	244 ± 59[2]
Nortriptyline	294 ± 4[1]	5 ± 0.3[2]	8.5 ± 3.7[2]
Reboxetine	18000 ± 3000[5]	7300 ± 400[5]	1500 ± 500[5]
Tomoxetine	10900 ± 100[1]	> 1000[6]	> 1000[6]

[1]human [59], [2]rat [62], [3]human [54], [4]rat data in IC$_{50}$ [49], [5]human [52], [6]human (Bymaster, unpublished observation). Abbreviation: S.E.M., standard error of the mean.

Table 5
Affinity of duloxetine and venlafaxine for human 5-HT receptor subtypes

Receptor subtype	Duloxetine	Venlafaxine
	K$_i$, nM ± S.E.M.	
5-HT$_{1A}$	> 5000	> 10000
5-HT$_{1B}$	3959 ± 810	> 10000
5-HT$_{1D}$	> 3000	> 10000
5-HT$_{1E}$	3733 ± 618	> 10000
5-HT$_{1F}$	4447 ± 30	> 10000
5-HT$_{2A}$	504 ± 87	2230 ± 723
5-HT$_{2B}$	2100 ± 206	> 10000
5-HT$_{2C}$	916 ± 190	2004 ± 808
5-HT$_4$	> 1000	> 1000
5-HT$_6$	419 ± 89	2792 ± 431

All 5-HT receptor subtypes were human except for 5-HT$_4$ which was from guinea pig striatum [54].

Table 6
Duloxetine and venlafaxine have low affinity (> 1 μM) for other neuronal receptors.[*]

Receptor	Receptor
Neurotransmitter receptors	
Adenosine, A1, A2	Glutamate, NMDA, glycine (Stry-insens.)
Adrenergic, α1A α1B	Glycine, strychnine-sensitive
Adrenergic, α2A (Human), α2B	Histamine, H1, H2
Adrenergic, β1, β2	Melatonin
Dopamine, D1, D2	Muscarinic, M1 (human), M2 (human)
GABA$_A$, agonist Site	Nicotinic (α-bungarotoxin insens.)
GABA$_A$, benzodiazepine, Cent.	Opiate, delta 1, kappa 1, Um
Glutamate, AMPA, kainate site	Sigma 1, 2
Glutamate, NMDA agonist site	
Ion channels	
Calcium channel, Type L, N	Glutamate, NMDA, PCP
GABA, chloride, TBOB site	Potassium channel, ATP-sense.
Glutamate, chloride site	Potassium channel, Ca^{2+} act. volt sense.
Glutamate, MK-801 site	Sodium, site 1, 2
Second messengers	
Adenylate cyclase, forskolin	NOS (neuronal-binding)
Inositol triphosphate	Protein kinase C, PDBu
Transporters	
Choline transporter	Adenosine transporter
GABA transporter	
Brain/gut peptides	
Cholecystokinin, CCK1(A), CCK2(B)	Neuropeptide, NPY1 (human)
Neurokinin, NK1, NK2(A) (human)	Neurotensin
Neurokinin, NK3 (NKB)	Somatostatin, non-selective
Enzyme activity	
Monoamine oxidase A, B	

[*]< 50% inhibition of receptors by 1 μM concentration of duloxetine or venlafaxine [54].

The newly developed antidepressant compounds, including SSRIs and NA uptake inhibitors, have in common low affinity for neuronal receptors and overall greater tolerability (Tabs. 3, 4). The knowledge of potential side-effects produced by neuronal receptor interactions of antidepressants gives the opportunity to design therapy to best benefit individual patients.

Since the 5-HT and NA uptake inhibitors have marked affinity for two monoamine transporters, the interaction of these compounds with neuronal receptors is of interest. Duloxetine, venlafaxine and milnacipran all had very

Table 7
Blockade of *ex vivo* transporter binding, *ex vivo* and *in vivo* monoamine uptake by duloxetine and venlafaxine

Measurement	Duloxetine	Venlafaxine
	ED_{50}, mg/kg (µmoles/kg), route	
[^{3}H]-Paroxetine *ex vivo* binding	0.03 (0.09), s.c.	2.0 (6.37), s.c.
[^{3}H]-Nisoxetine *ex vivo* binding	0.70 (2.10), s.c.	54 (172), s.c.
[^{3}H]-5-HT *ex vivo* uptake	12.2 ± 1.6 (36.5), p.o.	ND
	2.0 (6.0), s.c.	
[^{3}H]-NA *ex vivo* uptake	14.6 ± 2.3 (43.7), p.o.	ND
	3 (9.0), s.c.	
[^{3}H]-DA *ex vivo* uptake	> 40 (> 120), p.o.	ND
5-HT depletion by p-CA in rat brain	2.3 (6.9), i.p.	5.9 (18.8), i.p.
NA depletion by 6-OHDA in rat hypo.	12 (35.9), i.p.	94 (299), i.p.

Abbreviations: hypo., hypothalamus; ND, not determined. Data derived from [54].

low affinity for α_1-and α_2-adrenergic, histamine H_1, muscarinic and DA D_2 receptors (Tab. 3), suggesting a favorable side-effect profile due to potentially weak interaction with these receptors. Duloxetine and venlafaxine had low affinity for a number of 5-HT receptor subtypes (Tabs. 4, 5) and did not inhibit monoamine oxidase A or B (Tab. 6). We expanded the receptor profiling of duloxetine and venlafaxine to over 50 receptors and binding sites and found that these compounds are remarkably selective for 5-HT and NA transporters (Tab. 6) [54].

4 Inhibition of 5-HT and NA uptake *in vivo* by duloxetine and venlafaxine

The brain penetrance and *in vivo* selectivity for 5-HT and NA transporters of duloxetine and venlafaxine were investigated after systemic administration using well-characterized and selective techniques. Duloxetine and venlafaxine penetrated into the brain and dose-dependently inhibited *ex vivo* binding of [^{3}H]-paroxetine to 5-HT transporters in rat cerebral cortical homogenates with ED_{50} values of 0.03 and 2.0 mg/kg s.c., respectively (Tab. 7) [54]. The *ex vivo* binding of [^{3}H]-nisoxetine to the NA transporter was inhibited in a dose-dependent manner with ED_{50} values of 0.7 and 54 mg/kg s.c., respectively, for duloxetine and venlafaxine. Duloxetine inhibited 5-HT *ex vivo* uptake processes with ED_{50} values of 12.2 ± 1.6 mg/kg p.o. and 2.0 mg/kg s.c., respectively, and NA *ex vivo* uptake processes with ED_{50} values of 14.6 ± 2.3 p.o. and 3 mg/kg s.c., respectively (Tab. 7) [47]. Thus, duloxetine was 66 and 77 times more potent at inhibiting 5-HT and NA transporters *in vivo* than venlafaxine.

Several neurotoxins have been found to be neurotoxic due to cellular penetration *via* monoamine transporters. Inhibitors of transporters block the effects of these neurotoxins including monoamine depletion, thus demonstrating functional antagonism of the transporters *in vivo*. The depletion of 5-HT concentrations in rat brain induced by the 5-HT transporter-dependent neurotoxin p-chloramphetamine was antagonized dose-dependently by duloxetine and venlafaxine with ED_{50} values of 2.3 and 5.9 mg/kg i.p., respectively (Tab. 7) [54]. The depletion of NA levels in rat hypothalamus induced by the catecholamine transporter-dependent neurotoxin 6-hydroxy-dopamine was dose-dependently blocked by duloxetine and venlafaxine with ED_{50} values of 12 and 94 mg/kg i.p., respectively (Tab. 7). These data are consistent with the *in vitro* binding profiles of duloxetine and venlafaxine, suggesting that duloxetine would inhibit 5-HT and NA transporters at similar doses, whereas venlafaxine would be of lower potency and require up to 15-fold higher doses to inhibit NA transporters than 5-HT transporters. Milnacipran has not been characterized in these assays.

5 Alteration of extracellular monoamine levels by dual uptake inhibitors

5.1 Venlafaxine microdialysis

Measurement of extracellular levels of monoamines using the microdialysis technique in conscious, freely moving rats is a direct technique to demonstrate that blockade of monoamine uptake enhances interstitial levels of the monoamine(s) in question. The effects of the dual uptake inhibitors have been extensively studied using microdialysis techniques in several brain regions. In freely moving rats, subcutaneous administration of venlafaxine (10 mg/kg) elevated extracellular $_{(ex)}$ levels of 5-HT, NA and DA in microdialysates of frontal cortex to approximately 160, 400 and 200% of baseline levels, respectively (Tab. 8A). However, the increases in NA_{ex} and DA_{ex} were significantly different from baseline levels, while those of $5\text{-}HT_{ex}$ were not

Table 8A
Acute effect of venlafaxine on extracellular levels of monoamines in rat brain.

Drug	Dose, route mg/kg	Brain area	5-HT	NA	DA	Refs.
			% of baseline (100%)			
venlafaxine	10, s.c.	n. cortex	160	400*	200*	[63]
venlafaxine	3, s.c.	f. cortex	NC	140	–	[44]
	10, s.c.	f. cortex	NC	240*	–	
	30, s.c.		NC	400*	–	
	50, s.c.		NC	745*	–	
WAY 100635	0.3, s.c.	f. cortex	NC	NC	–	
+ venlafaxine	3, s.c.		160	160	–	
	10, s.c.		280**	250*	–	
	30, s.c.		384**	400*	–	
venlafaxine	10, s.c.	f. cortex	140	(240*)	–	
+ WAY 100635	0.01, s.c.		160	(240*)	–	
	0.03, s.c.		190**	(240*)	–	
	0.1, s.c.		230**	(240*)	–	
	0.3, s.c.		260**	(240*)	–	
GR 127935	3, s.c.	f. cortex				
+ venlafaxine	10, s.c.		NC	NC		
GR 127935	3, s.c.	f. cortex				
+ WAY 100635	0.3, s.c.					
+ venlafaxine	10, s.c.		429**	250*	–	
prazosin	0.3, s.c.	f. cortex				
+ WAY 100635	0.3, s.c.		70*	NC	–	
prazosin	0.3, s.c.	f. cortex				
+ WAY 100635	0.3, s.c.					
+ venlafaxine	10, s.c.		190**	NC	–	
idazoxan	0.2, s.c.	f. cortex				
+ WAY 100635	0.3, s.c.		NC	137	–	
idazoxan	0.2, s.c.	f. cortex				
+ venlafaxine	10, s.c.		143	605**	–	
idazoxan	0.2, s.c.	f. cortex				
+ WAY 100635	0.3, s.c.					
+ venlafaxine	10, s.c.		356**	605**	–	
(±)-pindolol	10, s.c.	f. cortex				
+ venlafaxine	10, s.c.		171	NC	–	
venlafaxine	5, i.p.	f. cortex	155	–	–	[73]
		hippoc.	210	–	–	
	10, i.p.	f. cortex	193	–	–	
		hippoc.	210	–	–	
	20, i.p.	f. cortex	364*	–	–	
		hippoc.	1400*	–	–	
(±)-pindolol	10, s.c.					
+ venlafaxine	5, i.p.	f. cortex	248	–	–	
		hippoc.	868**	–	–	
+ venlafaxine	10, i.p.	f. cortex	248	–	–	
		hippoc.	898**	–	–	

Significantly different from baseline (*) and from levels after administration of venlafaxine alone (**).
Abbreviations: NC, no change; –, not determined; n. cortex, neocortex; f. cortex, frontal cortex; hippoc., hippocampus in this and subsequent tables.

Table 8B.
Acute effects of milnacipran on extracellular levels of monoamines in brain.

Drug	Dose, route mg/kg	Brain area	5-HT	NA	DA	Refs.
				% of baseline (100%)		
Guinea pig						
milnacipran	10, i.p.	hypothalamus	200*	200*	–	[75]
	40, i.p.		450*	500*	–	
(–)-pindolol	10, s.c.		100	100	–	
(–)-pindolol	10, s.c.					
+ milnacipran	10, i.p.		690*	410*	–	
Rat						
milnacipran	1–30, s.c.	raphe nuclei	NC	–	–	[76]
	60, s.c.		202*			
milnacipran	60, s.c.		250*			
+ WAY 100635	1, s.c.		365**			
milnacipran	1–30, s.c.	f. cortex	NC	–	–	
	60, s.c.		213*			
milnacipran	60, s.c.		250*			
+ WAY 100635	1, s.c.		250*			
milnacipran	10, s.c.	hypothalamus	172*	–	–	

Significantly different from baseline (*) and from levels after administration of milnacipran alone (**).

[63]. Although venlafaxine probably does not block DA transporters *in vivo*, the increase of cortical DA levels is consistent with NA uptake processes heterologously taking up DA in cortical areas [64]. Venlafaxine levels in tissues were also determined in the treated rats. The tissue contained high concentrations of venlafaxine: 468 nmol/L in serum, 2600 pmol/g in neocortex and 2090 pmol/g in mesencephalon-pons, while extracellular concentrations of venlafaxine reached 175 nmol/L [63]. In a separate study, various doses of venlafaxine were administered by the same route. Consistent with the previous study, venlafaxine (3–50 mg/kg s.c.) dose-dependently increased NA_{ex} levels but produced no significant changes in 5-HT_{ex} levels (Tab. 8A) [44]. However, it has been noted that by acute, constant infusion, venlafaxine at 10 mg/kg s.c. significantly elevated both 5-HT_{ex} and NA_{ex} levels in microdialysates of frontal cortex above baseline levels without a significant change in DA_{ex} levels [65]. In anaesthetized rats, venlafaxine (0.8 mg/kg i.v.) failed to change extracellular NA levels in the dorsal raphe nucleus, whereas the NA_{ex} levels significantly double upon treatment with desipramine (5 mg/kg i.v.) [66].

Table 8C.
Acute effects of duloxetine on extracellular monoamine levels in rat brain.

Drug	Dose, route mg/kg	Brain area	5-HT	NA	DA	Refs.
			% of baseline (100%)			
duloxetine	3.1, p.o.	f. cortex	145*	170*	170*	[57]
	6.3, p.o.		180*	250*	240*	
	12.5, p.o.		240*	300*	260*	
amitriptyline	6.3, p.o.	f. cortex	NC	NC	NC	
	12.5, p.o.		NC	150*	150	
	25, p.o.		NC	215*	250*	
duloxetine	6.3, p.o.	n. accumbens	–	–	130*	
	12.5, p.o.		–	–	150*	
	25, p.o.		–	–	180*	
amitriptyline	50, p.o.	n. accumbens	–	–	130	
duloxetine	5, s.c.	f. cortex	220*	470*	180*	[85]
WAY 100635	0.16, s.c.	f. cortex	NC	NC	NC	
+ duloxetine	5, s.c.		450*	490*	170	
duloxetine	4, i.p.	hypothalamus	NC	NC	–	[84]
	7, i.p.		NC	200*	–	
	15, i.p.		240*	1100*	–	
duloxetine	4, i.p.	hypothalamus				
+ LY206130	3, s.c.		669**	579**	404**	[86]
LY206130	3, s.c.	hypothalamus	NC	160*	134*	
duloxetine	5.0, s.c.	f. cortex	230*	500*	165*	[87]
fluoxetine	10.0, s.c.		210*	190*	160*	
buspirone	2.5, s.c.		50*	260*	200*	
buspirone	2.5, s.c.					
+ duloxetine	5.0, s.c.		NC#	850**	550**	
buspirone	2.5, s.c.					
+ fluoxetine	10.0, s.c.		NC#	500**	300**	
atipamezole	0.16, s.c.	f. cortex	NC	280*	230*	[89]
duloxetine	5.0, s.c.		250*	500*	225*	
atipamezole	0.16, s.c.					
+ duloxetine	5.0, s.c.		350**	1130**	470**	
fluoxetine	10.0, s.c.		220*	200*	155*	
atipamezole	0.16, s.c.					
+ fluoxetine	10.0, s.c.		430**	315**	270**	
1-PP	2.5, s.c.		NC	285*	190*	
+ duloxetine	5.0, s.c.		390**	1320**	700**	

# denotes % of baseline at 180 min. Significantly different from baseline (*) and from levels after administration of duloxetine alone (**). Abbreviations: n. accumbens, nucleus accumbens.

Pharmacological manipulations of the venlafaxine-induced increases of extracellular levels of monoamines have provided insight into the 5-HT and NA releasing mechanisms. The combination of treatment with a selective 5-HT_{1A} antagonist, WAY 100635 at 0.3 mg/kg s.c., and venlafaxine (3, 10 or 30 mg/kg s.c.) dose-dependently elevated 5-HT_{ex} in frontal cortex to 160, 280 and 384%, respectively, of basal levels with significant increases with the two higher doses of venlafaxine (Tab. 8A) [44]. In rats treated with a constant dose of venlafaxine at 10 mg/kg s.c. that increased 5-HT_{ex} to about 140% of basal levels, WAY 100635 (0.01, 0.03, 0.1 and 0.3 mg/kg s.c.) dose-dependently enhanced the 5-HT_{ex} levels to 160, 190, 230 and 260%, respectively, of basal levels with significant effects from the three higher doses of WAY 100635. The augmentation suggests that WAY 100635 had effectively blocked the soma-todendritic 5-HT_{1A} autoreceptors, which upon activation by endogenously derived 5-HT would inhibit activity of 5-HT neurons in the raphe areas [67, 68] causing a ceiling effect on 5-HT_{ex} release in forebrain areas of rats treated with 5-HT uptake inhibitors [69, 70]. On the other hand, combined admin-istration of WAY 100635 did not significantly change the venlafaxine-induced increases of NA levels (Tab. 8A) [44].

Combined treatment with either (±)-pindolol (10 mg/kg s.c.), a 5-$HT_{1A/B}/\beta$-adrenergic receptor antagonist, or GR 127935 (3 mg/kg s.c.), a 5-$HT_{1B/D}$ recep-tor antagonist, and venlafaxine at 10 mg/kg s.c. failed to significantly change 5-HT_{ex} levels or the venlafaxine-induced increases in NA_{ex} levels (Tab. 8A) [44]. However, when WAY 100635 at 0.3 mg/kg s.c. was added to the com-bined treatment with GR 127935 and venlafaxine, 5-HT_{ex} levels significantly increased to 429%, a magnitude significantly greater than the 260% of base-line levels observed in rats treated with WAY 100635 and venlafaxine (Tab. 8A), suggesting a greater 5-HT release resulting from concomitant block-ade of presynaptic 5-$HT_{1B/D}$ and somatodendritic 5-HT_{1A} autoreceptors (see [44] for further discussion). However, the venlafaxine-induced increases of NA_{ex} did not change in these treatment combinations.

The role of α_1- and α_2-adrenoceptors on the venlafaxine-induced increases of 5-HT_{ex} and NA_{ex} levels in frontal cortex was investigated [44]. Co-administration of an antagonist of α_1-adrenoceptors, prazosin, attenu-ated increases of 5-HT_{ex}, but was without an effect on NA_{ex} in the WAY 100635- and venlafaxine-treated rats. On the other hand, when an antago-nist at α_2-adrenoceptors, idazoxan, was co-administered with venlafaxine, NA_{ex} levels significantly increased to 605% of basal levels without an effect on 5-HT_{ex} in frontal cortex nor an effect on the WAY 100635-induced increase of 5-HT_{ex} in venlafaxine-treated rats (Tab. 8A) [44]. These findings are consistent with the known stimulatory role of α_1-adrenoceptors on activity of 5-HT neurons in dorsal raphe that has been demonstrated in tissue slices [42] and *in vivo* [45, 71]. The lack of effect of idazoxan on the WAY 100635/venlafaxine-induced increase of 5-HT_{ex} shows 5-HT neurons are not under tonic control from the α_2-adrenoceptors [44, 72]. On the other hand, α_2-adrenoceptors exert an inhibitory control on NA release, as shown by the robust increases of NA_{ex} levels upon administering idazoxan in venlafaxine-treated rats.

By intraperitoneal injection, venlafaxine at 5, 10 and 20 mg/kg dose-dependently elevated 5-HT_{ex} levels to 155, 193 and 364%, respectively, in frontal cortex and 210, 210 and 1400%, respectively, in hippocampus (Tab. 8A) [73]. However, using two marginal doses of venlafaxine, 5 and 10 mg/kg i.p., and combining with a single acute dose of (±)-pindolol (10 mg/kg s.c.), the investigators observed robust increases of 5-HT levels by 768 and 798%, respectively, above basal levels in hippocampus, but without significant increases above basal levels in frontal cortex [73]. The augmentation of 5-HT levels in hippocampal microdialysates resulting from combining a marginally effective dose of venlafaxine with a single dose of (±)-pindolol suggests effective blockade of the somatodendritic 5-HT_{1A} autoreceptors and concomitant blockade of 5-HT uptake in hippocampus [73]. However, the augmentation was not detected in frontal cortex of rats treated with the combinations of venlafaxine and (±)-pindolol.

It appears that effective increases of 5-HT_{ex} in frontal cortex depends on the route of administration of venlafaxine, suggesting involvement of an active metabolite(s). The greater responsiveness in frontal cortex to venlafaxine administration following an intraperitoneal [73] compared to a subcutaneous route of administration [44, 63] suggests involvement of metabolic conversion of venlafaxine. Active metabolites of venlafaxine have been shown to produce some of the pharmacological responses of venlafaxine. For example, the O-desmethylated compound (Wy-45,233), a major metabolite of venlafaxine in rat and human, reversed the reserpine-induced hypothermia in mouse with a minimum effective dose 1/3 that of venlafaxine. The N-desmethylated compound (Wy-45,494), a minor metabolite in human, and the hydroxylated compound (Wy-47,877), a major metabolite in rat, were as effective as the parent compound [74].

While the O-desmethylated metabolite inhibited synaptosomal 5-HT and NA uptake with comparable potency of venlafaxine, the other two metabolites were less effective as uptake inhibitors *in vitro*. It is also interesting to note that the ability of venlafaxine to increase release of 5-HT$_{ex}$ appears to be more robust in hippocampus than in frontal cortex following an intraperitoneal injection of venlafaxine [73].

By intraperitoneal injection, venlafaxine at 5 mg/kg daily for 4 weeks failed to change 5-HT$_{ex}$ and NA$_{ex}$ levels in frontal cortex and hippocampus (Tab. 9) [73]. Following two weeks of continuous infusion of venlafaxine (10 mg/kg s.c. osmotic minipump), 5-HT$_{ex}$ and NA$_{ex}$ levels in frontal cortex significantly increased to 194 and 200%, respectively, of the saline-treated rats, indicating a sustained effect with chronic treatment (Tab. 9) [65].

5.2 Milnacipran microdialysis

In guinea pig, another dual inhibitor of 5-HT and NA uptake, milnacipran, at 10 and 40 mg/kg i.p. significantly elevated 5-HT$_{ex}$ levels to 200 and 450% of baseline and NA$_{ex}$ to 200 and 500%, respectively, in hypothalamus (Tab. 9) [75]. When co-administered with (–)-pindolol (10 mg/kg s.c.), milnacipran at the lower dose further enhanced the increase of 5-HT$_{ex}$ and NA$_{ex}$ levels to 690 and 410%, respectively, of basal levels. Since guinea pig possesses 5-HT$_{1D}$ receptors, but not 5-HT$_{1B}$ receptors (current nomenclature is 5-HT$_{1D\alpha}$ and 5-HT$_{1D\beta}$, respectively), in brain, the augmentation of 5-HT$_{ex}$ release is most likely associated with the effective blockade of somatodendritic 5-HT$_{1A}$ autoreceptors [75]. Moreover, the robust NA$_{ex}$ release resulting from the combined treatment with milnacipran and (–)-pindolol was most likely produced by the large increase in endogenous 5-HT, which may activate subtypes of 5-HT receptors to release NA in the forebrain.

Consistent as an inhibitor of 5-HT uptake, milnacipran locally infused through the dialysis probe at 10 μmol/l–1 mmol/l by reverse dialysis significantly increased the Ca^{2+}-dependent and the tetradotoxin-sensitive release of 5-HT$_{ex}$ to 7- and 10-fold in rat frontal cortex and raphe nuclei, respectively [76]. The potency of milnacipran was comparable to that of imipramine [77]. By subcutaneous administration, milnacipran at 60 mg/kg increased 5-HT$_{ex}$ to about 200% of baseline in both frontal cortex and raphe nuclei, while at lower doses of 1–30 mg/kg s.c. milnacipran had no significant effects in

Table 9.
Effect of long-term treatment with venlafaxine, milnacipran and duloxetine on levels of extracellular monoamines

Drug	Dose, route mg/kg	Brain area	5-HT	NA	DA	Refs.
			% of baseline (100%)			
venlafaxine daily for 4 wk	5, i.p.	f. cortex	NC	–	–	[73]
		hippoc.	NC	–	–	
venlafaxine, daily for 2 wk	10, s.c.	f. cortex	194*	200*	88	[65]
milnacipran daily for 2 wk	30, s.c.	d. raphe	NC	–	–	[76]
	60, s.c.		NC	–	–	
milnacipran daily for 2 wk	30, s.c.	f. cortex	61*	–	–	
	60, s.c.		NC	–	–	
duloxetine daily for 2 wk	6.3, p.o.	f. cortex	NC	NC	NC	[57]
+ duloxetine on 15th day	6.3, p.o.	f. cortex	137	NC	–	
	12.5, p.o.	n. accumbens	–	–	NC	

Significant differences from baseline (*). Abbreviations: d. raphe, dorsal raphe nucleus; wk, weeks.

either brain area (Tab. 8B) [76]. In hypothalamus, milnacipran at 10 mg/kg s.c. increased 5-HT_{ex} levels to 172% of baseline levels. Upon combination with WAY 100635 at 1 mg/kg s.c., milnacipran at 60 mg/kg s.c. elevated 5-HT_{ex} in raphe nuclei merely by 115% over that seen with milnacipran alone. In frontal cortex, 5-HT_{ex} levels did not increase further when WAY 100635 was administered after milnacipran. Long-term administration of milnacipran did not significantly increase 5-HT_{ex} in the raphe or frontal cortex (Tab. 9).

Judging from the smaller 5-HT output in raphe nuclei relative to that in frontal cortex in milnacipran-treated rats in comparison with SSRI-treated rats, the smaller potentiation by WAY 100635, and the lack of an enhancement of the 5-HT output following repeated administration, the investigators suggested that the clinical action of milnacipran was not mediated by an enhancement of the serotonergic function and is likely to involve other neurotransmitters [76].

Recently, milnacipran has been shown to exhibit micromolar affinity at N-methyl-D-aspartate (NMDA) receptors using [^{3}H]-MK801 binding in rat cortical membranes and antagonistic properties for NMDA receptor-expressing oocytes [78]. Moreover, milnacipran at 20 and 40 mg/kg i.p. effectively protected mice from NMDA-induced lethality by 60 and 100%, respectively (see behavioral section) [79]. Based on these findings, milnacipran at the doses that raised 5-HT_{ex} levels in raphe nuclei and frontal cortex would very likely be effective in blocking NMDA receptors in rat brain. Indeed, NMDA antagonists are known to modulate turnover of monoamines [80, 81] and to reduce immobility in the forced-swim test in mice [82] and have been proposed as potential antidepressant agents [83]. It would not be surprising that milnacipran exerts its clinical effects by multiple mechanisms, including inhibition of NA and 5-HT uptake and NMDA receptor antagonism.

5.3 Duloxetine microdialysis

The dual inhibitor of 5-HT and NA uptake, duloxetine (3.2, 6.3 and 12.5 mg/kg p.o.), dose-dependently and significantly increased 5-HT_{ex} to 145, 180 and 240%, respectively, NA_{ex} to 170, 250 and 300%, respectively, and DA_{ex} to 170, 240 and 260%, respectively, of their basal levels in frontal cortex of freely moving and conscious rats (Tab. 8C) [57]. Although duloxetine increases DA_{ex} to about the same magnitude as NA_{ex} in frontal cortex, duloxetine has relatively low affinity for dopamine uptake processes and transporters and the cortical increases of dopamine are probably due to blockade of NA transporters which regulate DA extracellular levels in cortical areas [64]. The increases of extracellular monoamine levels in frontal cortex caused by duloxetine were determined in separate groups of rats [57] rather than simultaneously analyzed in the same microdialysates from hypothalamus [84].

In hypothalamus, 5-HT_{ex} levels increased to 240% of basal levels after acute administration of duloxetine at 15 mg/kg i.p. and NA_{ex} levels increased to 200 and 1,100% of basal levels after administration of duloxetine at 7 and 15 mg/kg i.p., respectively (Tab. 8C) [84]. The magnitude of the duloxetine-induced increases of NA_{ex} in rat hypothalamus [84] was comparable to that observed in guinea pig hypothalamus following treatment with milnacipran [75].

Duloxetine also dose-dependently increased DA_{ex} levels in nucleus accumbens, but the magnitude of increase was lower than those observed in frontal cortex (Tab. 8C) [57]. Amitriptyline, on the other hand, at the two higher doses increased only the catecholamines, NA_{ex} and DA_{ex}, in frontal cortex [57] and this is consistent with amitriptyline *in vivo* being predominantly an inhibitor of NA uptake [56]. Repeated oral administration of duloxetine for 2 weeks did not change basal levels of $5\text{-}HT_{ex}$, NA_{ex} and DA_{ex} in frontal cortex (Tab. 9) [57], but an additional administration of a low dose of duloxetine (6.25 mg/kg p.o.) during the course of the microdialysis experiment increased only $5\text{-}HT_{ex}$ levels significantly in frontal cortex. However, there was no change in DA_{ex} in nucleus accumbens after additional administration of a low dose of duloxetine (6.25 mg/kg p.o.) [57]. Therefore, duloxetine continued to increase monoamine extracellular levels upon subchronic treatment.

Pharmacological manipulations provide further appreciation of the complexity of duloxetine-induced elevations of monoamines and insights into potential avenues of drug development. Following combined treatment with duloxetine and an antagonist of $5\text{-}HT_{1A}$ receptors, either WAY 100635 [85] or LY206130 (a pindolol derivative) [86], $5\text{-}HT_{ex}$ levels in frontal cortex and hypothalamus increased more than twice of those observed with duloxetine alone. However, the combinations did not bring further increases of NA_{ex} or DA_{ex} levels in frontal cortex and NA_{ex} in hypothalamus. Thus, effective blockade of somatodendritic $5\text{-}HT_{1A}$ receptors can augment 5-HT output without altering NA_{ex} and DA_{ex} outputs in forebrain areas following administration of the dual 5-HT and NA uptake inhibitor, duloxetine, as is observed with venlafaxine.

Pretreatment of rats with buspirone, a $5\text{-}HT_{1A}$ autoreceptor receptor agonist, in combination with duloxetine or fluoxetine, caused transient decreases of $5\text{-}HT_{ex}$ levels before reaching the levels caused by treatment with duloxetine or fluoxetine alone (Tab. 8C) [87]. The increases of NA_{ex} in frontal cortex showed additive effects from the combined administration of buspirone (260%) and duloxetine (500 to 850%) or fluoxetine (190 to 500%) (Tab. 8C) [87]. However, when the effects of buspirone and duloxetine administered alone were compared with the coadministration, the combination produced synergistic effects on DA_{ex} levels (165 and 200 to 550%) in frontal cortex (Tab. 8C) [87]. The synergism may involve the excitatory 5-HT receptors on dopaminergic terminals in the frontal cortex as well as their interactions at the dopaminergic cell bodies [87, 88]. However, buspirone is also known to be an antagonist of dopamine receptors. The authors suggested that antagonism of the inhibitory DA D_2 and D_3 autoreceptors may also contribute to the increase of DA levels in frontal cortex [87].

The co-administration of the α_2-adrenergic receptor antagonist atipamezole with duloxetine produced synergistic increases in NA_{ex} levels (280 and 500% with drug alone, respectively, to 1130% in combination) in frontal cortex (Tab. 8C) [89]. The effects on DA_{ex} levels in frontal cortex were additive (230, 225 and 470%, respectively) (Tab. 8C). Likewise, another α_2-adrenergic receptor antagonist, 1-(2-pyrimidinyl)piperazine (1-PP) and duloxetine increased NA_{ex} levels (285 and 500%, respectively) and DA_{ex} levels (190 and 225%, respectively) in frontal cortex (Tab. 8C) [89]. When the two drugs were combined, they synergistically elevated NA_{ex} levels (1320%) and DA_{ex} levels (700%) in frontal cortex (Tab. 8C). Both α_2-adrenergic receptor antagonists had no effect on basal 5-HT_{ex} levels and the duloxetine-induced increases of 5-HT_{ex} levels. Atipamezole in combination with fluoxetine produced small increases of 5-HT_{ex}, NA_{ex} and DA_{ex} levels in frontal cortex (Tab. 8C) [89]. These data clearly indicate that α_2-adrenergic autoreceptors limit the magnitude of increase of NA_{ex} produced by NA transporter inhibitors.

In conclusion, both venlafaxine and duloxetine, combined inhibitors of 5-HT and NA uptake, can effectively elevate extracellular 5-HT, NA and DA levels in forebrain areas of rat brain. Based on the studies conducted in different laboratories, the potencies of venlafaxine and duloxetine were approximately comparable. With a single study reported in guinea pig and rat, milnacipran appears effective in producing increases in 5-HT_{ex} and NA_{ex} without showing the effects on DA_{ex} levels in hypothalamus of guinea pig. Pharmacological manipulations in animals treated with venlafaxine, duloxetine and milnacipran produced results consistent with the mechanism of inhibitors of 5-HT and NA uptake *in vivo*.

6 Electrophysiological studies with dual uptake inhibitors

6.1 Venlafaxine electrophysiology

Antidepressant drugs with 5-HT uptake-inhibiting properties are known to suppress 5-HT cell firing in dorsal raphe nuclei [67, 68, 90, 91]. Inhibitors of

5-HT uptake, including chlorimipramine, amitriptyline, indalpine, citalopram, fluoxetine, paroxetine, duloxetine and venlafaxine, dose-dependently inhibited 5-HT cell firing (Tab. 10A) [66, 92–96]. There was a high correlation between the potency to suppress 5-HT cell firing *in vivo* and the ability to inhibit binding at 5-HT transporter sites among most of the 5-HT uptake inhibitors, except for venlafaxine [95].

Venlafaxine inhibited firing activity of 5-HT neurons in dorsal raphe with comparable potency reported by a number of investigators (Tab. 10A) [66, 74, 95]. In view of venlafaxine being 53 times less potent than paroxetine as an inhibitor of 5-HT uptake, venlafaxine is surprisingly potent at inhibiting firing of 5-HT neurons with ED_{50} values ranging from 160 to 280 µg/kg i.v., which is comparable to the potency of paroxetine (Tab. 10A) [66, 95]. In fact, in comparison with eight other 5-HT uptake inhibitors, venlafaxine failed to meet the correlation between the potency to inhibit binding to 5-HT transporter sites and the potency to suppress 5-HT cell firing [95].

Desipramine, a selective NA uptake inhibitor, at a relatively high dose had only a slight inhibitory effect on 5-HT cell firing (Tab. 10A) [66, 90, 97]. Consistent with these findings, venlafaxine inhibited 5-HT cell firing with potency in 6-hydroxydopamine-lesioned rats as effectively as seen in intact rats (Tab. 10A) [95]. Thus, inhibition of NA uptake had no effect on 5-HT cell firing or on the effectiveness of 5-HT uptake inhibitors to suppress 5-HT cell firing [95].

The selective $5-HT_{1A}$ antagonist, WAY 100635, effectively reversed the inhibitory effects on 5-HT cell firing caused by treatment with venlafaxine and other 5-HT uptake inhibitors, which themselves do not have affinity at $5-HT_{1A}$ receptors [66, 95]. This is consistent with the interpretation that the inhibition of 5-HT neuronal activity during the treatment with 5-HT uptake inhibitors is most likely caused by the resultant increase of 5-HT, which in turn activates the somatodendritic $5-HT_{1A}$ inhibitory autoreceptors.

However, prazosin suppressed 5-HT cell firing in a manner insensitive to administration of WAY 100635 (Tab. 10A) [66]. Activity of 5-HT neurons in tissue slices from the dorsal raphe is known to be dependent on activation of α-adrenoceptors [42] and similar observations have been made *in vivo* [98, 99]. Despite the known affinity and antagonism at α_1-adrenoceptors by TCAs including chlorimipramine and amitriptyline [37, 59], their inhibitory effects on 5-HT neuronal activity were completely reversed by WAY 100635 (Tab. 10A), indicative of the inhibition being mediated by the

Table 10A.
Effects of venlafaxine and other compounds on 5-HT and NA cell firing

Drug	Neuronal 5-HT	Activity NA		Refs.
	ED_{50}, µg/kg, i.v.			
venlafaxine	–	680 ± 100		[104]
desipramine	–	190 ± 30		
venlafaxine	280	680		[74]
Wy-45,233	2200	3000 (40% inhibition)		
			Reversal by WAY 100635	
venlafaxine	160 ± 23 (6)	–	yes	[66]
paroxetine	254 ± 71 (6)	–	yes	
chlorimipramine			yes	
amitriptyline	$1,330 \pm 170$ (3)	–	yes	
8-OH-DPAT	2.7 ± 0.5 (6)	–	yes	
prazosin	268 ± 58 (9)	–	no	
desipramine	$> 5,000$	–	–	
venlafaxine	233 ± 12	737 ± 68		[95]
in 6-OHDA-lesion	264 ± 42	–		
in 5,7-DHT-lesion	–	285 ± 49		
paroxetine	211 ± 11	$> 10,000$		
fluoxetine	–	$> 5,000$		
desipramine	–	240 ± 54		

in parentheses is number of determinations. Abbreviations: 6-OHDA, 6-hydroxydopamine; 5-7-DHT, 5,7-dihydroxytryptamine.

activation of the somatodendritic 5-HT$_{1A}$ autoreceptor, but not through α_1-adrenoceptor interactions.

Consistent with selective NA uptake-inhibition properties, desipramine dose-dependently inhibited the basal firing activity of NA neurons in locus coeruleus with an ED$_{50}$ value of 240 ± 54 µg/kg i.v. (Tab. 10A). Venlafaxine was unexpectedly potent in suppressing the firing activity of NA neurons with an ED$_{50}$ value of 737 ± 68 µg/kg i.v., despite venlafaxine being a weak inhibitor of NA uptake with a K_i value over two orders of magnitude greater than that of desipramine. Thus, for venlafaxine there is little correlation between potency to inhibit NA uptake *in vitro* and potency to suppress firing of NA neurons as observed with other NA uptake inhibitors [95]. Whereas desipramine fully inhibited NA cell firing, the inhibitory effects of venlafaxine reached only to 90%, even with doses five times higher than its ED_{50} dose. The administration of the α_2-adrenoceptor antagonist, piperoxane, effectively reversed the desipramine- and venlafaxine-induced suppression of NA neuronal activity [95]. The piperoxane-restored activity of NA neurons was attenuated by the i.v. administration of WAY 100635 [95]. In fact, venlafaxine suppressed NA neuronal activity with greater potency as indicated by a lower ED_{50} value of 285 ± 49 µg/kg i.v. in 5,7-dihydroxytryptamine-lesioned rats [95]. These findings are consistent with inhibitory 5-HT inputs at NA neurons of locus coeruleus [100].

Despite venlafaxine lacking the correlation between its potencies for inhibiting 5-HT and NA uptake *in vitro* and the potencies suppressing firing activities of 5-HT neurons in dorsal raphe and NA neurons in locus coeruleus, the latter potencies may still be indicative of the potencies *in vivo* inhibiting 5-HT and NA uptake [95, 101]. However, venlafaxine was found to inhibit *in vivo* uptake of NA at least 15-fold less potently than *in vivo* 5-HT uptake (Tab. 7). Perhaps the pharmacokinetics and the central concentrating properties of venlafaxine may have contributed to the unexpected potencies *in vivo* of venlafaxine [63]. Moreover, metabolism of venlafaxine may also be a contributing factor, since i.p. administration appears to be more effective than subcutaneous administration for venlafaxine to induce increases in extracellular 5-HT and NA levels in frontal cortex (Tab. 8A) [44, 63, 73].

6.2 Duloxetine electrophysiology

Consistent with the effects of known 5-HT uptake inhibitors, duloxetine suppressed the firing activity of dorsal raphe 5-HT neurons with an ED_{50} value of 99 µg/kg i.v. in anaesthetized rats (Tab. 10B) [94]. Duloxetine was twice as effective as citalopram and paroxetine and over six times more effective than fluoxetine [96, 102]. The inhibitory effect of duloxetine on activity of 5-HT neurons was reversed by the subsequent administration of a 5-HT_{1A} antagonist, spiperone, suggesting that the inhibitory effect of duloxetine was mediated by an activation of the somatodendritic 5-HT_{1A} autoreceptors. Since duloxetine does not have significant affinity for 5-HT_{1A} receptors (Tabs. 4, 5), duloxetine most likely inhibited 5-HT cell firing by producing a greater availability of endogenous 5-HT resulting from the inhibition of its uptake by

Table 10B.
Effects of duloxetine on 5-HT cell and NA cell firing.

Drug	Neuronal 5-HT	Activity NA	Refs.
	ED_{50}, µg/kg, i.v.		
duloxetine	99 ± 38	475 ± 58	[94]
desipramine	5,000	–	
reversible by	yes	yes	
(antagonist)	(spiperone)	(idazoxan)	
in 5,7-DHT lesioned rat		475 ± 42	[94]
citalopram	230	–	[68]
fluoxetine	600	–	[102]
fluoxetine	1,230	–	[96]

Abbreviation: 5-7-DHT, 5,7-dihydroxytryptamine.

duloxetine. Consistent with duloxetine being a potent inhibitor of NA uptake with low affinity for α-adrenoreceptors (Tabs. 1, 3), it inhibited firing activity of NA neurons in locus coeruleus with an ED_{50} value of 475 µg/kg i.v. (Tab. 10B) [94]. The inhibitory effect of duloxetine was reversed by a subsequent injection of the α$_2$-adrenoceptor antagonist, idazoxan, suggesting that the duloxetine-induced suppressive effect was due to activation of somatodendritic α$_2$-adrenoceptors by the increased availability of endogenous NA resulting from NA uptake inhibition. Desipramine was about two times more effective than duloxetine in the suppression of firing activity of NA neurons in locus coeruleus, while desipramine was weak in suppressing the firing activity of 5-HT neurons in dorsal raphe.

6.3 Milnacipran electrophysiology

The third dual inhibitor of 5-HT and NA uptake, milnacipran, inhibited activity of dorsal raphe 5-HT neurons in anaesthetized rat with an ED_{50} value of $5,700 \pm 150$ µg/kg i.v. (Tab. 10C) [103]. Thus, in comparison with duloxetine and venlafaxine, milnacipran is most weak in its ability to suppress 5-HT cell firing (Tabs. 10A, 10B and 10C). In contrast to the suppressive effects of duloxetine, venlafaxine and the well-known inhibitory effects of SSRIs, the

Table 10C.
Effects of milnacipran on 5-HT cell and NA cell firing.

Drug	Neuronal Activity 5-HT ED_{50}, µg/kg, i.v.	NA	Refs.
milnacipran	$5,700 \pm 1,500$	–	[103]
reversible by (antagonist)	no (spiperone)	–	
	yes (idazoxan)	–	
in 6-OHDA lesioned (2 weeks) 20 mg/kg s.c.	abolished	–	
for 2 days	decrease	decrease	
1 week	part. recov.	no recov.	
2 weeks	comp. recov.	no recov.	

Abbreviation: recov., recovery; 6-OHDA, 6-hydroxydopamine;.part., partial; comp., complete.

milnacipran-induced suppression of 5-HT neuronal activity was insensitive to spiperone, an antagonist of 5-HT$_{1A}$ receptors, suggesting it was not mediated by the activation of the somatodendritic 5-HT$_{1A}$ autoreceptor. However, the suppressive effects of milnacipran were sensitive to the administration of idazoxan, an antagonist of α_2-adrenergic receptors, and was abolished in 6-hydroxydopamine (6-OH-DA)-lesioned rats.

Both the activities of 5-HT neurons in the dorsal raphe nucleus and NA neurons in locus coeruleus were suppressed following administration of milnacipran at 20 or 60 mg/kg/day s.c. for 2 days (Tab. 10C) [103]. The suppressive effects on NA neurons persisted during continued treatment for 7 and 14 days. However, the inhibitory effects on 5-HT neurons recovered partially after 7 days and totally after 14 days of treatment. In contrast to the progressive recovery following long-term treatment with SSRIs and duloxetine, however, the sensitivity to the administration of 5-HT or 8-OH-DPAT (8-hydroxy-2-(di-n-propylamino)tetralin) on the activity of dorsal raphe 5-HT neurons was not reduced following treatment with milnacipran at 60 mg/ kg/day s.c. for 14 days, indicating the absence of desensitization of the somatodendritic 5-HT$_{1A}$ autoreceptor. The investigators suggested that the restoration of normal firing of 5-HT neurons during chronic milnacipran treatment appeared to involve the NA system [103]. Milnacipran was recently recognized to have moderate affinity at the NMDA receptor [79] and as an antagonist, as well as an ability to protect animal from NMDA-induced lethality [78]. Thus, the influence of milnacipran as an antagonist at NMDA receptors on activity of 5-HT and NA neurons requires further investigations.

The potencies of duloxetine for inhibiting firing activities of 5-HT neurons in dorsal raphe nucleus and NA neurons in locus coeruleus are comparable to their relative affinities at the 5-HT and NA transporter. However, such correlation is difficult to achieve with venlafaxine. Although duloxetine appears to be numerically superior to venlafaxine, without conducting the comparative electrophysiological studies side-by side, their potencies are considered comparable. Based on these electrophysiological studies, milnacipran exerts its effects on the activity of NA and particularly 5-HT neurons differently from those of duloxetine and venlafaxine.

7 Alteration of animal behavior by dual uptake inhibitors

The three dual uptake inhibitors show pharmacological effects in behavioral responses consistent with enhanced neurotransmission of noradrenergic and serotonergic pathways in the central nervous system. Venlafaxine at a moderate dose (10 mg/kg i.p.) was minimally effective in reversing the reserpine-induced hypothermia in mouse, while desipramine was more potent with a minimal effect dose (MED) 0.4 mg/kg i.p. in mouse (Tab. 11A) [105]. Amitriptyline also antagonized the reserpine-induced hypothermia with ED_{50} values of 8.7 and 28.4 mg/kg p.o. in mouse and rat, respectively [106]. In the same tests, duloxetine had ED_{50} values of 12.1 and 14.3 mg/kg p.o., respectively.

Moreover, a wide range of doses of venlafaxine (2–64 mg/kg i.p.) reversed the hypothermia induced by the DA agonist, apomorphine, in mouse [107]. Milnacipran and desipramine showed comparable potency in reversing the apomorphine-induced hypothermia (Tab. 11A) [108]. Thus, the reversal of reserpine- or apomorphine-induced hypothermia induced by venlafaxine and milnacipran was most likely associated with inhibition of NA uptake *in vivo*, since SSRIs showed relatively weak antagonism in both of these tests [53, 109]. Milnacipran and duloxetine showed comparable

Table 11A.
Behavioral studies with dual uptake inhibitors – reversal of hypothermia and cholinergic effects

Behavioral test	Animal	Treatment	Drug	Dose, mg/kg, route	Response	Refs.
hypothermia reserpine-induced	mouse, male	acute acute	venlafaxine desipramine	10, i.p.(MED) 0.4, i.p.(MED)	reversed reversed	[105]
hypothermia reserpine-induced	mouse, male rat, male	acute acute	duloxetine amitriptyline duloxetine amitriptyline	12.1, p.o. (ED_{50}) 8.7, p.o. (ED_{50}) 14.3, p.o. (ED_{50}) 28.4, p.o. (ED_{50})	reversed reversed reversed reversed	[106]
hypothermia apomorphine-induced	mouse, male	acute	venlafaxine	2–64, i.p.	reversed	[107]
hypothermia apomorphine-induced	mouse, male	acute	milnacipran desipramine	0.2, p.o. (ED_{50}) 0.3, p.o. (ED_{50})	reversed reversed	[108]
hypothermia oxotremorine-induced	mouse, male	acute	milnacipran desipramine	0.7, p.o. (ED_{50}) 4.8, p.o. (ED_{50})	reversed reversed	
hypothermia oxotremorine-induced	mouse, male	acute chronic, 14 d	venlafaxine	10, p.o. 10, p.o. × 2 daily	NE NE	[113]
tremor, salivation, and lacrimation-induced by oxotremorine	mouse, male	acute	duloxetine amitriptyline	> 200, p.o. 6, 536 & 31, p.o. (ED_{50})	NE increased	[106]

Abbreviations: MED, minimum effective dose; ED_{50}, dose required to produce 50% response; NE, no effect.

Table 11B.
Behavioral studies with dual uptake inhibitors – locomotor and reversal of NMDA-induced lethality

Behavioral test	Animal	Treatment	Drug	Dose, mg/kg, route	Response	Refs.
locomotor activity	mouse, male	acute	venlafaxine	16, 32, 64, i.p.	increased	[107]
locomotor activity	rat, male	repeated at 23.5, 5, & 1h before test	fluoxetine	10, s.c. × 3(23.5h)	decreased	[115]
			desipramine	10, s.c. × 3(23.5h)	decreased	
			fluoxetine	10, s.c.	decreased	
			+ desipramine	10, s.c. × 3(23.5h)		
			bupropion	10, s.c. × 3(23.5h)	NE	
			fluoxetine	10, s.c.	decreased	
			+ bupropion	10, s.c. × 3(23.5h)		
			venlafaxine	80, s.c. × 3(23.5h)	decreased	
			duloxetine	40, s.c. × 3(23.5h)	decreased	
			milnacipran	40, s.c. × 3(23.5h)	decreased	
locomotor activity d-amphetamine-induced	rat, male	acute	venlafaxine	10, p.o.	NE	[113]
		14 d	venlafaxine	10, p.o. × 2 daily	increased	
locomotor activity - apomorphine-induced		acute	venlafaxine	10, p.o.	NE	
		14 d	venlafaxine	10, p.o. × 2 daily	NE	
locomotor activity - quinpirole-induced		acute	venlafaxine	10, p.o.	decreased	
		14 d	venlafaxine	10, p.o. × 2 daily	NE	
- (±)-7-OH-DPAT-induced		14 d	venlafaxine	10, p.o. × 2 daily	increased	
NMDA-lethality	mouse, male	acute	milnacipran	20, i.p.	60% protected	[79]
				40, i.p.	100% protected	

Abbreviations: NE, no effect.

Table 11C.
Behavioral studies with dual uptake inhibitors – forced-swim test

Behavioral test	Animal	Treatment	Drug	Dose, mg/kg, route	Response	Refs.
immobility in forced-swim [116]	mouse, male	acute	venlafaxine	8, 16, 32, 64, i.p.	decreased	[107]
		acute	(±)-pindolol	32, i.p.	potentiated	
			+ venlafaxine	1, 2, i.p.		
		acute	RU 24969	1, i.p.	potentiated	
			+ venlafaxine	1, 2, 4, i.p.		
		acute	8-OH-DPAT	1, i.p.	potentiated	
			+ venlafaxine	4, i.p.		
		acute	NAN 190	0.5, i.p.	decreased	
			+ venlafaxine	8, 16, 32		
		acute	clonidine	0.06, i.p.	potentiated	
			+ venlafaxine	1, i.p.		
		repeated	PCPA	300, i.p. x 3 daily	attenuated	
		acute	+ venlafaxine			
		acute	DSP-4	50, i.p.	attenuated	
		acute	+ venlafaxine	16, i.p.		
immobility in forced-swim	mouse, male	acute	milnacipran	10, i.p. (ED$_{50}$)	decreased	[108]
			desipramine	20, i.p. (ED$_{50}$)	decreased	
immobility in forced-swim	mouse, male	acute	duloxetine	27.6, p.o. (ED$_{50}$)	decreased	[106]
			amitriptyline	33.2, p.o. (ED$_{50}$)	decreased	
immobility in forced-swim	rat, male	acute	venlafaxine	10, i.p.	NE	[117]
		acute	desipramine	7.5, i.p.	decreased	
		acute	paroxetine	7.5, i.p.	NE	

Abbreviation: ED$_{50}$, dose required to produce 50% response; NE, no effect.

Table 11C.
Behavioral studies with dual uptake inhibitors – forced-swim test (continued)

Behavioral test	Animal	Treatment	Drug	Dose, mg/kg, route	Response	Refs.
immob., swimming and climbing	rat, male	repeated at 23.5, 5, & 1h before test	desipramine	1, 3.2, 10, s.c.*	decr./NE/incr#.	[115]
			fluoxetine	1, 3.2, 10, s.c.	decr./incr./NE	
			fluoxetine	3.2, s.c.		
			+ desipramine	1, s.c.	decr./incr./incr.	
			fluoxetine	3.2, s.c.		
			+ desipramine	3.2, s.c.	decr./incr./incr.	
			fluoxetine	3.2, s.c.		
			+ desipramine	10, s.c.	decr./NE/incr.	
			fluoxetine	10, s.c.		
			+ desipramine	3.2, s.c.	decr./incr./incr.	
			fluoxetine	10, s.c.	decr./incr./incr.	
			fluoxetine	10, s.c.		
			+ desipramine	10, s.c.	decr./NE/incr.	
			venlafaxine	10, 20, 40, s.c.	decr./incr./NE	
			venlafaxine	80, s.c.	decr./incr./incr.	
			duloxetine	10. 20, 40, s.c.	decr./NE/NE	
			milnacipran	20, 40, s.c.	decr./NE/incr.	
			bupropion	10, s.c.	decr./NE/incr.	
			fluoxetine	10, s.c.		
			+ bupropion	10, s.c.	decr./incr./incr.	

*Each dose was administered 3 times within 23.5 h. Abbreviation: h, hour.
#Behavioral responses are listed in the order of immobility, swimming and climbing indicating decr., decrease; incr., increase; or NE, no effect.

Table 11D.
Behavioral studies with dual uptake inhibitors – aggression, potentiation of serotonin agents and food intake

Behavioral test	Animal	Treatment	Drug	Dose, mg/kg, route	Response	Refs.
resident aggression	rat, male	acute	venlafaxine	7.78, s.c. (ED$_{50}$) (24.87, µmol/kg)	decreased	[119]
aggression	mouse, male	7, 14 d.	venlafaxine	20 µmol/kg s.c.daily	increased	
		acute	venlafaxine	10, p.o.	NE	
		14 d	venlafaxine	10, p.o. × 2 daily	increased	
syndrome 8-OH-DPAT-induced	rat, male	acute	venlafaxine	10, p.o.	NE	[113]
		14 d	venlafaxine	10, p.o. × 2 daily	NE	
head twitches L-5-HTP-induced	rat, male	acute	venlafaxine	10, p.o.	NE	[113]
		14 d	venlafaxine	10, p.o. × 2 daily	decreased	
head twitches L-5-HTP-induced	mouse, male	acute	duloxetine	17.1, p.o. (ED$_{50}$)	increased	[106]
			amitriptyline	> 200, p.o.	NE	
	rat, male	acute	duloxetine	6.9, p.o. (ED$_{50}$)	increased	
			amitriptyline	> 200, p.o.	NE	
head weaving + tranylcypromine + l-tryptophan	rat, male	acute	milnacipran	50–100, p.o.	increased	[108]
food intake 8 h dark period	rat, male	acute	venlafaxine	100, 300, p.o.	decreased	[120]
		acute	duloxetine	30, p.o.	decreased	
		acute	fluoxetine	30, p.o.	NE	
		acute	nisoxetine	30, p.o.	NE	
		acute	fluoxetine + nisoxetine	30, p.o.	decreased	

Abbreviations: ED$_{50}$, dose required to produce 50% effect; NE, no effect.

Table 11E.
Behavioral studies with dual uptake inhibitors – other behaviors

Behavioral test	Animal	Treatment	Drug	Dose, mg/kg, route	Response	Refs.
ptosis induced by tetrabenazine	mouse, male	acute	duloxetine	4, p.o. (ED_{50})	reversed	[106]
			amitriptyline	3.4, p.o. (ED_{50})	reversed	
	rat, male	acute	duloxetine	14, p.o. (ED_{50})	reversed	
			amitriptyline	67, p.o. (ED_{50})	reversed	
ptosis induced by tetrabenazine	mouse, male	acute	milnacipran	0.5, p.o. (ED_{50})	reversed	[108]
			desipramine	2.5, p.o. (ED_{50})	reversed	
			imipramine	5.0, p.o. (ED_{50})	reversed	
			clomipramine	8.8, p.o. (ED_{50})	reversed	
place preference	rat, male	acute	venlafaxine	5, 10, i.p.	NE	[112]
			cocaine	5, i.p.	increased	
			sertraline	2.5–10, i.p.	increased	
			fluoxetine	5, 10, i.p.	increased	
			paroxetine	15, i.p.	increased	
analgesia, hotplate	mouse	acute	venlafaxine	46.7, i.p. (ED_{50})	increased	[110]
stereotypes apomorphine-induced	mouse, male	acute	venlafaxine	2–64, i.p.	NE	[107]
stereotypes amphetamine or apomorphine	rat, male	acute 14 days	venlafaxine	10, p.o. 10, p.o. × 2 daily	NE NE	[113]

Abbreviations: ED_{50}, dose required to produce 50% response; NE, no effect.

potencies with the TCAs, desipramine, imipramine and chlorimipramine, in reversing the ptosis induced by tetrabenazine in mouse and rat (Tab. 11E) [106, 108].

Venlafaxine exhibited analgesic effects with an ED_{50} value of 46.7 mg/kg i.p. using the hotplate test in mouse (Tab. 11E) [110]. Duloxetine at doses that inhibit 5-HT and NE uptake significantly attenuated formalin-induced, late-phase paw-licking behavior in this model of persistent pain [111]. Furthermore, duloxetine was also active in the partial sciatic nerve ligation and L5/L6 spinal nerve ligation models of neuropathic pain. In the place-preference test in rat, venlafaxine at 5 and 10 mg/kg i.p. did not produce any effect, while place-preference behavior was increased by administration of several drugs (mg/kg i.p.) including cocaine (5), sertraline (2.5–10), fluoxetine (5, 10) and paroxetine (15) (Tab. 11E) [112]. Venlafaxine at doses between 2 and 64 mg/kg i.p. had no effect on the apomorphine-induced stereotypical behaviors in mouse (Tab. 11E) [107] and at a dose of 10 mg/kg p.o., venlafaxine acutely or chronically for 2 weeks had no effect on the stereotypical behaviors induced either by apomorphine or amphetamine [113].

Consistent with the weak affinity at muscarinic acetylcholine receptors, venlafaxine acutely or with twice-daily dosing for 14 days at 10 mg/kg p.o. failed to antagonize hypothermia induced by the muscarinic agonist oxotremorine (Tab. 11A) [113]. Unexpectedly, milnacipran was seven times more effective than desipramine in blocking the oxotremorine-induced hypothermia in mouse, but was ineffective at blocking oxotremorine-induced tremor or pilocarpine-induced salivation [108]. Duloxetine at doses greater than 200 mg/kg p.o. failed to antagonize the oxotremorine-induced tremor, salivation and lacrimation in mice, while amitriptyline showed antagonism with ED_{50} values of 6, 536 and 31 mg/kg p.o., respectively, in these responses [106].

Venlafaxine at high doses (16–64 mg/kg i.p.) acutely caused significant increases in locomotor activity to 30–60% above baseline levels in mouse (Tab. 11B) [107]. The increased locomotor activity by venlafaxine is consistent with its ability to inhibit DA uptake [114]. However, after three consecutive administrations of venlafaxine at 80 mg/kg s.c. within 24 h in rat, locomotor activity was significantly reduced (Tab. 11B) [115]. The two dual 5-HT and NA uptake inhibitors, duloxetine and milnacipran, as well as fluoxetine and desipramine alone, and the combination of the latter two uptake inhibitors caused significant decreases in locomotor activity in rat (Tab. 11B)

[115]. A similar dosing regimen with bupropion, an inhibitor of DA uptake, had no effect, whereas its combination with fluoxetine significantly decreased locomotor activity in rat [115]. Venlafaxine administered at 10 mg/kg p.o. twice daily for two weeks, but not after a single dose, in rat, increased locomotor activity induced by d-amphetamine, a catecholamine-releasing agent and (±)-7OH-DPAT, an agonist at DA D_3 receptors (Tab. 11B) [113]. Venlafaxine at the same dosing regimen, acutely and chronically, did not change the apomorphine-induced locomotor activity, but only acute dosing would decrease the quinpirole-induced locomotor activity in rat (Tab. 11B) [113].

It is of interest to note that milnacipran at 20 and 40 mg/kg i.p. effectively protected against NMDA-induced lethality in mouse by 60 and 100%, respectively (Tab. 11B) [79]. This is consistent with the findings that milnacipran exhibits micromolar affinity at NMDA receptors [79] and acts as an antagonist [78].

In the forced-swim model of antidepressant activity [116], venlafaxine at a dose range of 8–64 mg/kg i.p. decreased immobility in mice (Tab. 11C) [107]. Despite the increase in locomotor activity at a higher dose range (16–64 mg/kg i.p.), the reduction of immobility by venlafaxine occurred at a non-stimulant dose of 8 mg/kg i.p. [107]. Combined treatment with an antagonist, pindolol (5-$HT_{1A/1B}$, β-adrenoceptor antagonist), or RU 24969, an agonist at 5-$HT_{1A/1B}$ receptors, potentiated the decrease in immobility time in mouse treated with venlafaxine at a dose as low as 1 mg/kg i.p. (Tab. 11C) [107]. The co-administration of 8-OH-DPAT, an agonist at 5-HT_{1A} receptors, also potentiated the anti-immobility effects of venlafaxine at 4 mg/kg i.p. (Tab. 11C). The administration of pindolol, RU 24969 or 8-OH-DPAT alone had no effect. In rats pretreated with para-chlorophenylalanine (PCPA), an inhibitor of 5-HT synthesis which lowered 5-HT levels in whole brain by 61%, the anti-immobility effects of venlafaxine at 8 and 16 mg/kg i.p. were attenuated, suggesting a response depending on presynaptic 5-HT levels. These findings are consistent with the interpretation that the potentiation of venlafaxine responses by the antagonist, pindolol, may be associated with higher presynaptic 5-HT levels resulting from effective blockade of somatodendritic 5-HT_{1A} autoreceptors [76].

Reduction of brain NA levels 28% by the noradrenergic neurotoxin, DSP-4, attenuated the anti-immobility effects of venlafaxine (16 mg/kg i.p.) in the forced-swim test in mouse (Tab. 11C) [107]. Co-administration with clonidine, an α_2-adrenoceptor agonist, potentiated the venlafaxine-induced decrease in immobility in mouse (Tab. 11C), suggesting a role of NA in the effects of venlafaxine in the forced-swim test. Milnacipran and desipramine decreased immobility with ED_{50} values of 10 and 20 mg/kg i.p. in mouse (Tab. 11C) [108] and duloxetine and amitriptyline had ED_{50} values of 27.6 and 33.2 mg/kg p.o. in the same test [106]. However, venlafaxine at 10 mg/kg i.p. and paroxetine at 7.5 mg/kg i.p. had no effect on immobility time, while desipramine decreased immobility time in rat (Tab. 11C) [117]. Using a modified procedure of the forced-swim test in rat, venlafaxine at 80 mg/kg s.c. was found to decrease immobility, increase swimming and increase climbing behaviors as observed in rats treated with the combination of fluoxetine and desipramine (Tab. 11C) [115]. In the same paradigm, milnacipran at 20 and 40 mg/kg s.c. decreased immobility and increased climbing behavior, whereas rats treated with duloxetine at 10, 20 or 40 mg/kg s.c. showed only a decrease in immobility [115].

Consistent with the anti-aggressive effects of 5-HT uptake inhibitors [118], venlafaxine acutely decreased aggressive behavior of the resident rat with an ED_{50} value of 7.78 mg/kg s.c. (Tab. 11D) [119]. However, upon chronic administration for 1 or 2 weeks, venlafaxine increased aggressive behavior. Chronic treatment with venlafaxine at 10 mg/kg p.o. daily for 2 weeks in mouse also increased aggressive behavior [113]. The 8-OH-DPAT-induced "5-HT syndrome" in rat was not changed by either acute or chronic treatment with venlafaxine for 2 weeks. Although chronic treatment with venlafaxine at 10 mg/kg p.o. twice daily for 2 weeks decreased L-5-hydroxytryptophan (L-5-HTP, the immediate precursor of 5-HT synthesis) induced rat head twitches, acutely administered venlafaxine had no effect (Tab. 11D) [113]. Duloxetine increased the head twitches induced by L-5-HTP, with an ED_{50} value of 17.1 and 6.9 mg/kg p.o. in mouse and rat, respectively, while amitriptyline at doses up to 200 mg/kg p.o. had no effect (Tab. 11D) [106]. Milnacipran at 50–100 mg/kg p.o. increased rat head-weaving behavior induced by L-tryptophan, a precursor amino acid of 5-HT synthesis (Tab. 11D) [108]. These findings are consistent with the enhanced availability of presynaptic 5-HT as a result of inhibition of 5-HT uptake by the three dual 5-HT and NA uptake inhibitors.

In rats accustomed to feeding during the 8 dark hours on a reversed light cycle, venlafaxine at 100 and 300 mg/kg p.o. decreased food intake (Tab. 11D) [120]. Duloxetine, an inhibitor of 5-HT and NA uptake, at 30 mg/kg p.o. also decreased feeding behavior. Neither fluoxetine, a selective 5-HT uptake inhibitor, nor nisoxetine, a selective NA uptake inhibitor, alone at 30 mg/kg p.o. during the 8-hour dark period had an effect on food consumption, but their combination decreased feeding behavior. Thus, it appears that the increased activity in the 5-HT and NA neuronal pathways by inhibition of their respective uptake processes have in concert contributed to the anorectic response in the feeding paradigm.

8 Clinical studies with dual uptake inhibitors

The introduction of SSRIs has brought an improved side-effect profile over those of the earlier generation of TCAs, while the SSRIs and TCAs are generally considered comparable in antidepressive efficacy. The convenience of use for a once-a-day dosage of the SSRIs is another advantage. However, the limited percentage of responders, rate of remission and the delayed onset of antidepressive effects of both SSRIs and TCAs are challenges in the treatment of depression. Therefore, there is a continuous quest to search for practical evidence of medications for treatment of depression with one or more of these improved features [8, 9, 13–15, 121–123]. However, it is generally agreed that these analyses are based mainly on clinical investigations intended to establish the efficacy and side-effect profile of the newly introduced antidepressant drugs. Therefore, there are insufficient studies that are specifically designed to establish evidence of improved medications.

The limitations of the current medications and the clinical quest for improved medications have prompted interest in developing antidepressant drugs which may fill the void of one or more of the aforementioned limitations and medical concerns. Moreover, the clinical research demonstrating that both serotonergic and noradrenergic pathways can independently be responsible for the antidepressive effects of the SSRIs and the NA uptake-inhibiting TCAs [18, 29, 124, 125], respectively, gives further support for developing the next generation of antidepressant drugs bearing the mechanisms of inhibiting uptake of both 5-HT and NA in single molecules. The present review describes the pharmacology of three dual 5-HT and NA uptake inhibitors, venlafaxine, duloxetine and milnacipran. While the clinical experience of these three dual uptake inhibitors is still limited, they provide opportunities to assess if they indeed bring greater efficacy by conducting appropriate clinical investigations. Of the three dual 5-HT and NA uptake inhibitors, venlafaxine and milnacipran have been studied more extensively than duloxetine.

Since the initial antidepressive efficacy of venlafaxine was demonstrated in two open-label dose-ranging studies [126, 127] and the first placebo-controlled trial [128], venlafaxine has been repeatedly shown to be efficacious in inpatients and in outpatient placebo-controlled trials. Based on meta-analysis of the comparator-controlled trials, the venlafaxine-treated patients had greater improvement than the patients treated with the comparators, including chlorimipramine, dothiepin, amineptine, maprotiline, trazodone or imipramine, but generally without statistical significance. According to the Hamilton Rating scale for Depression (HAM-D) total score at 6 weeks, however, venlafaxine showed significant advantage in one study [121]. In a separate study, among outpatients with DSM-III-R major depression, those who increased their dose of venlafaxine to 150 mg/day (43 patients) or fluoxetine to 40 mg/day after 3 weeks (54 patients) showed a trend of superiority with venlafaxine over fluoxetine on HAM-D, Montgomery-Asberg Depression Rating Scale (MADRS), Clinical Global Impression (CGI) scores and global response rates [129].

In a double-blind trial, sixty-seven hospitalized patients who suffered from major depression with melancholia were treated with venlafaxine (200 mg/day) or fluoxetine (40 mg/day) for 6 weeks. Significantly more patients responded to venlafaxine than to fluoxetine using a decline of 50% or more on the MADRS, HAM-D or CGI scales [130]. However, in another study, fluoxetine was statistically superior to placebo in patients with melancholia according to the MADRS score, response rates and remission rates [131]. Moreover, analysis of pooled data from multiple, double-blind trials, in patients with mild, moderate and severe depression, showed statistically significant superior efficacy in fluoxetine-treated patients compared to placebo-treated patients in rate of response and remission and overall the results were comparable to those of TCA-treated patients within the three severity subgroups [132]. Consistent with these findings, SSRIs and TCAs are considered to have comparable effectiveness in the treatment of severe or melancholic depression (8). A recent meta-analysis of pooled data from eight randomized, double-blind studies of major depressive disorder showed that remission rates were significantly higher in patients treated with venlafaxine than those treated with a SSRI [133]. In five out of the six published studies included in the meta-analysis, venlafaxine was compared to fluoxetine, while in one study paroxetine was the comparator [133]. Thus, in the limited number of direct comparative studies between venlafaxine and SSRIs, venlafaxine appears to be more efficacious than SSRIs for the treatment of severe depression [8, 9, 130].

Based on placebo-controlled trials that employed rapid dose escalation to 200 mg or higher a day, venlafaxine showed an early onset of action. In one study, forty-six severely depressed inpatients with melancholia were treated with venlafaxine and forty-seven with placebo [134]. The dose of venlafaxine was increased to a maximum of 375 mg/day within the first week and the average dose was 350 mg/day. Venlafaxine was shown to have statistically significant benefit over placebo after 4 days of treatment according to the MADRS total score and after one week of treatment on the HAM-D total score [121, 134]. In a double-blind, randomized, parallel study, 167 patients with major depression and melancholia were treated with rapidly escalating doses of venlafaxine to 375 mg/day over 5 days, maintained for 10 days and returned to 150 mg/day, or were given imipramine with escalating doses to 200 mg/day over 5 days, then maintained throughout the study. Median time to response based on HAM-D scores was 14 days for the venlafaxine-treated group compared with 21 days for the imipramine-treated group, but there were no statistically significant differences based on MADRS scores [135]. However, the results were considered ambiguous [14]. Moreover, in some patients treated with venlafaxine at doses higher than 300 mg/day, cardiovascular side-effects have been reported and the effects were dose-dependent [136, 137]. Perhaps specifically designed studies will resolve the question on improved onset of clinically meaningful antidepressive effects of venlafaxine.

Milnacipran has been extensively investigated in clinical trials [138]. In a double-blind, placebo-controlled study, milnacipran was given at a dose of 50 mg twice a day in 58 patients hospitalized for severe depression [139]. Milnacipran was shown to be more effective than placebo based on MADRS and HAM-D scales at 2 weeks and at 4 weeks. Additional double-blind, placebo-controlled trials in major depression showed significant superiority for milnacipran compared to placebo on either HAM-D or MADRS scores [140]. In a multicenter 6-week study, two doses of milnacipran (50 mg and 100 mg/day) were compared with amitriptyline (150 mg/day) in three parallel groups of 45 major depressive inpatients [141]. Significant superiority of both milnacipran at 100 mg/day and amitriptyline over milnacipran at 50 mg/day was demonstrated at the end of the treatment period according to HAM-D, MADRS and CGI scores. Results from meta-analysis of the original pooled data involving mostly hospitalized patients showed that milnacipran at 50 mg twice a day and imipramine at 150 mg/day have comparable efficacy based on HAM-D and MADRS scores [142].

In a double-blind, randomized comparison, milnacipran at 50 mg twice a day reduced the HAM-D score in patients with endogenous depression to a greater extent than fluoxetine at 20 mg once a day [138]. In patients with moderate to severe depression, milnacipran at 50 mg twice a day showed a significantly greater reduction in MADRS, HAM-D and CGI scores than fluvoxamine at 100 mg twice a day [143]. Based on these studies, milnacipran showed superiority over the SSRIs to treat patients with moderate to severe depression.

After showing efficacy in two open-label trials [144, 145], duloxetine at 5, 10 and 20 mg/day doses in an 8-week double-blind, placebo-controlled study was investigated in 124 patients meeting DSM-III-R criteria for major depression. However, the response rates of the duloxetine-treated group and the placebo group were un-separable [146]. Most recently, in an 8-week double-blind, placebo-controlled study, 173 patients were randomly allocated to placebo (n = 70), duloxetine (n = 70) or a fluoxetine at 20 mg daily group (n = 33). Duloxetine was titrated from 20 mg twice daily to a maintenance dose of 60 mg twice daily in weekly dose increments [147]. Based on the HAM-D-17 total score as the primary efficacy outcome, duloxetine demonstrated statistically significant superiority to placebo and was numerically superior to fluoxetine. Duloxetine also demonstrated statistically significant response on the MADRS scale and on the anxiety, core factor, retardation, and sleep subscales of the HAM-D-17. The response and remission rate for duloxetine was 64 and 56%, respectively, which was numerically superior to fluoxetine which had response and remission rates of 52 and 32%, respectively. It also showed favorable tolerability with only insomnia and asthenia observed as treatment-emergent adverse events statistically greater than placebo [147]. The authors concluded that duloxetine is a safe and efficacious treatment of major depressive disorder.

Results from these clinical trials consistently show that venlafaxine and milnacipran are effective as antidepressant drugs, while one recent double-blind, placebo-controlled trial showed the antidepressive efficacy of duloxetine. The majority of data show that efficacy of venlafaxine and milnacipran is comparable to the TCAs, and they tend to be superior to the SSRIs, especially for treating patients with moderate to severe depression.

9   Conclusions

In general, the pharmacology of the dual uptake inhibitors venlafaxine, milnacipran and duloxetine are consistent with blockade of 5-HT and NA transporters. However, the discrepancy with venlafaxine between widely different relative affinities for 5-HT and NA transporters *in vitro* and more close relative potencies *in vivo* is unexplained. Milnacipran has some inconsistent effects *in vivo* that may be explained by affinity for neuronal receptors such as NMDA receptors. The pharmacology of duloxetine seems to be the most consistent with dual uptake inhibition.

The clinical results of the dual uptake inhibitors suggest robust efficacy, possibly even superior to SSRIs. However, more specifically designed trials of these new antidepressant drugs are required in order to ascertain if they indeed can deliver higher percentages of responders, a broader spectrum of efficacy, rapid onset of clinically meaningful antidepressive effects and greater remission rates. Moreover, it would be a greater challenge to address the question of whether any superiority in antidepressive efficacy is indeed a consequence of the dual inhibition of 5-HT and NA uptake, as has been so elegantly demonstrated with the SSRIs and the selective NA uptake inhibitors [18, 19, 29]. Overall, the pharmacological and clinical studies suggest that dual uptake inhibition is indeed promising as an improved antidepressant therapy and not just redundancy of two pharmacological effects that produce antidepressant effects. Furthermore, the use of these agents in other disorders, including anxiety, panic disorders, obsessive compulsive disorders, bulimia, anorexia nervosa and persistent pain, needs to be explored.

Acknowledgements

We gratefully acknowledge our many colleagues at Eli Lilly and Company who have worked closely with us over the last 30 years in our continued search for improved antidepressant compounds. We especially acknowledge Dr. David L. Nelson and Penny G. Threlkeld for supplying monoamine transporter binding data.

References

1   C.L. Bowden, A.F. Schatzberg, A. Rosenbaum, S.A. Contreras, J.A. Samson, E. Dessain and M. Sayler: J. Clin. Psychopharmacol. *13*, 305 (1993).
2   R.A. Remick, J. Claman, R. Reesal, R.E. Gibson, M.O. Agbayewa, R.W. Lam and F.D. Keller: Current Therapeutic Res. *53*, 457 (1993).
3   P.E. Stokes: Clin. Therapeutics *15*, 216 (1993).
4   D.C. Steffens, K.R. Krishnan and M.J. Helms: Depress. Anxiety *6*, 10 (1997).
5   C.B. Nemeroff, in: J.M. Gorman and C.B. Nemeroff (chairs): The Role of Norepinephrine in the Treatment of Depression (Academic Highlights). J Clin Psychiatry *60*, 623 (1999).
6   C.M. Beasley, Jr, S.L. Holman and J.H. Potvin: Ann. Clin. Psychiatry *5*, 199 (1993).
7   J.D. Armsterdam: J. Psychopharmacol. *12*, S99 (1998).
8   R.M.A. Hirschfield: J. Clin. Psychiatry *60*: 326 (1999).
9   A.F. Schatzberg: J. Clin. Psychiatry *60* (Suppl. 4), 14 (1999).
10   M. Briley: Human Psychopharmacol. *13*, 99 (1998).
11   J. Cookson: Brit. J. Psychiatry *163* (Suppl. 20), 20 (1993).
12   M.M. Katz, C. Bowden, P. Stokes, R. Casper, A. Frazer, S.H. Koslow, J. Kocsis, S. Secunda, A. Swann and N.Berman: Neuropsychopharmacol. *17*, 110 (1997).
13   D. Hackett: Eur. Psychiatry *13*, 117 (1998).
14   A.J. Gelenberg and C.L. Chesen: J. Clin. Psychiatry *61*, 712 (2000).
15   A. Sambunaris, J.K. Hesselink, R. Pinder, J. Panagides and S.M. Stahl: J. Clin. Psychiatry *58* (Suppl. 6) 40 (1997).
16   D.T. Wong, D.W. Robertson, F.P. Bymaster, J.H. Krushinski and L.R. Reid: Life Sci. *43*, 2049 (1988).
17   D.T. Wong: Exp. Opin. Invest. Drugs *7*, 1 (1998).
18   P.L. Delgado, D.S. Charney, L.H. Price, G.K. Aghajanian, H. Landis and G.R. Heninger: Arch. Gen. Psychiatry *47*, 411 (1990).
19   P.L. Delgado, H.L. Miller, R.M. Salomon, J. Licinio, J.H. Krystal, F.A. Moreno, G.R. Heninger and D.S. Charney: Biol. Psychiatry *46*, 212 (1999).
20   P.L. Delgado and F.A. Moreno: J. Clin. Psychiatry *61* (Suppl. 1), 5 (2000).
21   D.T. Wong, J.S. Horng, F.P. Bymaster, K.L. Hauser and B.B. Molloy: Life Sci. *15*, 471 (1974).
22   D.T. Wong, J.S. Horng and F.P. Bymaster: Life Sci. *17*, 755 (1975).
23   R.W. Fuller and D.T. Wong: Fed. Proc. *36*, 2154 (1977).
24   A. Coppen: Brit. J. Psychiatry *113*, 1237 (1967).
25   H. Weil-Malherbe and S.I. Szara (eds): The biochemistry of functional and experimental psychosis. C.C. Thomas Publisher, Springfield, IL (1971), pp 57.
26   J.J. Schildkraut: Am. J. Psychiatry *122*, 509 (1965).
27   W.E. Bunney, Jr. and J.M. Davis: Arch. Gen. Psychiatry *13*, 483 (1965).
28   P.L. Delgado, H.L. Miller, R.M. Salomon, J. Licinio, G.R. Heninger, A.J. Gelenberg and D.S. Charney: Psychopharmacol. Bull. *29*, 389 (1993).
29   H.L. Miller, P.L. Delgado, R.M. Salomon, R. Berman, J.H. Krystal, G.R. Heninger and D.S. Charney: Arch. Gen. Psychiatry *53*, 117 (1996).
30   W.Z. Potter, H.M. Calil, I. Extein, P.W. Gold, T.A. Wehr and F.K. Goodwin: Acta Psychiatr. Scand. *290* (Suppl.), 152 (1981).
31   A. Aberg: Acta Psychiatr. Scand. 290 (Suppl.), 244 (1981).

32   J.B. Weilburg, J.F. Rosenbaum, J. Biederman, G.S. Sachs, M.H. Pollack, and K. Kelly: J. Clin. Psychiatry 50, 447 (1989).

33   J.C. Nelson, C.M. Mazure, M.B. Bowers Jr. and P.I. Jatlow: Arch. Gen. Psychiatry 48, 303 (1991).

34   R. Seth, A.L. Jennings, J. Bindman, J. Phillips and K. Bergmann: Brit. J. Psychiatry 161, 562 (1992).

35   J. Vetulani, R.J. Stawarz, J.V. Dingell and F. Sulser: Naunyn-Schmiedebergs Arch. Pharmacol. 293, 109 (1976).

36   R. Mishra, A. Janowsky and F. Sulser: Eur. J. Pharmacol. 60, 379 (1979).

37   D.T. Wong, L.R. Reid, F.P. Bymaster and P.G. Threlkeld: J. Neural. Transm. 64, 251 (1985).

38   N. Brunnello, M.L. Barbaccia, D.M. Chuang and E. Costa: Neuropharmacol. 21, 1145 (1982).

39   V.L. Nimgaonkar, G.M. Goodwin, C.L. Davies and A.R. Green: Neuropharmacol 24, 279 (1985).

40   C.A. Stockmeier, A.M. Matino and K.J. Kellar: Science 230, 323 (1985).

41   B.M. Baron, A.-M. Ogden, B.W. Siegel, J. Stegeman, R.C. Ursillo and M.W. Dudley: Eur. J. Pharmacol. 154, 125 (1988).

42   J.M. Baraban and G.K. Aghajanian: Neuropharmacol. 19, 355 (1980).

43   C.P. VanderMaelen and G.K. Aghajanian: Brain Res. 289, 109 (1983).

44   L.A. Dawson, H.Q. Nguyen and A. Geiger: Neuropharmacol. 38, 1153 (1999).

45   S. Hjorth, H.J. Bengtsson, S. Milano, J.F. Lundberg and T. Sharp: Neuropharmacol. 34, 615 (1995).

46   J.M. Baraban and G.K. Aghajanian: Eur. J. Pharmacol. 66, 287 (1980).

47   D.T. Wong, F.P. Bymaster, D.A. Mayle, L.R. Reid, J.H. Krushinski and D.W. Robertson: Neuropsychopharmacol. 8, 23 (1993).

48   C. Bolden-Watson and E. Richelson: Life Sci. 52, 1023 (1993).

49   C. Moret , M. Charveron , J.P.M. Finberg, J.P. Couzinier and M. Briley: Neuropharmacol. 24, 1211 (1985).

50   C. Sanchez and J. Hyttel: Cell. Mol. Neurobiol. 19, 467 (1999).

51   D.T. Wong, F.P. Bymaster, L.R. Reid, D.A. Mayle, J.H. Krushinski and D.W. Robertson: Neuropsychopharmacol. 8, 337 (1993).

52   E.H.F. Wong, M.S. Sonders, S.G. Amara, P.M. Tinholt, M.F.P. Piercey, W.P. Hoffmann, D.K. Hyslop, S. Franklin, R.D. Porsolt, A. Bonsignori et al.: Biol. Psychiatry 47, 818 (2000).

53   D.T. Wong, F.P. Bymaster and E.A. Engleman: Life Sci. 57, 411 (1995).

54   F.P. Bymaster, L.J. Dreshfield-Ahmad, P.G. Threlkeld, J.L. Shaw, L. Thompson, D.L.G. Nelson, S.K. Hemrick-Luecke and D.T Wong: Neuropsychopharmacol. 25, 871–880 (2001).

55   M. Tatsumi, K. Groshan , R.D. Blakely and E. Richelson: Eur. J. Pharmacol. 340, 249 (1997).

56   D.T. Wong and F.P. Bymaster: Res. Comm. Chem. Pathol. Pharmacol. 15, 221(1976).

57   T. Kihara and M. Ikeda: J. Pharmacol. Exp. Ther. 272, 177 (1995).

58   D.T. Wong, F.P. Bymaster, L.R. Reid and P.G. Threlkeld: Biochem. Pharmacol. 32, 1287 (1983).

59   B. Cusack, A. Nelson and E. Richelson: Psychopharmacol. 114, 559 (1994).

60   A.I. Levey: Life Sci. 52, 441(1993).

61   T. Stanton, C. Bolden-Watson, B. Cusack and E. Richelson: Biochem. Pharmacol. 45, 2352 (1993).

62   E.-P., Pälvimäki, B.L. Roth, H. Majasuo, A.Laakso, M. Kuoppamäki, E. Syvälahti and J. Hietala: Psychopharmacol. *126*, 234, (1996).

63   C. Wikell, P.B.F. Bergqvist, S. Hjorth, G. Apelqvist, H. Bjork and F. Bengtsson: Clin. Neuropharmacol. *21*, 296 (1998).

64   E. Carboni, G.L. Tanda, R. Frau and G. Di Chiara: J. Neurochem. *55*, 1067 (1990).

65   C. Wikell, S. Hjorth, G. Apelqvist, J. Kullingsjo, J. Lundmark, P.B. Bergqvist and F. Bengtsson: Naunyn-Schmiedebergs Arch. Pharmacol. *363*, 448 (2001).

66   S.E. Gartside, V. Umbers and T. Sharp: Psychopharmacol. *130*, 261 (1997).

67   D.W. Gallager and G.K. Aghajanian: J. Pharmacol. Exp. Ther. *193*, 785 (1975).

68   Y. Chaput, C. de Montigny and P. Blier: Naunyn-Schmiedebergs Arch. Pharmacol. *333*, 342 (1986).

69   F. Artigas, L. Romero, C. de Montigny and P. Blier: Trends Neurosci. *19*, 378, (1996).

70   L.J. Dreshfield, D.T. Wong, K.W. Perry and E.A. Engleman: Neurochem. Res. *21*, 557(1996).

71   T. Sharp, V. Umbers and S. Hjorth: Neuropharmacol. *35*, 735 (1996).

72   R. Tao and S. Hjorth: Naunyn Schmiedebergs Arch. Pharmacol. *345*, 137 (1992).

73   E. Gur, E. Dremencov, B. Lerer and M.E. Newman: Eur. J. Pharmacol. *372*, 17 (1999).

74   E.A. Muth, J.A. Moyer, J.T. Haskins, T.H. Andree and G.E.M. Husbands: Drug Dev. Res. *23*, 191 (1991).

75   C. Moret and M. Briley: J. Neurochem. *69*, 815, (1997).

76   N. Bel and F. Artigas: Neuropsychopharmacol. *21*, 745 (1999).

77   N. Bel and F. Artigas: J. Pharmacol. Exp. Ther. *278*, 1064 (1996).

78   S. Shuto, S. Ono, Y. Hase, Y. Ueno, T. Noguchi, K. Yoshii and A. Matsuda: J. Med. Chem. *39*, 4844 (1996).

79   S. Shuto, H. Takada, D. Mochizuki, R. Tsujita, Y. Hase, S. Ono, N. Shibuya and A. Matsuda: J. Med. Chem. *38*, 2964 (1995).

80   W. Loscher, R. Annies and D. Honack: Neurosci Lett. *128*, 191 (1991).

81   J.M. Mathe, G.G. Nomikos, K.H. Blakemen and T.H. Svensson: Neuropharmacol. *38*, 121 (1999).

82   R. Trullas and P. Skolnick: Eur. J. Pharmacol. *185*, 1 (1990).

83   P. Skolnick, B. Legutko, X. Li and F.P. Bymaster: Pharmacological Research *43*, 411 (2001).

84   E.A. Engleman, K.W. Perry, D.A. Mayle and D.T. Wong: Neuropsychopharmacol. *12*, 287 (1995).

85   M.J. Millan, M. Brocco, S. Veiga, L. Cistarelli, C. Melon and A. Gobert: Eur. J. Pharmacol. *341*, 165 (1998).

86   E.A. Engleman, D.W. Robertson, D.C. Thompson, K.W. Perry and D.T. Wong: J. Neurochem. *66*, 599 (1996).

87   A. Gobert, J.-M. Rivet, L. Cistarelli and M.J. Millan: J. Neurochem. *68*, 1326 (1997).

88   G. Tanda, E. Carboni, R. Frau and G. Di Chiara: Psychopharmacol. *115*, 285(1994).

89   A. Gobert, J-M Rivet, L. Cistarelli, C. Melon and M.J. Millan: J. Neurochem. *69*, 2616 (1997).

90   J.J. Scuvee-Moreau and A.E. Dresse: Eur. J. Pharmacol. *57*, 219 (1979).

91   M. Hajos, S.E. Gartside and T. Sharp: Naunyn-Schmiedebergs Arch. Pharmacol. *351*, 624(1995).

92   P. Blier, C. de Montigny and D. Tardif: Psychopharmacol. *84*, 242 (1984).

93   C. de Montigny, Y. Chaput and P. Blier: J. Clin. Psychiatry *51* (Suppl. B), 4 (1990).

94   K. Kasamo, P. Blier and C. de Montigny: J. Pharmacol. Exp. Ther. *277*, 278 (1996).

95   J.C. Beique, C. de Montigny, P. Blier and G. Debonnel: Synapse 32, 198 (1999).

96   J.F. Czachura and K. Rasmussen: Naunyn-Schmiedebergs Arch. Pharmacol. *362*, 266 (2000).

97   M.H. Sheard, A. Zolovick, and G.K. Aghajanian: Brain Res. *43*, 690 (1972).

98   T.H. Svensson, B.S. Bunney and G.K. Aghajanian: Brain Res. *92*, 291 (1975).

99   F. Lejeune, V. Audinot, A. Gobert, J.-M. Rivet, M. Spedding and M.J. Millan: Eur. J. Pharmacol. *260*, 79 (1994).

100   N. Haddjeri, C. de Montigny and P. Blier: Brit. J. Pharmacol *120*, 865 (1997).

101   N. Quinaux, J. Scuvee-Moreau and A. Dresse: Naunyn Schmiedebergs Arch. Pharmacol. *319*, 66 (1982).

102   M. Salter, R. Hazelwood, C.I. Pogson, R. Iyer, D.J. Madge, H.T. Jones, B.R. Cooper, R.F. Cox, C.M. Wang and R.P. Wiard: Neuropharmacol. *34*: 217 (1995).

103   R. Mongeau, M. Weiss, C. de Montigny and P. Blier: Neuropharmacol. 37, 905 (1998).

104   J.T. Haskins, J.A. Moyer, E.A. Muth and E.B. Sigg: Eur. J. Pharmacol. *115*, 139 (1985).

105   J.P. Yardley, G.E.M. Husbands, G. Stack, J. Butch, J. Bicksler, J.A. Moyer, E.A. Muth, T. Andree, H. Fletcher 3rd, M.N. James et al.: J. Med. Chem. *33*, 2899 (1990).

106   A. Katoh, M. Eigyo, C. Ishibashi, Y. Naitoh, M. Takeuchi, N. Ibii, M. Ikeda and A. Matsushita: J. Pharmacol. Exp. Ther. *272*, 1067 (1995).

107   J.P. Redrobe, M. Bourin, M.C. Colombel and G.B. Baker: Psychopharmacol. *138*, 1 (1998).

108   A. Stenger, J.P. Couzinier and M. Briley: Psychopharmacol. *91*, 147 (1987).

109   I.H. Slater, R.C. Rathbun and R. Kattau: J. Pharm. Pharmacol. *31*, 108 (1979).

110   S. Schreiber, M.M. Backer and C.G. Pick: Neurosci. Lett. *273*, 85 (1999).

111   S. Iyengar, D.L. Li, D.H. Lee, R.M.A. Simmons: World Biol. Psychiatry 2, 325S (2001).

112   F. Subhan, P.N. Deslandes, D.M. Pache and R.D.E. Sewell: Eur. J. Pharmacol. *408*, 257, (2000).

113   J. Maj and Z. Rogoz: J. Neural Transm. *106*, 197 (1999).

114   E.A. Muth, J.T. Haskins, J.A. Moyer, G.E. Husbands, S.T. Nielsen and E.B. Sigg: Biochem. Pharmacol. *35*, 4493 (1986).

115   J.-P. Reneric and I. Lucki: Psychopharmacol. *136*, 190 (1998).

116   R.D. Porsolt, M. Le Pichon and M. Jalfre: Nature *266*, 730 (1977).

117   T.J. Connor, P. Kelliher, Y. Shen, A. Harkin, J.P. Kelly and B.E. Leonard: Pharmacol. Biochem. Behav. *65*, 591 (2000).

118   V. Molina, L. Ciesielski, S. Gobaille, F. Isel and P. Mandel: Pharmacol. Biochem. Behav. *27*, 123 (1987).

119   P.J. Mitchell and A. Fletcher: Neuropharmacol. *32*, 1001 (1993).

120   H.C. Jackson, A.M. Needham, L.J. Hutchins, S.E. Mazurkiewicz and D.J. Heal: Brit. J. Pharmacol. *121*, 1758 (1997).

121   S.A. Montgomery: Intl. Clin. Psychopharmacol. *10* (Suppl. 2), 21 (1995).

122   R.C. Shelton: J. Clin. Psychiatry 60 (Suppl. 4), 57 (1999).

123   J.C. Nelson: J. Clin. Psychiatry 61 (Suppl. 2), 13 (2000).

124   P.L. Delgado, L.H. Price, H.L. Miller, R.M. Salomon, G.K. Aghajanian, G.R. Heninger and D.S. Charney: Arch. Gen. Psychiatry *51*, 865 (1994).

125   J.C. Nelson: Biol. Psychiatry *46*, 1301 (1999).

126   H.L. Goldberg and R. Finnerty: Psychopharmacol. Bull. *24*, 198 (1988).

127   E. Schweizer, C. Clary, I. Fox and C. Weise and K. Rickels: Psychopharmacol. Bull. *24*, 195 (1988).

128   E. Schweizer, C. Weise, C. Clary and K. Rickels: J. Clin. Psychopharmacol. *11*, 233 (1991).

129   J.C. Costa e Silva: J. Clin. Psychiatry *59*, 352 (1998).

130   G.E. Clerc, P Ruimy and J. Verdeau-Pailles: Int Clin Psychopharmacol. *9*, 139 (1994).

131   J.H. Heiligenstein, G.D. Tollefson and D.E. Faries: Int. Clin. Psychopharmacol. *8*, 247 (1993).

132   A.C. Pande and M.E. Sayler: Int. Clin. Psychopharmacol. *8*, 243 (1993).

133   M. Thase, A.R. Entsuah and R.L. Rudolph: Brit. J. Psychiatry *178*, 234 (2001).

134   J.D. Guelfi, C. White, D. Hackett, J.Y. Guichoux and G. Magni: J. Clin. Psychiatry *56*, 450 (1995).

135   O. Benkert, G. Grunder, H. Wetzel and D. Hackett: J. Psychiatr. Res. *30*, 441 (1996).

136   M.A. Scott, P.S. Shelton and W.Gattis: Pharmacotherapy *16*, 352 (1996).

137   Wyeth-Ayerst: Venlafaxine (Effexor) package insert, Philadelphia, PA (1995).

138   J.D. Guelfi, M. Ansseau, E. Corruble, J.C. Samuelian, I. Tonelli, A. Tournoux and Y. Pletan: Int. Clin. Psychopharmacol. *13*, 121 (1998).

139   J.P.Macher, J.P. Sichel, C. Serre, R. Von Frenckell, J.C. Huck and J.P. Demarez: Neuropsychobiology *22*, 77(1989).

140   Y. Lecrubier, Y. Pletan, A. Solles, A. Tournoux and V. Magne: Int. Clin. Psychopharmacol. *11* (Suppl. 4), 29 (1996).

141   M. Ansseau, R. von Frenckell, C. Mertens, J. de Wilde, L. Botte, J.-M. Devoitille, J.-L. Evrard, A. De Nayer, P. Darimont, G. Dejaiffe et al.: Psychopharmacol. *98*, 163 (1989).

142   A. Puech, S.A. Montgomery, J.F. Prost, A. Solles and M. Briley: Int. Clin. Psychopharmacol. *12*, 99 (1997).

143   G. Clerc and the Milnacipran/Fluvoxamine Study Group: Int. Clin. Psychopharmacol. *16*, 145 (2001).

144   J. Ishigooka, E. Nagata, A. Takahashi, T. Sugiyama, M. Uchiumi, T. Tsukahara, M. Murasaki, S. Mura, T. Oguma and Y. Yano: Curr. Ther. Res. *58*, 679 (1997).

145   M. Berk, A. du Plessis, M. Birkett and D. Richardt, on behalf of the Lilly Duloxetine study group: Int. Clin. Psychopharmacol. *12*, 137 (1997).

146   A.F. Joubert, A.D. du Plessis, D. Faries and C.A. Gagiano: Biol. Psychiatry *42* (Suppl. 1), Abstr 86 (1997).

147   D.J. Goldstein, C. Mallinckrodt, Y. Lu and M.A. Demitrack: World J. Biol. Psychiatry *2* (suppl 1), 331S (2001).

Progress in Drug Research, Vol. 58 (E. Jucker, Ed.)
© 2002 Birkhäuser Verlag, Basel (Switzerland)

Advances in QSAR studies of HIV-1 reverse transcriptase inhibitors

By Satya P. Gupta

Department of Chemistry, Birla
Institute of Technology and Science,
Pilani 333031, India

Satya P. Gupta

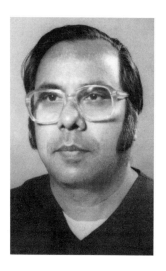

Satya P. Gupta is at present a professor of Chemistry at Birla Institute of Technology and Science (BITS), Pilani. He obtained his D.Phil. degree in quantum chemistry in 1971 from the University of Allahabad, Allahabad, India. For his doctoral degree, he worked with Professor Bal Krishna in quantum chemistry, leading to the development of a new molecular orbital method, known as the IOC-ω-technique. Dr. Gupta then spent a couple of years at Tata Institute of Fundamental Research (TIFR), Mumbai, working with Professor Girjesh Govil on the structure and functions of biomembranes. He joined BITS in 1973 and stayed there, working on theoretical aspects of drug design. He has made notable contributions in this area, for which he has been given the Ranbaxy Research Foundation Award, a coveted national award, and elected as a Fellow of the National Academy of Sciences, India. He is currently an advisory member of the Technical Resource Group on Research and Development on HIV/AIDS, constituted by the Ministry of Health and Welfare, Government of India, and a member of the Editorial Advisory Board of Current Medicinal Chemistry: Cardiovascular and Hematological Agents, *Bentham Science Publishers BV, The Netherlands.*

Summary

A review is presented of the recent advances in quantitative structure–activity relationship (QSAR) studies of HIV-1 reverse transcriptase (RT) inhibitors. These inhibitors have been put into two classes: nucleoside RT inhibitors (NRTIs), which are 2′,3′-dideoxynucleoside analogues (ddNs), and non-nucleoside RT inhibitors (NNRTIs). For NRTIs (ddNs), which act as competitive inhibitors or alternate substrates of RT and hence interact at the substrate binding site of the enzyme, QSARs have pointed out the major role of the electronic factors governing their activity. For NNRTIs, which bind to a site entirely distinct from the substrate binding site, the activity has been shown to be largely dependent upon the hydrophobic nature of the compounds or substituents. The hydrophobic nature of the active site in the receptor with which the NNRTIs interact provides relatively few possibilities for the molecules to have polar interactions or hydrogen bondings, but QSARs have indicated that NNRTIs do involve some polar interactions and hydrogen bondings with some pockets of the enzyme. QSARs also indicate the significant roles of steric interactions and conformational shape of the molecule.

Contents

Key words

HIV-1 reverse transcriptase inhibitors, nucleoside reverse transcriptase inhibitors, non-nucleoside reverse transcriptase inhibitors, 2',3'-dideoxynucleoside analogues, HEPT derivatives, TIBO derivatives, TSAO derivatives, α-APA derivatives, nevirapine analogues, pyridine derivatives, quantitative structure-activity relationships.

Glossary of abbreviations

AIDS, acquired immunodeficiency syndrome; HIV-1, human immunodeficiency virus of type 1; RT, reverse transcriptase; FDA, Food and Drug Administration; ddN, 2',3'-dideoxynucleoside; NNRTIs, non-nucleoside reverse transcriptase inhibitors; NRTIs, nucleoside reverse transcriptase inhibitors; QSAR, quantitative structure-activity relationship; IC_{50}, the minimum concentration of the compound leading to 50% inhibition of the enzyme HIV-1 RT; EC_{50}, the concentration (mol/L or mol/g) of the compound required to achieve 50% protection of MT-4 or CEM cell against the cytopathic effect of the virus; CC_{50}, the concentration of the compound required to reduce by 50% the number of mock-infected MT-4 or CEM cells; P, octanol-water partition coefficient; π, hydrophobic constant; HEPT, 1-[(2- hydroxyethoxy)methyl]-6-(phenylthio)thymine; TIBO, 4,5,6,7-tetrahydro-5-methylimidazo[4,5,1-jk][1, 4]benzodiazepin-2(1H)-one; TSAO, 1-[2',5'-bis-O-(tert-butyldimethylsilyl)-β-D-xylo- or ribofuranosyl]-3'-spiro-5"-[4"-amino-1", 2"-oxathiole-2", 2"-dioxide]; α-APA, α-anilinophenylacetamide; σ, σ⁻,σ⁺, Hammett's electronic constants applied to aromatic substituents; σ*, Taft's electronic constant applied to aliphatic substituents; Es, Taft's steric parameter; MW, molecular weight; MR, molar refractivity; B1, Verloop's sterimol parameter for the width of the first atom of a substituent; B5, Verloop's sterimol parameter to define the maximum width of a substituent; L, Verloop's sterimol parameter for the length of the substituent; V_w, van der Waals volume; C log P, calculated log P; R, resonance electronic parameter; F, field or inductive electronic constant; n, number of data points; r, correlation coefficient; s, standard deviation; $F_{x, y}$, F-ratio between the variances of calculated and observed activities (x: number of independent variables; y = n–x–1); q^2, Cramer's statistics to account for the variance in the activity.

1 Introduction

The acquired immunodeficiency syndrome (AIDS), which is the most fatal disorder of the present era and for which no complete successful chemotherapy has been developed so far, is caused by a retrovirus of the *Lentiviridae* family [1, 2]. Originally referred to as HTLV-III or LAV, this enveloped single-stranded RNA virus is now called human immunodeficiency virus (HIV) [3, 4] and two genetically distinct subtypes, HIV-1 and HIV-2, have been characterized [5–7], of which the former has been found to be prevalent in causing the disease.

The replicative cycle of HIV-1 presents several viable targets that could be exploited for the development of anti-HIV chemotherapy. One of the most important of them is the process of reverse transcription of genomic RNA into double-stranded DNA which is mediated by the enzyme called reverse transcriptase (RT). Therefore, the inhibitors of this enzyme have been widely studied and most of the compounds approved so far by the FDA in the United States for the treatment of HIV infections are RT inhibitors [8]. For the design and development of still more successful RT inhibitors, an in-depth knowledge of the mechanism of RT inhibition is required, which can be essentially provided by a comprehensive quantitative structure-activity relationship (QSAR) study on RT inhibitors.

2 RT inhibitors: classification

RT inhibitors are put basically into two main classes: (1) nucleoside RT inhibitors (NRTIs) and (2) non-nucleoside RT inhibitors (NNRTIs). The NRTIs are 2',3'-dideoxynucleoside analogues (ddNs) that mimic normal nucleoside substrates but lack the 3'-OH group required for DNA chain elongation. They compete with native nucleosides and effectively stall polymerase activity by

1
Zidovudine

2
Zalcitabine

3
Didanosine

4
Stavudine

5
Lamivudine

6
Abacavir

becoming incorporated into the growing DNA strand, thereby causing premature termination [9, 10]. Compounds **1–6** represent a few important ddN analogues that have been approved by FDA for the treatment of HIV infections.

The ddN inhibitors are first metabolized to the corresponding 5′-phosphates and then act as competitive inhibitors/alternate substrates of the enzyme. Binding at the substrate binding site, they act as chain terminators since their incorporation into the growing DNA chain does not permit further chain elongation [11].

ddN analogues, however, have been found to be associated with some side-effects, which is assumed to be due to the interference of their metabolites (5′-mono-, di- and triphosphates) with 2′-deoxynucleoside metabolism and, in particular, of their triphosphate metabolites with the cellular DNA polymerization process.

NNRTIs do not interact with the substrate binding site of DNA polymerases, whether DNA dependent or RNA dependent; hence they do not cause any side-effects that compromise the clinical utility of the ddN analogues [12, 13]. NNRTIs interact noncompetitively with an allosteric site of the enzyme and thus do not directly impair the function of the substrate binding site [14]. In fact, NNRTIs have a comparatively higher binding affinity for the enzyme-substrate complex than for the free enzyme itself. Their interaction with the enzyme leads to a conformational change in the enzyme, resulting in a decrease in the affinity of the active site for the substrate. However, NNRTIs are active against the RT of only HIV-1 and not of HIV-2 or any other retrovirus. This specificity of NNRTIs for HIV-1 RT is due to the presence in HIV-1 RT, and not in other RTs or DNA polymerases, of a flexible highly hydrophobic pocket in which a nonsubstrate analogue can fit snugly [15–17].

The hydrophobic pocket in HIV-1 RT is formed by the hydrophobic residues of the Y181–Y188 region. The hydrophilic residues, in particular the D184-D186 dipeptide, which are essential for nucleotide substrate binding, are located at the outside of the pocket.

Several classes of compounds could be considered as NNRTIs, which are specifically targeted at HIV-1 RT. They can be put into the following categories: (1) tetrahydroimidazobenzodiazepinone (TIBO) derivatives [18, 19], (2) hydroxyethoxymethylphenylthiothymine (HEPT) derivatives [20, 21], (3) dihydropyridodiazepinone, such as nevirapine, derivatives [22], (4) pyridinone derivatives [23], (5) bis(heteroaryl)piperazine (BHAP) derivatives [24], (6) tertiarybutyldimethylsilylspiroaminooxathioledioxide (TSAO) pyrimidine nucleosides [25], and (7) α-anilinophenylacetamide (α-APA) derivatives [26]. The FDA has approved several NNRTIs, as given in Chart 1, for the treatment of HIV infection.

3 QSAR results and discussion

In the QSAR studies that we present here – 2-dimensional or 3-dimensional – the dependant variable, i.e., the biological activity of the compounds, is expressed as IC_{50} or EC_{50}. The IC_{50} refers to the minimum concentration of the compound leading to 50% inhibition of the enzyme HIV-1 RT, and EC_{50} (or ED_{50}) refers to the concentration (mol/L or mol/g) of the compound

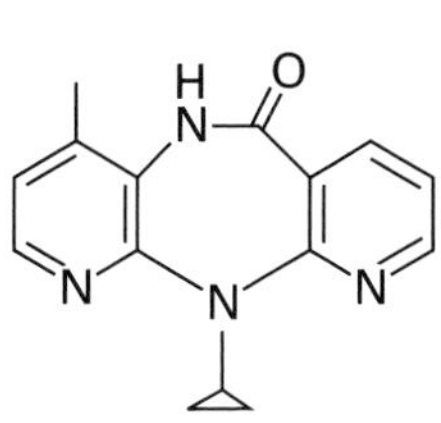

7
Nevirapine

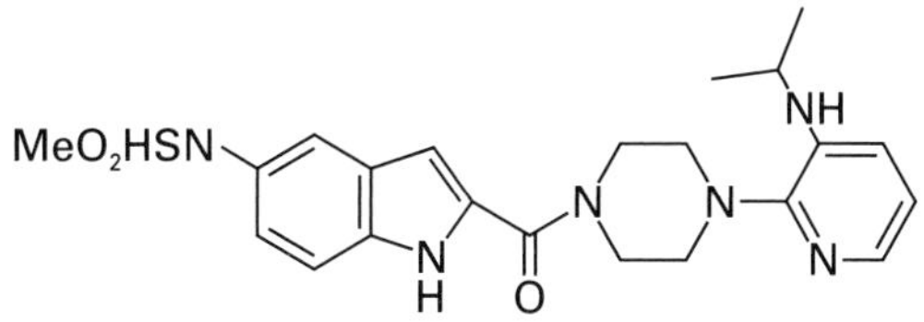

8
Delavirdine

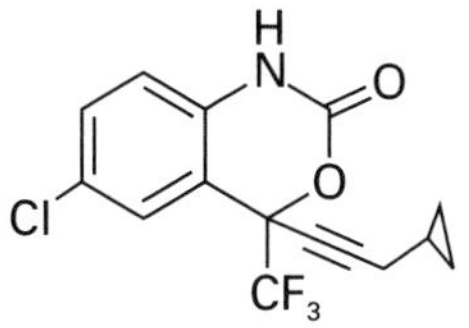

9
Efavirenz

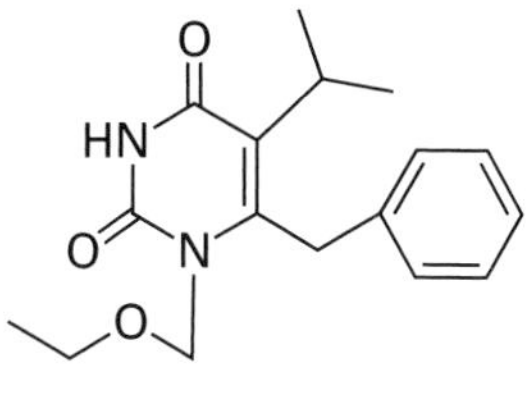

10
MKC-442 (HEPT derivative)

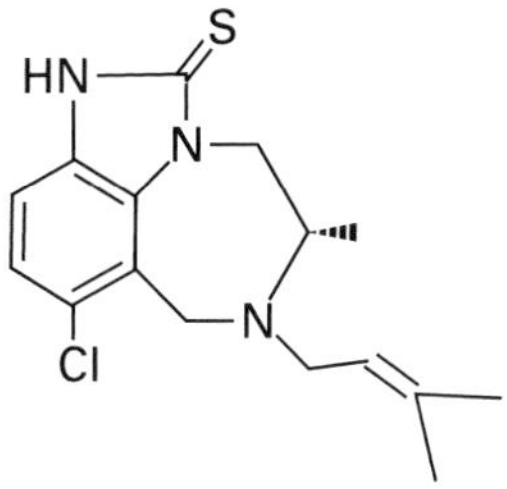

11
Tivirapine

Chart 1

required to achieve 50% protection of MT-4 or CEM cells against the cyto-pathic effect of the virus. For the selectivity of the compounds, their cyto-toxic effect has also been analyzed, which has been expressed in terms of CC_{50}, the concentration of the compound required to reduce by 50% the number of mock-infected MT-4 or CEM cells. The logarithms of the inverse of these parameters refer to the biological end-points in QSAR studies. The correlates of these biological parameters are various physiochemical, elec-tronic and steric parameters. They are experimentally obtained log P or cal-culated log P (C log P), where P is the octanol-water partition coefficient; the hydrophobic constant of the substituents π; the electronic parameters (Ham-

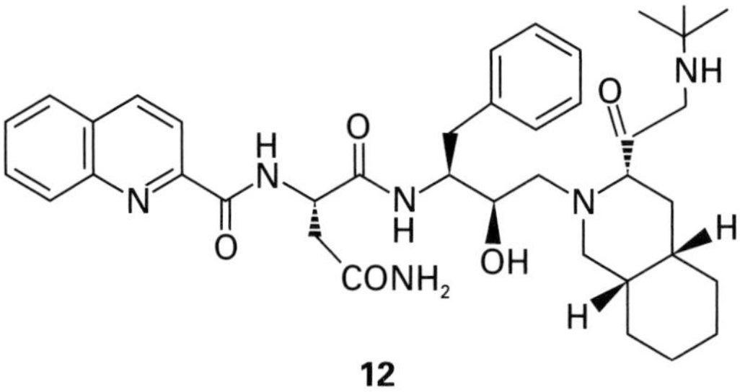

12
Saquinavir

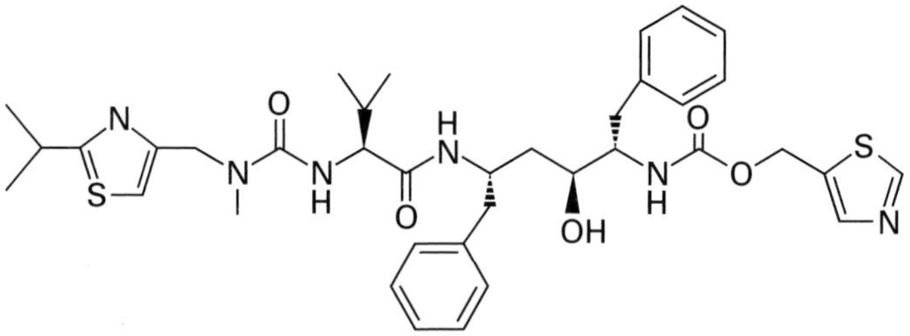

13
Ritonavir

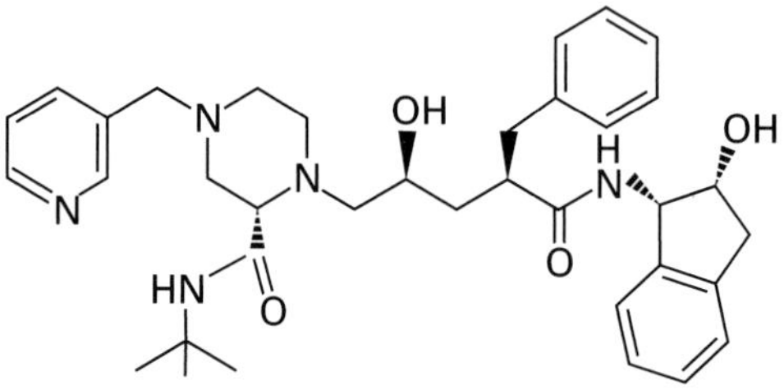

14
Indinavir

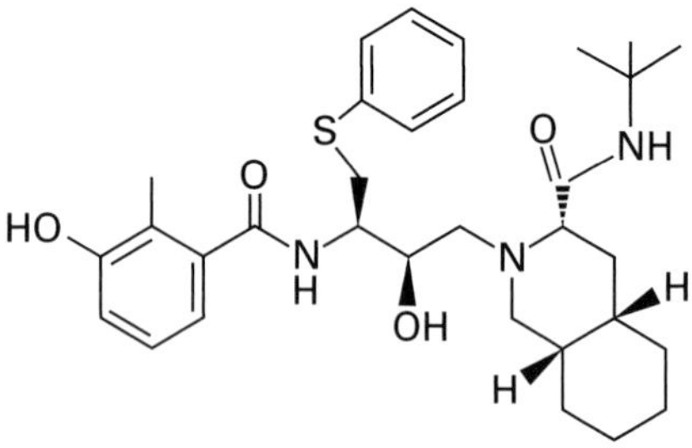

15
Nelfinavir

Chart 1 (continued)

mett constants) σ, σ^-, σ^+; Taft's electronic parameter σ^*, applicable to aliphatic substituents; molar refractivity MR (CMR: calculated MR); Taft's steric parameter Es; McGowan volume MgVol, van der Waals volume V_w; molecular weight MW; Verloop's sterimol parameters B1, B5 and L, where B1 and B5 refer to the minimum and maximum width of a substituent, respectively, and L to the length of the substituent.

In all the QSAR equations that follow, n refers to the number of data points, r is the correlation coefficient, s is the standard deviation, q^2 is Cramer's coefficient to account for the variance in the activity, and data within the parentheses are 95% confidence intervals.

3.1 Nucleoside analogues

As NRTIs, 2',3'-dideoxypyrimidine nucleoside (**16, 17**) and purine nucleoside (**18**) analogues have been well studied. However, QSAR studies could be only recently reported on some series of these analogues. For a very small series of **16** (uridine derivatives) studied by Balzarini et al. [27], where Y = F and X = H, Cl, Br, I, or Me, the anti-HIV activities against both HIV-1 and HIV-2 were shown by Garg et al. [28] to be significantly correlated with the electronic constant σ^+ of the X-substituents as

$$\log (1/ED_{50})_{HIV-1} = 7.26 \ (\pm 0.32) - 5.51 \ (\pm 1.87) \ \sigma^+ \tag{1}$$
$$n = 5, \ r^2 = 0.967, \ s = 0.23, \ q^2 = 0.907$$
$$\log (1/ED_{50})_{HIV-2} = 6.80 \ (\pm 0.34) - 3.26 \ (\pm 1.95) \ \sigma^+ \tag{2}$$
$$n = 5, \ r^2 = 0.904, \ s = 0.24, \ q^2 = 0.784$$

16   **17**   **18**

In these equations ED_{50} refers to the effective dose of the compound required for 50% inhibition of virus-induced cytopathicity in MT-4 cells. Since the negative value of σ^+ refers to the electron-donating ability of substituents *via* resonance, both Equations (1) and (2) suggest that electron donation by X-substituents to N1 might be important for the activity.

The electron-donating effect (not necessarily by resonance) of the X-substituents was also shown to be important in another uridine series (16), studied by Herdewijn et al. [29, 30], when Garg et al. [28] derived Equation (3) for it.

$$\log (1/EC_{50}) = 7.79\ (\pm\ 1.79)\ F_Y - 5.63\ (\pm\ 1.24)\ \sigma_X$$
$$+ 0.55\ (\pm\ 0.41)\ C \log P + 4.62\ (\pm\ 0.64) \tag{3}$$
$$n = 12,\ r^2 = 0.953,\ s = 0.39,\ q^2 = 0.798$$

In this series, the Y-substituents were also varied, for which Equation (3) demonstrated that they would also affect the activity through their field or inductive effect (F_Y). An added effect of overall hydrophobicity of the molecule expressed by $C \log P$ on activity has been shown.

For a still larger series of uridine derivatives (16), studied by several authors [31–33] in human PBM cells varying both X- and Y-substituents, Garg et al. [28] had obtained a correlation as

$$\log (1/EC_{50}) = 3.06\ (\pm\ 1.68) - 5.11\ (\pm\ 2.49)\sigma_{I,\ X} - 0.95\ (\pm\ 0.52)\ L_X$$
$$+ 3.52\ (\pm\ 1.62)\ B1_X + 1.88\ (\pm\ 0.92)\ I_Y \tag{4}$$
$$n = 16,\ r^2 = 0.804,\ s = 0.63,\ q^2 = 0.549$$

This correlation showed that the X-substituents could also have, along with the electronic effect, some negative steric effects as accounted for by the sterimol length parameter L_X. However, their width parameter $B1_X$ was shown to be conducive to the activity. In this correlation, the effect of Y-substituents was described by only an indicator parameter I_Y which was used with a value of unity for $Y = N_3$ and zero for other Y-substituents.

For a series of pyrimidine derivatives (17) studied by Herdewijn et al. [34] in MT-4 cells, where the variation was in nucleic acid bases (B) (i.e., B = thymin-1-yl*, adenin-9-yl, guanine-9-yl, uracil-1-yl, cytosine-1-yl, N^4-methylcytosin-1-yl*, 4-(hydroxyamino)-5-methyl-1,2-dihydro-2-pyrimidin-1-yl, 5-methoxycytosin-1-yl, and N^4-5-dimethylcytosin-1-yl), the activity was shown [28] to be correlated with the McGowan volume of the molecule as

$$\log (1/EC_{50}) = 14.12 \ (\pm 4.03) - 4.62 \ (\pm 2.18) \ \text{MgVol} \tag{5}$$
$$n = 7, \ r^2 = 0.856, \ s = 0.21, \ q^2 = 0.747$$

which suggested that increasing the size of the molecule will be unfavourable to the activity. In deriving Equation (5), the derivatives marked with an asterisk were not included, as they had exhibited the aberrant behaviour.

The FDA-recommended anti-HIV drug stavudine (D4T) (**4**) is a uridine nucleoside analogue. Recently in a communication [35], Siddiqui et al. reported a series of substituted-aryl phosphoramidate derivatives of this analogue (**19**) as membrane-soluble intracellular prodrugs for the free bioactive phosphate to study their structure-activity relationships. Extending this series further [36], these authors made a QSAR study of it to find that the anti-HIV-1 activity of the compounds against CEM cells could be significantly correlated with log P as

$$\log (1/EC_{50}) = 5.157 \ (1.117) \ \log P - 1.499 \ (0.395) \ (\log P)^2 - 2.440 \tag{6}$$
$$n = 21, \ r^2 = 0.807, \ Q^2 = 0.745, \ \log P_o = 1.72$$

where the figures within the parentheses are standard errors of the coefficient rather than 95% confidence intervals and Q^2 is the cross-validated, squared correlation coefficient. This correlation is consistent with cellular transport

20

21

by passive diffusion being a major determinant of the *in vitro* activity. Since the correlation is parabolic in nature, a reasonable estimate of the optimum prodrug lipophilicity could be made (log P_o = 1.72).

Siddiqui et al. had failed to find any effective role of electronic characters of aryl ring substituents in the activity of **19**, but for a series of uridine nucleoside phosphates as represented by **20**, and studied by McGuigan et al. in C8166 cells [37], Garg et al. [28] had found a significant electronic effect on the activity of the substituents of the aryl rings as shown by Equation (7). Equation (7) suggests that electron withdrawal by the ring substituents can favour nucleophilic attack of the receptor site on the phosphorus atom.

$$\log (1/EC_{50}) = 1.42 \ (\pm 0.23) \ \sigma_X + 6.47 \ (\pm 0.21) \tag{7}$$
$$n = 7, \ r^2 = 0.981, \ s = 0.17, \ q^2 = 0.961$$

In the case of purine nucleoside derivatives (**18**), the substituents of the base were found to produce only the steric effects. For a series of **18** with $Y = NH_2$ and $Z = N_3$, the enzyme inhibition data reported by Freeman et al. [38] were found to be correlated with Verloop's width parameter of the X-substituents as [28]

$$\log (1/IC_{50}) = 5.96 \ (\pm 0.29) - 0.29 \ (\pm 0.07) \ B5_X \tag{8}$$
$$n = 16, \ r^2 = 0.837, \ s = 0.17, \ q^2 = 0.761$$

Similarly for another series of **18** with $Y = H$ or NH_2 and $Z = H$, the anti-viral activity reported by Murakami et al. in ATH8 cells [39] was shown to be correlated with Verloop's width parameter B1 of the X-substituents as [28]

$$\log (1/ED_{50}) = 6.47 \ (\pm 0.40) - 0.68 \ (\pm 0.22) \ B1_X \tag{9}$$
$$n = 7, \ r^2 = 0.924, \ s = 0.07, \ q^2 = 0.835$$

Thus, both Equations (8) and (9) suggest that any substituents at the 6-position of the base will not be conducive to the activity because of its steric effect.

3.2 Non-nucleoside analogues

3.2.1 HEPT derivatives

Among the NNRTIs, the HEPT derivatives have drawn more attention than any other class of compounds; hence we start with the QSARs of the HEPT derivatives. Hansch and Zhang [40] were the first to report a QSAR study on a series of **21** studied by Tanaka et al. [41]. This QSAR was, however, later modified by Garg et al. [28] to include the log P term and was reported as shown by Equation (10). This equation suggests that while the overall lipophilicity of the compounds will enhance the activity, the R-substituents at the ortho and meta positions will have the detrimental effects. The Y-substituents, which were only alkyl groups, are, however, shown to produce the favourable effects due to their length, but the parameter L_Y, describing their length, would have an optimum value of 3.7.

$$\log (1/EC_{50}) = 14.58 \ (\pm 3.97) \ L_Y - 1.97 \ (\pm 0.53) \ (L_Y)^2$$
$$- 1.25 \ (\pm 0.77) \ B1_{R,m} + 0.94 \ (\pm 0.36) \ C \log P + 1.51 \ (\pm 0.73) \ Es_{R,o}$$
$$- 20.03 \ (\pm 7.32) \tag{10}$$
$$n = 32, \ r^2 = 0.911, \ s = 0.45, \ q^2 = 0.863$$

Using the same data of Tanaka et al. on the series of **21** with a few more compounds, Garg et al. [42] had tried to show the lipophilic effect of the Y-substituents, with an additional effect of a Y-substituent being an isopropyl group (Eq. 11).

$$\log (1/EC_{50}) = 12.215 \ (\pm 4.297) \ \pi_Y - 5.716 \ (\pm 2.197) \ (\pi_Y)^2$$
$$+ 1.876 \ (\pm 0.808) \ I_{i\text{-}Pr} + 1.305 \ (\pm 0.411) \ I_{m,m'}$$
$$- 0.955 \ (\pm 0.521) \ I_{o,p} - 0.018 \tag{11}$$
$$n = 36, \ r = 0.949, \ s = 0.46, \ F_{5,30} = 54.80$$

Equation (11) shows that although the lipophilic factor of Y-substituents (π_Y) will have an optimum value equal to 1.07, an isopropyl group having the π-value (1.53) greater than this optimum value can favour the activity. This effect of the isopropyl group is shown by an indicator parameter $I_{i\text{-Pr}}$ used for it in the equation with a value of unity.

Equation (11) describes a more detailed effect of R-substituents also. From the indicator parameter $I_{m,m'}$, which has been used with a value of 1 for an R-substituent present at both the meta positions, it is indicated that a substituent present at both the meta positions identically will have a favourable, rather than a detrimental, effect. A detrimental effect will be produced only by an ortho or para substituent as exhibited by the negative coefficient of the indicator parameter $I_{o,p}$ used for them with a value of 1. In Equation (11), F is the F-ratio between the variances of calculated and observed activities.

In neither of their studies could Garg et al. find any relative preference of O or S at the position of X.

All the activity data of **21** reported by Tanaka et al. [40] were in MT-4 cells. For another series of HEPT derivatives (**22**) studied by Tanaka et al. [43] in the same system, Garg et al. first derived Equation (12) [42] and then Equation (13) [28], in which some outliers were not included. In this series, the variation in the substituents at the N1-position (Z-substituents) was also studied. Equation (12) demonstrates an exclusive effect of the molecular size, as measured by van der Waals volume (V_w), of the Z-substituents, which is negative. This negative effect of the molecular size of the Z-substituents is inclusively described by the McGowan volume of the whole molecule in Equation (13).

$$\log (1/EC_{50}) = 2.325 \ (\pm 0.618) \ \pi_Y - 1.457 \ (\pm 0.883) \ V_{w,Z}$$
$$+ 1.562 \ (\pm 0.553) \ I_Z + 1.061 \ (\pm 0.447) \ I_{m,m'} + 5.444 \tag{12}$$
$$n = 35, \ r = 0.917, \ s = 0.47, \ F_{4,30} = 39.68$$

$$\log (1/EC_{50}) = 2.48 \ (\pm 0.66) \ MR_Y - 1.22 \ (\pm 0.88) \ MgVol$$
$$+ 1.44 \ (\pm 0.52) \ I_Z + 1.49 \ (\pm 0.50) \ I_{m,m'} + 6.99 \ (\pm 1.91) \tag{13}$$
$$n = 33, \ r^2 = 0.842, \ s = 0.47, \ q^2 = 0.783$$

The Z-substituents were mostly of the CH_2O-R type where R was an alkyl group or an alkylphenyl group. In both Equations (12) and (13), the I_Z parameter was used for a Z-substituent where R was an alkylphenyl group. An

22   **23**

essentially identical positive coefficient of I_Z in both the equations suggests that a Z-substituent containing an alkylphenyl group, or essentially a phenyl moiety, will be conducive to the activity, notwithstanding its molecular size.

Regarding the R-substituents, which were only H, 3,5-Me$_2$, or 3,5-Cl$_2$, in this series, both Equations (12) and (13) suggest, through the positive coefficient of $I_{m,m'}$, that, as exhibited in the series of **21**, a substituent present at both the meta positions will have a conducive effect in this series also. However, as far as Y-substituents in **22** are concerned, which again were varying alkyl groups, Equation (12) describes a positive effect by them through their hydrophobic character and Equation (13) a positive effect by them through their molar refractivity. Since for alkyl groups, π and MR may be intercorrelated, and since in the series of **21**, only hydrophobic character has been shown to play a role, it seems plausible to attribute the positive effect of the Y-substituents to only their hydrophobic character. The role of the hydrophobic character of Y-substituents was reaffirmed when Garg et al. [42] derived Equation (14) for a series of HEPT derivatives (**23**) studied by Tanaka et al. [44], where the 6-phenylthio group was replaced by a benzyl group.

$$\log (1/EC_{50}) = 2.017 \ (\pm 0.982) \ \pi_Y - 9.051 \ (\pm 8.325) \ V_{w,Z}$$
$$+ 1.511 \ (\pm 0.655) \ I_{m,m'} + 10.556 \tag{14}$$
$$n = 13, \ r = 0.939, \ s = 0.48, \ F_{3,9} = 22.56$$

However, for the same series, Garg et al. [28] later found, by deriving Equation (15), that the hydrophobic character of Y-substituents may have an inclusive effect with total hydrophobicity of the molecule, but their molar refractivity may have an exclusive effect.

$$\log (1/EC_{50}) = 0.46 \ (\pm \ 0.43) \ C \log P + 1.19 \ (\pm \ 0.73) \ I_{m,m'}$$
$$+ 1.71 \ (\pm \ 1.20) \ MR_Y + 3.75 \ (\pm \ 1.31) \tag{15}$$
$$n = 13, \ r^2 = 0.887, \ s = 0.48, \ q^2 = 0.739$$

Regarding the effects of R- and Z- substituents, Equation (12) derived for the series of **22** and Equation (14) derived for the series of **23** agree well with each other. The absence of the parameter I_Z in Equation (14) was due to the absence in the series of **23** of the kind of substituents related to this parameter.

In most of the QSAR studies on HEPT derivatives, however, the overall lipophilicity of the molecule has been found to be the major governing factor. For another series of **22** studied by Baba et al. [45] in MT-4 cells, Garg et al. [28] had derived Equation (16), and for a series of **24** studied by Pontkis et al. [46] in CEM-SS infected cells, the correlation obtained by these authors was as shown by Equation (17). Even against different mutant strains of the HIV-1, the activity of a set of HEPT derivatives (**25**) studied by Balzarini et al. [47] in CEM cells was found to be largely governed by the lipophilicity of the molecules (Eqs.18–24) [28]. The specific roles of various substituents were delineated by some indicator parameters such as I_5, $I_{m,m'}$ and D_6. I_5 is equivalent to $I_{i\text{-}Pr}$ of Equation (11) and $I_{m,m'}$ has the same meaning as in Equations (12) to (14). Now the presence of I_5 with a negative coefficient in Equations (18), (21) and (24) indicates an adverse effect of a isopropyl group at the 5-position which is not consistent with what $I_{i\text{-}Pr}$ indicates in Equation (11). However, $I_{m,m'}$ reaffirms a favourable effect of the presence of a substituent at both the meta positions of the 6-benzyl or 6-thiophenyl ring. The parameter D_6 has been used for the 6-benzyl group ($W = CH_2$), and with a positive coefficient it indicates that a 6-benzyl group is preferred to a thiophenyl group, but it occurs only in Equations (22) and (23).

$$\log (1/EC_{50}) = 0.55 \ (\pm \ 0.22) \ C \log P + 1.15 \ (\pm \ 0.40) \ B5_Z$$
$$+ 2.35 \ (\pm \ 0.99) \tag{16}$$
$$n = 19, \ r^2 = 0.894, \ s = 0.37, \ q^2 = 0.860$$
$$\log (1/EC_{50}) = 3.66 \ (\pm \ 1.49) \ C \log P - 0.48 \ (\pm \ 0.20) \ (C \log P)^2$$
$$+ 0.18 \ (\pm \ 2.29) \tag{17}$$
$$n = 8, \ r^2 = 0.889, \ s = 0.42, \ q^2 = 0.725, \ \log P_o = 3.81$$

Against HIV-1 wild type

24, X = Ph/Py   **25**, W = S/CH$_2$

$$\log (1/EC_{50}) = 4.25\ (\pm 1.67)\ C \log P - 0.50\ (\pm 0.22)\ (C \log P)^2$$
$$- 0.41\ (\pm 0.28)\ I_5 + 0.43\ (\pm 0.28)\ I_{m,m'} - 0.32\ (\pm 3.12) \tag{18}$$
$$n = 18,\ r^2 = 0.839,\ s = 0.26,\ q^2 = 0.650,\ \log P_o = 4.23$$

Against HIV-1 mutant strain 100-Leu → Ile

$$\log (1/IC_{50}) = 2.80\ (\pm 1.52)\ C \log P - 0.30\ (\pm 0.20)\ (C \log P)^2$$
$$+ 0.47\ (\pm 0.28)\ I_{m,m'} + 1.47\ (\pm 2.76) \tag{19}$$
$$n = 21,\ r^2 = 0.813,\ s = 0.30,\ q^2 = 0.691,\ \log P_o = 4.60$$

Against HIV-1 mutant strain 103-Lys → Asn

$$\log (1/EC_{50}) = 0.29\ (\pm 0.16)\ C \log P + 0.86\ (\pm 0.23)\ I_{m,m'}$$
$$+ 4.81\ (\pm 0.61) \tag{20}$$
$$n = 18,\ r^2 = 0.864,\ s = 0.22,\ q^2 = 0.821$$

Against HIV-1 mutant strain 106-Val → Ala

$$\log (1/EC_{50}) = 2.45\ (\pm 1.38)\ C \log P - 0.26\ (\pm 0.18)\ (C \log P)^2$$
$$- 0.41\ (\pm 0.26)\ I_5 + 1.31\ (\pm 2.50) \tag{21}$$
$$n = 20,\ r^2 = 0.847,\ s = 0.26,\ q^2 = 0.721,\ \log P_o = 4.82$$

Against HIV-1 mutant strain 138-Glu → Lys

$$\log (1/EC_{50}) = 0.29\ (\pm 0.14)\ C \log P + 0.60\ (\pm 0.21)\ I_{m,m'}$$
$$+ 0.43\ (\pm 0.27)\ D_6 + 5.88\ (\pm 0.52) \tag{22}$$
$$n = 18,\ r^2 = 0.857,\ s = 0.19,\ q^2 = 0.798$$

Against HIV-1 mutant strain 181-Tyr → Cys

$$\log (1/EC_{50}) = 0.55\ (\pm 0.13)\ C \log P + 0.44\ (\pm 0.19)\ I_{m,m'}$$
$$+ 0.68\ (\pm 0.26)\ D_6 + 4.02\ (\pm 0.49) \tag{23}$$
$$n = 20,\ r^2 = 0.894,\ s = 0.19,\ q^2 = 0.817$$

Against HIV-1 mutant strain 181-Tyr → Ile

$$\log (1/EC_{50}) = 0.47\ (\pm 0.15)\ C \log P - 1.06\ (\pm 0.25)\ I_5$$
$$+ 0.23\ (\pm 0.23)\ I_{m,m'} + 4.20\ (\pm 0.57) \tag{24}$$
$$n = 18,\ r^2 = 0.910,\ s = 0.22,\ q^2 = 0.868$$

Not only the activity, but also even the toxicity of the compounds has been found to be largely governed by the lipophilicity of the molecules. The CC_{50} activity data for the series of **18** reported by Tanaka et al. [43] were shown to be correlated with $C \log P$ as shown by Equation (25) [28] and for another set of congeners of **18** reported by Baba et al. [45] as shown by Equation (26) [28]. Both the equations suggest the sole dependence of the toxicity on the lipophilicity of the molecule.

$$\log(1/CC_{50}) = 0.35\ (\pm 0.06)\ C \log P + 2.82\ (\pm 0.22) \tag{25}$$
$$n = 23,\ r^2 = 0.870,\ s = 0.14,\ q^2 = 0.841$$
$$\log (1/CC_{50}) = 0.47\ (\pm 0.09)\ C \log P + 2.49\ (\pm 0.26) \tag{26}$$
$$n = 14,\ r^2 = 0.919,\ s = 0.09,\ q^2 = 0.899$$

In certain cases the steric parameters have also been shown to play the dominant role. For a small set of congeners of **26** studied by Tanaka et al. [48], the anti-viral activity in MT-4 cells was shown to be correlated with only the sterimol width parameter B5 of the 6-position substituents (Eq. 27) [28] and for a larger set of congeners of **27** studied by Kim et al. [49] in CEM-SS infected cells, the activity was found to be correlated with both length and width parameters of Z-substituents (Eq. 28) [28]. Thus Equations (27) and (28) suggested that while the width of 6-position substituents may be favourable to the activity, the same of the Z-moiety of N1-substituent may not; rather, its length may, but with an optimum value of 6.44.

26   **27**

$$\log (1/EC_{50}) = 2.07 \ (\pm 0.85) \ B5_R - 7.88 \ (\pm 5.27) \tag{27}$$
$$n = 8, \ r^2 = 0.856, \ s = 0.29, \ q^2 = 0.734$$
$$\log (1/EC_{50}) = 1.23 \ (\pm 1.02) \ L_Z - 0.01 \ (\pm 0.08) \ (I_Z)^2$$
$$- 0.58 \ (\pm 0.15) \ B5_Z + 1.28 \ (\pm 0.32) \ \pi_{R\text{-}3,5} + 3.46 \ (\pm 3.32) \tag{28}$$
$$n = 27, \ r^2 = 0.841, \ s = 0.29, \ q^2 = 0.761, \ (L_Z)_o = 6.44$$

For a very large series of HEPT derivatives, which includes almost all sets of **22** discussed so far plus some new series of it taken from other sources [50–55], Luco and Ferretti [56] correlated the EC_{50} data with a number of structural parameters which were of little importance from the mechanistic point of view. Using the same parameters, however, Luco and Ferretti [56] had also performed a partial least-squares (PLS) analysis which had resulted in a significant three-component model with high predictive value with a cross-validated value of r (r_{cv}) equal to 0.927.

Later Garg et al. [28], however, found that the activity of this series could be correlated with fewer and simpler structural parameters along with C log P (Eq. 29). Although Equation (29) was not of as high a predictive value as the analysis made by Luco and Ferretti and although this equation was obtained excluding a few outliers, it exhibited more clearly the role of steric parameters of various substituents and of the overall lipophilicity of the molecule. Similarly, for a very large series of **21** that included all these compounds that we have already discussed and a few more compounds reported by Hopkins et al. [57], Kireev et al. [58] had obtained Equation (30), which demonstrated some role of electronic factors also along with the steric factors.

$$\log (1/IC_{50}) = 6.65 \ (\pm 2.79) - 1.67 \ (\pm 1.35) \ B1_{R,2'}$$
$$+ 1.06 \ (\pm 0.38) \ B5_{R,5'} - 1.92 \ (\pm 1.62) \ B1_Y + 2.80 \ (\pm 0.78) \ MR_Y$$
$$+ 0.24 \ (\pm 0.15) \ C \log P \tag{29}$$
$$n = 73, \ r^2 = 0.815, \ s = 0.60, \ q^2 = 0.783$$

$$\log (1/EC_{50}) = 1.64 - 1.92 \ (\pm 0.28) \ \Sigma(q-)_6 + 1.43 \ (\pm 0.11) \ (^{1/2}W_5)$$
$$- 0.47 \ (\pm 0.07) \ W_{cis} + 0.41 \ (\pm 0.05) \ (RB5)_{cis} \qquad (30)$$
$$n = 87, \ r^2 = 0.884, \ s = 0.46$$

The $\Sigma(q-)_6$ in Equation (30) refers to the total negative charge, calculated by using the AM1 method, over the atoms of the C6-substituent, W_5 refers to the width of the plane C5-substituent, W_{cis} is the width parameter of the whole molecule when the rotatable bond S-C1' is cis to N1-C6 bond, and $(RB5)_{cis}$ is the rotation barrier to the rotatable bond (S-C1' numbered as 5) when cis to the N1-C6 bond. Thus, besides the electronic and steric (molecular size) effects, the effect of conformational flexibility of the molecule is also shown.

A detailed conformational study of HEPT was studied by Lawtrakul et al. [59, 60], which was concerned with the dihedral angle α (rotation about the C6-S bond) that determines the position of the phenyl ring with respect to the thymine ring. Using the semi-empirical AM1 and *ab initio* HF/3-21G methods, these authors found that two energy minima existed, one for a dihedral angle α of ca. 65–76° and the other for an α value of about 244–250°. The energy barrier between these two minima due to the steric interactions between the phenyl ring and the side-chain, as well as the methyl group of the thymine ring (5-CH$_3$), was found to be 18–21 kJ/mol from AM1 and 36–38 kJ/mol from the *ab initio* method. The comparison of calculated ^{1}H NMR spectra with the experiment indicated that the first minimum is the preferred conformation in solution which corresponds to the geometry of the molecule when complexed with the enzyme as determined by X-ray diffraction.

Some detailed studies on the electronic effects on the activity of HEPT derivatives were also made by the Lawtrakul group [61–63]. For the series of **21** for which Equations (10) and (11) were reported, Hannongbua et al. [61] reported Equation (31) representing the best correlation among several equations derived by them.

$$\log (1/EC_{50}) = 0.198 \ (\pm 0.134) \ HE + 0.093 \ (\pm 0.052) \ MR$$
$$+ 45.797 \ (\pm 35.602) \ C5 + 38.482 \ (\pm 27.062) \ C6 + 14.418 \ (\pm 8.835) \qquad (31)$$
$$n = 35, \ r = 0.869, \ s = 0.743, \ q^2 = 0.665$$

In Equation (31) HE represents the hydration energy (kcal/mol) and MR the molar refractivity of the molecule, while C5 and C6 represent the atomic net charges on the C5 and C6 atoms, respectively. Thus, as far as electronic effects are concerned, the net charges on C5 and C6 atoms are suggested to be conducive to the activity, probably due to involvement of these atoms in some electrostatic interactions with the receptor. A significant improvement in this correlation was shown (Eq. 32) when an outlier was excluded [61], but then the coefficient of C5 had become insignificant at the 95% confidence level. All the electronic properties of the molecules were calculated using the semi-empirical AM1 method.

$$\log (1/EC_{50}) = 0.228 \ (\pm 0.121) \ HE + 0.118 \ (\pm 0.049) \ MR$$
$$+ 31.072 \ (\pm 33.111) \ C5 + 28.979 \ (\pm 24.851) \ C6 + 10.195 \ (\pm 8.339) \qquad (32)$$
$$n = 34, \ r = 0.902, \ s = 0.658, \ q^2 = 0.760$$

For the same series of compounds, however, when a comparative molecular field analysis (CoMFA) was performed by Hannongbua et al. [62], it was found that electrostatic interaction was of little importance as compared to the steric interaction, which could explain a majority (70%) of the variance in the activity. But in a recent CoMFA study on a very large series of HEPT derivatives belonging to **22** and **23**, Hannongbua et al. [63] supported their earlier QSAR model [61] that the atomic charge at C5 position plays an important role in the binding.

Using different quantum mechanical methods, Lawtrakul and Hannongbua [64] examined the electronic effects in the series of HEPT derivatives represented by **28**, where the X-substituents varied from a thiophenyl group to a variety of aliphatic groups [43]. In this examination, no consistency was, however, found in the role of the atomic charges, but the polarizability of the molecule was found to be a constant factor in all the correlations derived, irrespective of the method used to find the polarizability factor Pol. If only this factor, calculated by the AM1 method, was used, a correlation obtained was as shown by Equation (33), which demonstrates a significant effect of the polarizability of the molecule on the activity.

$$\log (1/EC_{50}) = 0.083 \ (\pm 0.035) \ Pol + 1.688 \ (\pm 1.103) \qquad (33)$$
$$n = 27, \ r = 0.701, \ s = 0.567, \ q^2 = 0.438$$

For the same set of compounds as treated by Luco and Ferretti [56], Jalali-Heravi and Parastar [65] had obtained equation (34) in which an electronic para-

28

meter C(+/–), representing the ratio of the partial charges on the most positive and the most negative atoms, was introduced.

$$\log (1/EC_{50}) = 3.307 \ (\pm 0.679) \ (1/S) + 2.013 \ (\pm 0.741) \ C \ (+/-)$$
$$+ 6.689 \times 10^{-3} \ (\pm 1.631 \times 10^{-3}) \ \Delta H_f + 0.141 \ (\pm 0.028) \ (N_{C-Y})^2$$
$$- 0.804 \ (\pm 0.171) \ N_{OH-Z} + 5.097 \times 10^{-3} \ (\pm 9.938 \times 10^{-4})(\Sigma x'_R)^3$$
$$+ 2.977 \ (\pm 1.335) \tag{34}$$
$$n = 80, \ r = 0.901, \ s = 0.607, \ F_{6,73} = 52$$

The significance of this parameter can be almost attached to the delocalization of the charge. Since for each molecule C(+/–) was taken negative, Equation (34) suggests that the presence of an atom with high positive charge or the presence of an atom with very low negative charge will not be favourable to the activity. The other parameters in Equation (34) have been defined as follows: the S stands for the standard shadow area on the Y-Z plane. The molecules are drawn in such a way that their two rings are in the X-Y plane. Therefore, for the molecules whose substituents are large and can be positioned out of the X-Y plane, the shadow area on the Y-Z plane is large and hence shows a smaller activity because of the smaller value of 1/S. ΔH_f refers to the heat of formation in kcal/mol. It has a negative value, therefore high heat of formation does not seem to be conducive to the activity. (N_{C-Y}) stands for the number of sp^3 carbon atoms in a 5-position substituent Y. A positive coefficient of this in the equation suggests that a more saturated Y-substituent may be more effective. The parameter N_{OH-Z} refers to the number of OH groups in a Z-substituent at the N1- position. The negative coefficient of it in the equation indicates that the presence of more hydroxyl groups in the Z-substituents may have an adverse effect. The last parameter, $\Sigma x'_R$, refers to the sum of the positions of R-substituents on the C6-aromatic ring, e.g., for a 3',5'-Me$_2$, $\Sigma x'_R = 6$, since 5' is equivalent to 3'. With a power of 3 and a positive coefficient in the equation, this parameter indicates that a highly substituted phenyl ring may be advantageous. It agrees well with the finding that a substituent present at both the meta positions will favour the activity (Eqs. 11–14).

Equation (34), however, does not allow us to discuss much about the nature of drug-receptor interactions. Lawtrakul et al. [60], while studying the conformational effect, pointed out that the pocket in which HEPT binds is characterized by a mainly hydrophobic surface. The binding force depends on the complementary molecular shape of the inhibitor molecules and results from a number of van der Waals and ring-stacking interactions and contributes to the electrostatic interactions as well as to the hydrogen bonding.

In their CoMFA study [63], Hannongbua et al. pointed out that one of the important binding modes of the HEPT derivatives is the interaction of an alkyl side-chain, positioned at C5, with Tyr 181 and Tyr 188 residues in the binding pocket of RT. It was also, however, pointed out that only a moderately sized group at C5 would be favourable to the activity. The C5-substituent is supposed to be involved in steric interactions. A smaller group may have insufficient steric requirements to push it into the binding pocket of the enzyme and a larger group may render the ligand too large for the pocket. The experiment has shown that an isopropyl group is the best to be substituted at the C5-position [43]. Garg et al. have confirmed this by deriving Equation (11), which exclusively accounts for the effect of the C5-isopropyl group by an indicator parameter $I_{i\text{-}Pr}$.

In HEPT derivatives, the substituents on the phenylthio (or benzyl) side-chain at C6 of the thymine ring increase the hydrophobicity of the molecules, which results in a favourable inhibition by the improvement of the interaction of the molecules with the hydrophobic binding pocket of HIV-1 RT.

The hydrophobic nature of the NNRTI pocket in the enzyme provides relatively few possibilities for polar interactions and hydrogen bondings. However, the geometry of interaction for HEPT analogues appears to be constrained by a strong hydrogen bond from the 3-NH of the thymine ring to the carbonyl oxygen of Lys 101.

3.2.2 TIBO derivatives

The derivates of 4,5,6,7-tetrahydro-5-methylimidazo[4,5,1-jk][1,4]benzodiazepin-2(1H)-one (TIBO) have also been quite extensively studied by a number of investigators [66-70]. Gupta and Garg [71] were the first to make a QSAR study on anti-HIV data of TIBO derivatives reported by some of these investigators. Three different series as represented by **29–31** and reported by Ho et al. [70], Kukla et al. [67] and Breslin et al. [69], respectively, were taken by Gupta and Garg. For the series of **29**, Gupta and Garg had obtained Equation (35) and then, combining a set of 21 compounds of the series of **30**, obtained Equation (36).

$$\log (1/EC_{50}) = 0.751 \ (\pm 0.389) \ \pi_X + 1.250 \ (\pm 0.574) \ I_Z$$
$$+ 0.601 \ (\pm 0.769) \ I_R + 0.800 \ (\pm 0.540) \ I_8 + 4.687 \tag{35}$$
$$n = 34, \ r = 0.883, \ s = 0.70, \ F_{4,29} = 25.57$$

$$\log (1/EC_{50}) = 0.694 \ (\pm 0.324) \ \pi_X + 1.337 \ (\pm 0.449) \ I_Z$$
$$+ 0.842 \ (\pm 0.487) \ I_R + 0.930 \ (\pm 0.421) \ I_8 + 4.279 \tag{36}$$
$$n = 55, \ r = 0.925, \ s = 0.62, \ F_{4,50} = 73.74$$

In both Equations (35) and (36), the indicator parameter I_Z is equal to 1 for $Z = S$ and zero for $Z = O$, and the parameter I_R is equal to 1 for $R = DMA$ (3,3-dimethylallyl) and zero for $R = CPM$ (cyclopropylmethyl) or DEA (3,3-diethylallyl). In Equation (35), I_R did not appear to be significant at the 95% confidence level but in Equation (36) it was found to be quite significant. It had become significant for Equation (35) also, when an outlier (the only compound having $R = DEA$) was excluded (Eq. 37). The exclusion of this outlier had also significantly improved the value of r.

$$\log (1/EC_{50}) = 0.635 \ (\pm 0.375) \ \pi_X + 1.311 \ (\pm 0.535) \ I_Z$$
$$+ 0.855 \ (\pm 0.746) \ I_R + 0.837 \ (\pm 0.502) \ I_8 + 4.408 \tag{37}$$
$$n = 33, \ r = 0.904, \ s = 0.65, \ F_{4,28} = 31.20$$

The third indicator variable I_8 was used, with a value of unity, for any substituent present at the 8-position of the aromatic ring. Thus, in all three equations (Eqs. 35–37) the positive coefficients of I_Z, I_R and I_8 suggested that at position 2, $Z = S$ will have better effect than $Z = O$, at position 6, $R = DMA$ will be better than $R = CPM$ or DEA, and the presence of any substituent at the 8-position of the phenyl ring will be advantageous. Thus, the 8-position substituents were shown to have an additional effect, as the occurrence of the hydrophobic parameter π_X in all three equations showed that any X-substituent present at any position of the phenyl ring will have a hydrophobic effect on the activity. All the activity data reported by Ho et al. [70] and Kukla et al. [67] were measured in MT-4 cells.

For the activity data in MT-4 cells reported by Breslin et al. [69] for the series of **31**, Gupta and Garg had obtained Equation (38) [71], which contained only the indicator variables. However, Gupta and Garg were able to combine this series of compounds also with those of **29** and **30** to obtain Equation (39) [71], where the additional parameter I_5 equal to 1 was for a 5-Me group with S-configuration. With a positive coefficient, this parameter indicated that at the 5-position a methyl group with S-configuration would be preferred. However, in Equation (38), which was derived for only the series of **31**, where the substitution in the diazepine ring at positions other than C5 and N6 (Y-substitution) was also examined, the presence of an indicator variable D, used with a value of 1 for a disubstitution excluding the N6-position, indicated, with a negative coefficient, that a disubstitution may have a detrimental effect, which, however, did not emerge in Equation (39) derived for the combined series. Instead of π_X, only a dummy variable I_X was used in Equation (38) for X-substituents, as X was only Cl or H. I_X was equal to 1 for X = Cl and 0 for X = H.

$$\log (1/EC_{50}) = 0.829 \ (\pm 0.531) \ I_X + 1.185 \ (\pm 0.484) \ I_Z$$
$$+ 0.874 \ (\pm 0.539) \ I_R + 0.851 \ (\pm 0.600) \ I_5 - 0.795 \ (\pm 0.631) \ D + 4.521 \qquad (38)$$
$$n = 36, \ r = 0.877, \ s = 0.65, \ F_{5,30} = 20.08$$

$$\log (1/EC_{50}) = 0.789 \ (\pm 0.297) \ \pi_X + 1.212 \ (\pm 0.308) \ I_Z$$
$$+ 0.706 \ (\pm 0.337) \ I_R + 0.991 \ (\pm 0.350) \ I_8 + 1.109 \ (\pm 0.518) \ I_5 + 4.352 \qquad (39)$$
$$n = 89, \ r = 0.900, \ s = 0.65, \ F_{5,83} = 70.57$$

For this combined series, Garg et al. [28] had reattempted a QSAR to find the effect of overall hydrophobicity of the molecule and obtained Equation (40).

In this equation the effect of 8-position substituents was accounted for by Verloop's width parameter B1, which did exhibit a positive role of these substituents. The overall hydrophobicity of the molecule was also shown to be important. However, in deriving Equation (40), a few outliers had to be excluded.

$$\log (1/EC_{50}) = 0.39\ (\pm 0.20)\ C \log P + 1.16\ (\pm 0.43)\ B1_8$$
$$+ 1.49\ (\pm 0.28)\ I_Z + 0.88\ (\pm 0.36)\ I_R + 1.80\ (\pm 0.78) \tag{40}$$
$$n = 82,\ r^2 = 0.861,\ s = 0.55,\ q^2 = 0.840$$

Garg et al. [28] found that the overall hydrophobicity of the molecule could be a common factor in the activity of different series of TIBO derivatives, as for one more series of **29** with sufficient variation in R-substituents [72], the correlation obtained was as

$$\log (1/EC_{50}) = 0.93\ (\pm 0.34)\ C \log P + 1.79\ (\pm 0.56)\ I_Z + 3.50\ (\pm 1.46) \tag{41}$$
$$n = 22,\ r^2 = 0.820,\ s = 0.57,\ q^2 = 0.767$$

However, for this series of the compounds studied by Pauwels et al. [72], the cytotoxic activity was found to be more influenced by hydrophobicity (Eq. 42) [28] than the anti-HIV activity (compare the coefficient of log P of Eq. 42 with that of Eq. 41), but the hydrophobicity had an optimum value for the cytotoxicity (log P_o = 5.55).

$$\log (1/CC_{50}) = 2.40\ (\pm 1.49)\ C \log P - 0.22\ (\pm 0.18)\ (C \log P)^2$$
$$- 1.88\ (\pm 3.02) \tag{42}$$
$$n = 19,\ r^2 = 0.813,\ s = 0.27,\ q^2 = 0.753,\ \log P_o = 5.55$$

For a selected set of 46 compounds from the series of **29–31**, Hannongbua et al. [73] reported a correlation as shown by Equation (43) to delineate the electronic effects on the anti-HIV activity of TIBO derivatives.

$$\log (1/EC_{50}) = 8.697\ (\pm 1.474) - 3.320\ (\pm 1.175)\ C2$$
$$- 6.506\ (\pm 2.489)\ C4 + 16.743\ (\pm 7.022)\ C8 + 6.473\ (\pm 3.866)\ C9$$
$$- 12.312\ (\pm 11.227)\ C13 \tag{43}$$
$$n = 46,\ r = 0.869,\ s = 0.662,\ q^2 = 0.677$$

In this equation C's refer to the net atomic charges at various carbon atoms; thus the equation exhibits the positive and negative effects of the charges at some atoms. Since the coefficient of C8 is largest, Hannongbua et al. argued that the presence of a strong electron-withdrawing substituent at the 8-position, which can increase the positive charge of C8 by withdrawing the electron, may be of great value for the activity. Although the set of compounds treated by Hannongbua et al. had only Cl at the 8-position, their finding is consistent with the finding of Gupta and Garg (Eqs. 35, 36 and 39) that an 8-position substituent will have an additional effect. An electron-withdrawing substituent at the 9-position is also shown to be advantageous. These observations of Hannongbua et al. or those of Gupta and Garg are in agreement with the empirical observation that compounds with 8-Cl and/or 9-Cl are more active than those without it.

In the same communication [73], Hannongbua et al. had also performed a CoMFA study, which revealed that one of the important binding sites of the TIBO derivatives was a dimethylallyl (DMA) side-chain substituted at N6, which could be involved in the steric interaction with Tyr 181 and Tyr 188 residues in the binding pocket of RT. The specific effect of this group was indicated in the studies made by Gupta and Garg (Eqs. 35, 36 and 39) and Garg et al. (Eq. 40) by the use of the indicator parameter I_R for this group.

From the CoMFA model [73], it was also suggested that a Cl atom substituted at 8- or/and 9-position(s) of the benzene ring can, by increasing the hydrophobicity of the molecule, improve the hydrophobic interactions of the molecule with the lipophilic binding pocket of the enzyme, thus making the molecule a better inhibitor.

3.2.3 Nevirapine derivatives

Nevirapine (7) is one of the NNRTIs which have been recommended by the FDA for the treatment of HIV infections. Therefore, its derivatives have been studied in detail for the anti-HIV activity. QSAR studies on nevirapine analogues have been recently reported by Garg et al. [28]. For a small series of 4-substituted nevirapines (32) studied by Kelly et al. [74], the enzyme inhibition activity against wild-type HIV-1 RT was found to be correlated with the hydrophobicity of the molecule and the molar refractivity index of the X-substituents as shown by Equation (44).

$$CH_2O-X$$

32

$$\log (1/IC_{50}) = 6.54 \ (\pm 0.62) - 0.84 \ (\pm 0.36) \ C \log P$$
$$+ 0.89 \ (\pm 0.31) \ MR_X \qquad (44)$$
$$n = 13, \ r^2 = 0.808, \ s = 0.25, \ q^2 = 0.595$$

In this series, the X-substituents were alkyl, benzyl, or substituted phenyl groups. The hydrophobicity of the molecule was controlled by only the X-substituent, whose molar refractivity seems to favour the activity. The negative effect of C log P, therefore, can be attributed to the limited bulk tolerance of the active sites of the enzyme. The hydrophobicity was otherwise shown to favour the enzyme inhibition activity, when Garg et al. obtained Equations (45a) for a series of pyridobenzodiazepin-5-ones (**33a**) and Equation (45b) for a series of dipyridodiazepin-6-ones (**33b**), both studied by Hargrave et al. [75].

$$\log (1/IC_{50}) = 0.94 \ (\pm 0.19) \ C \log P - 0.82 \ (\pm 0.21) \ B5_{11}$$
$$- 1.09 \ (\pm 0.41) \ I + 6.32 \ (\pm 0.67) \qquad (45a)$$
$$n = 28, \ r^2 = 0.847, \ s = 0.31, q^2 = 0.765$$
$$\log (1/IC_{50}) = 0.38 \ (\pm 0.11) \ C \log P - 1.54 \ (\pm 0.52) \ B1_{11}$$
$$- 0.51 \ (\pm 0.36) \ I_3 + 7.84 \ (\pm 0.86) \qquad (45b)$$
$$n = 20, \ r^2 = 0.840, \ s = 0.26, \ q^2 = 0.789$$

However, in both the cases, the 11-position substituents were found to produce some detrimental steric effects. Also in the series of **33a**, a detrimental effect of 2- and 3-substituents, too, was shown, through an indicator variable I (Eq. 45a), which was used with a value of unity for these substituents. Similarly, in the series of **33b**, an adverse effect of 3-Cl or 3-Me as described by the I_3 parameter used for them, with a value of unity, was also shown in Equation (45b). All substituents in both the series were comprised of small

33a

33b

34

35

but varying groups like Me, Et, c-Pr, OMe, NO_2, NH_2, SMe, $CHMe_2$, CF_3, Cl, etc.

Also for a series of pyridobenzoxazepinones (**34**), studied by Klunder et al. [76], the enzyme inhibition activity was shown to be governed by the hydrophobicity of the molecule (Eq. 46), but in a series of benzoxazepinones (**35**), studied by Klunder et al. [76], the role of hydrophobicity could not be demonstrated; rather, the molar refractivity of some substituents was shown to favour the activity (Eq. 47) [28].

$$\log (1/IC_{50}) = 0.67 \ (\pm 0.31) \ C \log P + 1.36 \ (\pm 0.68) \ B1_7$$
$$+ 0.75 \ (\pm 0.40) \ \alpha_7 + 3.59 \ (\pm 1.44) \tag{46}$$
$$n = 13, \ r^2 = 0.862, \ s = 0.23, \ q^2 = 0.608$$

$$\log (1/IC_{50}) = 0.55 \ (\pm 0.25) \ MR_{2,7,9} - 0.52 \ (\pm 0.23) \ MR_{8,10}$$
$$+ 6.94 \ (\pm 0.46) \tag{47}$$
$$n = 19, \ r^2 = 0.821, \ s = 0.22, \ q^2 = 0.727$$

However, Equation (47) shows that the molar refractivity of some substituents may have detrimental effects also. From a CoMFA study on a set of dipyridodiazepinones (**33b**) selected from the studies of Kelly et al. [74, 77] and Proudfoot et al. [78], Pungpo and Hannongbua [79] observed that both the steric and electrostatic interactions play important roles in RT inhibition, but found that in the inhibition of wild-type RT the former play a more significant role than the latter, while in the inhibition of mutant-type RT (Y 181 C) both have approximately equal contributions.

3.2.4 Pyridinone derivatives

Pyridinone derivatives were also found to act as HIV-1 RT inhibitors. Garg and Gupta [80] reported QSAR studies on four different series of pyridinone derivatives (36–39) studied by Hoffman et al. [81–84]. In 36–38, the R-substituents were only Me, Cl, F, OH, OMe, NO_2, or NH_2. For the series of 36, where the effect of variation was examined only in R-substituents [83], Garg and Gupta had obtained Equation (48), which showed a favourable hydrophobic effect of 4- and 7-substituents, although with an optimum value of $\pi_{4,7} = 1.49$, but a negative effect of hydrophobicity of 5- and 6-substituents. This negative effect of 5- and 6-substituents can be attributed either to the steric role played by these substituents or to the polar nature of the binding sites for these substituents in the receptor. All the substituents were, however, shown to have electronic effects also through the electron donation.

$$
\begin{aligned}
\log (1/IC_{50}) = {}&1.569 \ (\pm 0.389) \ \pi_{4,7} - 0.526 \ (\pm 0.403) \ (\pi_{4,7})^2 \\
&- 1.335 \ (\pm 1.210) \ \pi_{5,6} - 1.077 \ (\pm 0.678) \ \alpha_R + 6.544 \\
&n = 19, \ r = 0.926, \ s = 0.40, \ F_{4,14} = 20.97
\end{aligned}
\tag{48}
$$

For the series of 37, where the effect of change in the linker chain was also studied [84], the correlation obtained by Garg and Gupta was as

$$
\begin{aligned}
\log (1/IC_{50}) = {}&9.559 \ (\pm 1.811) \ V_{w,L} - 1.204 \ (\pm 0.233) \ (V_{w,L})^2 \\
&+ 0.408 \ (\pm 0.277) \ \pi_R - 1.141 \ (\pm 0.504) \ I_{5,6} - 11.565 \\
&n = 32, \ s = 0.39, \ r = 0.925, \ F_{4,27} = 40.09
\end{aligned}
\tag{49}
$$

which also demonstrated through the negative coefficient of an indicator variable $I_{5,6}$, that 5- and 6-substituents would have the detrimental effects, most probably due to their steric roles. The $I_{5,6}$ was given a value of 1 for 5- and 6-substituents and zero for other R-substituents. However, in totality all R-substituents were shown to produce the hydrophobic effect.

36

37

38

39

As far as the linker chain is concerned, its size was shown to be conducive to the activity, with an optimum value of $V_{w,L} = 3.97 \times 10^2$ Å^3. The change of X from O to S was found to have little effect.

In the series of **38**, L was changed only from CH_2CH_2 to $NHCH_2$ [83, 84], which could be shown to be of little importance in the study of Garg and Gupta. Similarly, in this series R was either 4,7-Cl_2 or H, whose effect could be described by a simple indicator parameter I_R, assigning a value of 1 for 4,7-Cl_2 and zero for H. The main variation was studied in Y-substituents at the pyridinone ring. A very simple equation (Eq. 50) was obtained for this series, demonstrating the hydrophobic effects of Y-substituents and a beneficial role of 4,7-substituents, which can also be due to the hydrophobic character of Cl groups, as such substituents in the series of **36** and **37** have been shown to have only hydrophobic effects.

$$\log (1/EC_{50}) = 0.553 \ (\pm 0.246) \ \pi_Y + 0.937 \ (\pm 0.524) \ I_R + 6.038 \qquad (50)$$
$$n = 24, \ r = 0.882, \ s = 0.57, \ F_{2,21} = 21.87$$

In the series of **39**, the variation in substituents at one more position of the pyridinone ring was studied, i.e., 6-position-substituents (Z-substituents), and the series also had more variation in the linker chain [82]. For this series of compounds, the equation obtained by Garg and Gupta [80] was as

$$\log (1/IC_{50}) = 3.452 \ (\pm \ 1.538) \ \pi_Y - 1.243 \ (\pm 0.704) \ (\pi_Y)^2$$
$$- 1.249 \ (\pm \ 1.250) \ \pi_Z + 3.209 \ (\pm 0.608) \ I_L + 2.590 \qquad (51)$$
$$n = 12, \ r = 0.982, \ s = 0.32, \ F_{4,7} = 48.36$$

which again demonstrated the hydrophobic role of Y-substituents, but with an optimum value of $\pi_Y = 1.39$. Equation (51), however, indicated a negative role of the Z-substituents, suggesting that no substituent at the 6-position of the pyridinone ring could be tolerated. A Z-substituent may have steric bulk effect and probably this may be the reason for the Y-substituents also to have the limited effect, being at the adjacent position (5-position).

Regarding these pyridinone derivatives, almost the same conclusions were drawn when Garg et al. reattempted a QSAR on them, taking into account the total hydrophobicity of the molecule [28].

3.2.5 TSAO derivatives

The anti-viral activity has also been found to be associated with ter-butyl-dimethylsilylspiroaminooxathioledioxide (TSAO) pyrimidine and pyrimidine –modified nucleosides (40, 41). Compound 40, having a thymine ring, is referred to as a TSAO-T nucleoside and compound 41, having a cytosine ring, as a TSAO-C nucleoside. Garg and Gupta [85] made a detailed QSAR study on some series of 40 and 41 studied by the Camarasa group [86–88]. For a series of 40, where X-substituents were like CH_3, C_2H_5, F, Br, Cl, CF_3, CN, $C(=NH)OCH_3$, H, etc., and Y-substituents were only alkyl or alkene groups, the activity (EC_{50} in MT-4 cells) was shown to be correlated with physicochemical parameters as

$$\log (1/EC_{50}) = 0.678 \ (\pm 0.248) \ \pi_X - 1.385 \ (\pm 0.668) \ \sigma_X$$
$$- 0.244 \ (\pm 0.241) \ \pi_Y + 6.548 \qquad (52)$$
$$n = 15, \ r = 0.925, \ s = 0.25, \ F_{3,11} = 21.64$$

Similarly, for a small set of 41, where Z-substituents were substituted or unsubstituted NH_2 groups, the correlation obtained was:

$$\log (1/EC_{50}) = 1.265 \ (\pm 1.260) \ \sigma_Z + 0.717 \ (\pm 0.402) \ I_X + 6.414 \qquad (53)$$
$$n = 7, \ r = 0.931, \ s = 0.18, \ F_{2,4} = 13.03$$

40   **41**

Equation (52) shows that while the hydrophobic character of X-substituents can favour the activity, the same of Y-substituents may not. To account for the effect of X-substituents in **41**, a dummy variable I_X was used, since there X was either a CH_3 group or H. With a value of 1 for CH_3, the presence of this variable with a positive coefficient in Equation (53) suggested a favourable role (essentially hydrophobic) of X-substituents in the series of **41** also. Equation (52), however, shows that X-substituents can be important electronically also, if they possess an electron-donating nature.

In equation (53), a positive coefficient of σ_Z suggested that a Z-substituent in the TSAO-C series (**41**) can be important because of its electron-withdrawing nature. However, σ_Z was only marginally significant at the 95% confidence level. Hence, when Garg and Gupta combined both TSAO-T and TSAO-C series (**40 and 41**) and obtained Equation (54), the role of σ_Z could not emerge.

$$\log (1/EC_{50}) = 0.696\ (\pm 0.229)\ \pi_X - 1.396\ (\pm 0.644)\ \sigma_X$$
$$- 0.247\ (\pm 0.233)\ \pi_Y + 0.213\ (\pm 0.296)\ D + 6.330 \tag{54}$$
$$n = 22,\ r = 0.900,\ s = 0.25,\ F_{4,17} = 18.20$$

In Equation (54), the dummy variable D was used, with a value of unity, for the TSAO-T series (**40**). Since the coefficient of D was not found to be statistically significant, a little advantage of a thymine ring over a cytosine ring could be demonstrated.

42

43

In their further study on these two series of compounds, Garg et al. [28] were able to show by the use of Verloop's L parameter that the negative hydrophobic effect of Y-substituents in the TSAO-T series (40) could be better attributed to their steric character (Eq. 55).

$$\log (1/EC_{50}) = 0.67 \ (\pm \ 0.24) \ \pi_X - 1.41 \ (\pm \ 0.66) \ \sigma_X$$
$$- 0.12 \ (\pm \ 0.11) \ L_Y + 6.81 \ (\pm \ 0.40) \tag{55}$$
$$n = 15, \ r^2 = 0.864, \ s = 0.24, \ q^2 = 0.30$$

For most of the compounds in the series of TSAO-T (40), as well as TSAO-C (41), the cytotoxic data were also reported by Camarasa et al. [86–88]. Adding to these series a few more TSAO-derivatives studied by Camarasa et al. for their cytotoxicity [86–88], Garg and Gupta [85] had obtained Equation (56) for the cytotoxicity data. In this equation, the parameter $I_{2'}$ was used for an O-tert-butyldimethylsilyl [Si-] group at the 2'-position and $I_{5'}$ for the same at the 5'-position of the sugar ring, each with a value of 1. The parameter $I_{X,Y}$ was used with a value of 1 for a thymine ring that had both X- and Y-substituents. For a thymine ring which had only one substituent, either X or Y, or no substituent at all, this parameter was equal to zero. Thus, Equation (56) suggested that while the presence of an [Si-] group at both 2'- and 5'-positions of the sugar ring will be favourable to the toxic activity, the presence of an X- and a Y-substituent simultaneously at the pyrimidine ring will have a high detrimental effect. A positive and statistically significant coefficient of D in this equation indicates that TSAO-T derivatives can have more cytotoxic effect than TSAO-C derivatives.

$$\log (1/CC_{50}) = 0.734 \ (\pm 0.446) \ I_{2'} + 1.135 \ (\pm 0.369) \ I_{5'}$$
$$- 1.124 \ (\pm 0.415) \ I_{X,Y} + 0.341 \ (\pm 0.319) \ D + 2.811 \tag{56}$$
$$n = 28, \ r = 0.900, \ s = 0.31, \ F_{4,23} = 24.19$$

In the set of additional compounds that were added to the series of **40** and **41** in the derivation of Equation (56), some compounds had their sugar ring in the β-D-xylo configuration and some compounds had their [Si-] groups replaced by H or OH. While configuration was not found to have any effect, Equation (56) shows that the replacement of an [Si-] group by H or OH will lead to a reduced toxicity since for both H and OH, $I_{2'}$ and $I_{5'}$ are equal to zero.

For a small series of TSAO derivatives as represented by **42**, the EC_{50} data were measured by Balzarini et al. [89] in four different cell systems, MOLT4, PBL, MT-4 and CEM, for which Garg et al. [28] obtained Equations (57) – (60), all showing a significant effect of the hydrophobicity of the molecule on the activity.

$$\log (1/EC_{50})_{MOLT4} = 4.18 \ (\pm 2.24) + 0.83 \ (\pm 0.61) \ C \log P \tag{57}$$
$$n = 5, \ r^2 = 0.860, \ s = 0.25, \ q^2 = 0.771$$
$$\log (1/EC_{50})_{PBL} = 6.47 \ (\pm 6.05) + 6.46 \ (\pm 3.13) \ C \log P$$
$$- 0.75 \ (\pm 0.39) \ (C \log P)^2 \tag{58}$$
$$n = 6, \ r^2 = 0.964, \ s = 0.15, \ q^2 = 0.860, \ \log P_o = 4.32$$
$$\log (1/EC_{50})_{MT-4} = 4.50 \ (\pm 4.79) + 5.66 \ (\pm 2.48) \ C \log P$$
$$- 0.68(\pm 0.31) \ (C \log P)^2 \tag{59}$$
$$n = 6, \ r^2 = 0.958, \ s = 0.12, \ q^2 = 0.681, \ \log P_o = 4.15$$
$$\log (1/EC_{50})_{CEM} = 7.71 \ (\pm 9.08) + 7.25 \ (\pm 4.70) \ C \log P$$
$$- 0.86 \ (\pm 0.59) \ (C \log P)^2 \tag{60}$$
$$n = 6, \ r^2 = 0.919, \ s = 0.22, \ q^2 = 0.745, \ \log P_o = 4.21$$

A series of TSAO-T_Z derivatives (**43**), where T_Z refers to a 1,2,3-triazole ring, was studied by Alvarez et al. [90], for which the activity data were measured in two different cell systems, MT-4 and CEM. For these data, Garg et al. [28] derived Equations (61) and (62) to suggest that in both the systems the X-substituents will have an electronic (inductive) effect on the activity, with a dominance in MT-4 cells. However, in MT-4 cells, these substituents are also found to have strong steric effects because of their width, while in CEM cells an X-substituent of only the 5-position will have a detrimental effect till its hydrophobicity reaches a value of 1.03.

$$\log (1/EC_{50})_{MT-4} = 3.10 \ (\pm 0.91) \ \Sigma\sigma_{I,X} - 0.28 \ (\pm 0.11) \ \Sigma B5_X$$
$$+ 1.21 \ (\pm 0.44) \ I_N + 0.49 \ (\pm 0.22) \ C \log P + 4.41 \ (\pm 0.85) \quad\quad (61)$$
$$n = 20, \ r^2 = 0.857, \ s = 0.24, \ q^2 = 0.777$$

$$\log (1/EC_{50})_{CEM} = 0.76 \ (\pm 0.58) \ \Sigma\sigma_{I,X} - 0.39 \ (\pm 0.12) \ \pi_{X,5}$$
$$+ 0.19 \ (\pm 0.08) \ (\pi_{X,5})^2 + 5.74 \ (\pm 0.16) \quad\quad (62)$$
$$n = 20, \ r^2 = 0.835, \ s = 0.20, \ q^2 = 0.748, \ (\pi_{X,5})_o = 1.03$$

The use of C log P in Equation (61) demonstrates that the overall hydrophobicity of the molecule can be beneficial to the activity in MT-4 cells. Also the use of an indicator parameter I_N with a value of 1 for $CONR_2$ substituent present at 4- or/and 5-position (s) suggests that such a substituent present at these positions will be of additional advantage to the activity in MT-4 cells.

3.2.6 α-APA derivatives

Pauwels et al. [91] reported anti-HIV and cytotoxic activities for a small series of α-anilophenylacetamide derivatives (44). Garg et al. [28] made a QSAR study of them and obtained Equations (63) and (64).

44

$$\log (1/EC_{50}) = 8.90 \ (\pm 1.05) - 2.16 \ (\pm 1.78) \ \sigma_{X,Y} - 2.47 \ (\pm 0.58) \ I \quad\quad (63)$$
$$n = 8, \ r^2 = 0.96, \ s = 0.26, \ q^2 = 0.889$$

$$\log (1/CC_{50}) = 14.99 \ (\pm 2.61) - 0.68 \ (\pm 0.40) \ ) \ \sigma_{X,Y}$$
$$- 1.22 \ (\pm 0.29) \ CMR \quad\quad (64)$$
$$n = 9, \ r^2 = 0.951, \ s = 0.13, \ q^2 = 0.885$$

In Equation (63), I is an indicator variable with a value of unity for dextrorotatory isomers. Its negative coefficient indicated that such isomers would be less effective as anti-HIV agents. However, the electron-releasing X- and Y-substituents on the phenyl ring were shown to produce strong electronic effects on anti-HIV activity. Such substituents were found to have some electronic effects on the cytotoxic activity also, but the bulk of the molecule appears to reduce this activity. The X-substituents were of the type OMe, NO_2 and COMe with dextro- and levorotatory characters in some molecules and Y-substituents were only CH_3 or H.

In addition to these important classes of NNRTIs, some miscellaneous groups of compounds were also investigated and their QSAR reported [28], but they contained so small a number of data points that their QSARs were of little importance.

4   An overview

Now it seems appropriate to draw an overall picture of all QSAR results on varying kinds of RT inhibitors. It would be worthwhile to do this in the light of the information available about the structure of HIV-1 RT. A high-resolution electron density map of HIV-1 RT complexed with nevirapine (**7**) has revealed its structure as an asymmetric dimer [17]. The enzyme is processed initially from the pol gene product as a 66-kDa (kilodalton) polypeptide that has both a pol and an RNAse H (ribonuclease H) domain. But a subsequent proteolytic cleavage of a homodimer of the 66-kDa subunits removes the RNase H domain from one subunit, leaving a heterodimer containing one 66-kDa subunit (p66) and one 51-kDa subunit (p51). The p66–p51 heterodimer appears to have only one pol active site, one RNase active site, one tRNA binding site, and one nevirapine binding site [17]. The p66 domain possesses a large cleft analogous to that of the Klenow fragment of *E. coli* DNA polymerase, but the p51 domain of an identical sequence has no such domain.

The ddN analogues act as competitive inhibitors or alternate substrates of RT, hence interact at the substrate binding site of the enzyme characterized by its catalytic triad (D110, D185, D186). This catalytic triad seems to be predominantly of an electronic nature, as for most of the ddN analogues the activity has been shown to be largely affected by the electronic nature of the compounds (Eqs. 1–4 and 7). Only for a series of phosphoramidates (**19**), which are membrane-soluble intracellular prodrugs for the free bioactive phosphate, was the activity found to be governed by the hydrophobicity of the compounds (Eq. 6), and this may be due to their membrane solubility. More than hydrophobicity, the steric factors were found to govern the activity of ddN analogues (Eqs. 5, 8, and 9), whose effects might have been definitely due to their interference in the electronic interactions of the molecules with the receptors.

Since NNRTIs bind to a site entirely distinct from the catalytic triad, their activity has been largely governed by the hydrophobic character of the molecules. For almost each class of NNRTIs, QSARs have revealed the important role of hydrophobicity, viz., Equations (10–12), (15–26), (28) and (29) (HEPT analogues), Equations (35–41) (TIBO derivatives), Equations (44–46) (nevirapine derivatives), Equations (48–51) (pyridinone derivatives) and Equations (52–55) and (57–62) (TSAO derivatives). Only in the case of α-APA derivatives could no hydrophobic effect be shown, but a lone series with a small number of data points severely limited the scope of detailed investigation.

The hydrophobic nature of the active site in receptors with which the NNRTIs interact provides relatively few possibilities for the molecules to have polar interactions or hydrogen bondings. However, most of the QSAR equations that have exhibited hydrophobic effects have also shown the electronic effects.

Several studies have revealed a common mode of binding for the chemically diverse NNRTIs with their target site at the HIV-1 RT [92]. NNRTIs cause a repositioning of the three-stranded β-sheet in the p66 subunit containing the catalytic triad [93]. This suggests that the NNRTIs inhibit the HIV-1 RT by locking the active catalytic site in an inactive conformation, reminiscent of the conformation observed in the inactive p51 subunit [93]. When bound into their pocket at the HIV-1 RT, NNRTIs acquire a very similar conformational "butterfly-like" shape [94–98]. The degree of butterfly-like configuration depends on the overall shape parameters, the polarizability and the lipophilicity of the molecule [98]. It was found that the butterfly-like shape fits well into a sizeable internal cavity of the allosteric area of the enzyme. Structurally diverse NNRTIs interact with different amino acid residues of the allosteric pocket and the number of amino acid residues interacting with an inhibitor is correlated with the degree of butterfly-like shape of the inhibitor. Thus, the drug affinity for the enzyme and the probability of drug-resistance development will be closely correlated with the degree of the butterfly-like shape of the drug.

Acknowledgement

The assistance rendered in the preparation of the manuscript by one of my students, Vineet Pande, is gratefully acknowledged.

References

1   F. Barre-Sinoussi, J.-C. Chermann, F. Rey, M.T. Nugeyre, S. Chamaret, J. Gruest, C. Dauget, C. Axler-Blin, F. Vezinet-Brun, C. Rouzioux et al.: Science *220*, 868 (1983).

2   (a) M. Popovic, M.G. Sarngadharan, E. Read and R.C. Gallo: Science *224*, 497 (1984). (b) R.C. Gallo, S.Z. Salahuddin, M. Popovic, G.M. Shearer, M. Kaplan, B.F. Haynes, T.J. Palker, R. Redfield, J. Oleske, B. Safai et al.: Science *224*, 500 (1984).

3   R.C. Gallo and L. Montagnier: Sci. Am. *259*, 40 (1988).

4   J. Coffin, A. Hasse, J.A. Levy, L. Montagnier, S. Oroszlan, N. Teich, H. Temin, K. Toyoshmia, H. Varmus, P. Vogt et al.: Science *232*, 697 (1986).

5   J.A. Levy: JAMA *261*, 2997 (1989) and references therein.

6   F. Clavel, M. Guyader, D. Guetard, M. Salle, L. Montagnier and M. Alizon: Nature (London) *324*, 691 (1986).

7   M. Guyader, M. Emerman, P. Sonigo, F. Clavel, L. Montagnier and M. Alizon: Nature (London) *326*, 662 (1987).

8   http://www.niaid.nih.gov/daids/dtpdb/fdadrug.html

9   E. De Clercq: Biochem. Pharmacol. *47*, 155 (1994).

10 C. Tantillo, J.P. Ding, A. Jacobomolina, R.G. Nanni, P.L. Boyer, S.H. Hughes, R. Pauwels, K. Andries, P.A.J. Janssen and E. Arnold: J. Biol. Chem. *243*, 369 (1994).

11 P. Huang, D. Farquhar and W. Plunkett: J. Biol. Chem. *265*, 11914 (1990).

12 E. De Clercq: Med. Res. Rev. *13*, 229 (1993).

13 E. De Clercq: AIDS Res. Human Retrov. *8*, 119 (1992).

14 I.W. Althaus, J.J. Chou, A.J. Gonzales, M.R. Deibel, K.C. Chou, F.J. Kezdy, D.L. Romero, R.C. Thomas, P.A. Aristoff, W.G. Tarpley et al.: Biochem. Pharmacol. *47*, 2017 (1994).

15 A. Jacobo-Molina, J. Ding, R.G. Nanni, A.D. Clark Jr., X. Lu, C. Tantillo, R.L. Williams, G. Kamer, A.L. Ferris, P. Clark et al.: Proc. Natl. Acad. Sci. USA *90*, 6320 (1993).

16 R.G. Nanni, J. Ding, M.A. Jacobo, S.H. Hughes and E. Arnold: Perspect. Drug Discov. Des. *1*, 129 (1993)

17 L.A. Kohlstaedt, J. Wang, J.M. Friedman, P.A. Rice and T.A. Steitz: Science *256*, 1783 (1992).

18 R. Pauwels, K. Andries, J. Desmyter, D. Schols, M.J. Kukla, H.J. Breslin, A. Raemaeckers, J. Van Gelder, R. Woestenborghs, J. Heykants et al.: Nature (London) *343*, 470 (1990).

19 Z. Debyser, R. Pauwels, K. Andries, J. Desmyter, M.J. Kukla, P.A.J. Janssen and E. De Clercq: Proc. Natl. Acad. Sci. USA *88*, 1451 (1991).

20 T. Miyasaka, H. Tanaka, M. Baba, H. Hayakawa, R.T. Walker, J. Balzarini and E. De Clercq: J. Med. Chem. *32*, 2507 (1989).

21 M. Baba, H. Tanaka, E. De Clercq, R. Pauwels, J. Balzarini, D. Schols, H. Nakashima, C.F. Perno, R.T. Walker and T. Miyasaka: Biochem. Biophys. Res. Commun. *165*, 1375 (1989).

22   U.J. Merluzzi, K.D. Hargrave, M. Labadia, K. Grozinger, M. Skoog, J.C. Wu, C.-K. Shih, K. Eckner, S. Hattox, J. Adams et al.: Science *250*, 1411 (1990).

23   M.E. Goldman, J.H. Nunberg, J.A. O'Brien, J.C. Quintero, W.A. Schleif, K.F. Freund, S.L. Gaul, W.S. Saari, J.S. Wai, J.M. Hoffman et al.: Proc. Natl. Acad. Sci. USA *88*, 6863 (1991).

24   D.L. Romero, M. Busso, C.K. Tan, F. Reusser, J. R. Palmer, S.M. Poppe, P.A. Aristoff, K.M. Downey, A.G. So, L. Resnick et al.: Proc. Natl. Acad. Sci. USA *88*, 8806 (1991).

25   J. Balzarini, M.-J. Péréz-Péréz, A. San-Felix, D. Schols, C.F. Perno, A.M. Vandamme, M.J. Camarasa and E. De Clercq: Proc. Natl. Acad. Sci. USA *89*, 4392 (1992).

26   R. Pauwels, K. Andries, Z. Debyser, P. Van Daele, D. Schols, P. Stoffels, K. De Vreese, R. Woestenborghs, A.M. Vandamme, C.G.M. Janssen et al.: Proc. Natl. Acad. Sci. USA *90*, 1711 (1993).

27   J. Balzarini, A. van Aerschot, R. Pauwels, M. Baba, D. Schols, P. Herdewijn and E. De Clercq: Mol. Pharmacol. *35*, 571 (1989).

28   R. Garg, S.P. Gupta, H. Gao, M.S. Babu, A.K. Debnath and C. Hansch: Chem. Rev. *99*, 3525 (1999).

29   P.A.M. Herdewijn, A. van Aerschot, J. Balzarini and E. De Clercq: Med. Chem. Res. *1*, 9 (1991).

30   J. Balzarini, M. Baba, R. Pauwels, P. Herdewijn and E. De Clercq: Biochem. Pharmacol. *37*, 2847 (1988).

31   M. Mahmoudian: Pharm. Res. *8*, 43 (1991).

32   K.C. Chu, R.F. Schinazi, M.K. Ahn, G.V. Ultas and Z.P. Gu: J. Med. Chem. *32*, 612 (1989).

33   T.-S. Lin, J.-Y. Guo, R.F. Schinazi, C.K. Chu, J.-N. Xiang and W.H. Prusoff: J. Med. Chem. *31*, 336 (1988).

34   P. Herdewijn, J. Balzarini, M. Baba, R. Pauwels, A. van Aerschot, G. Janssen and E. De Clercq: J. Med. Chem. *31*, 2040 (1988).

35   A.Q. Siddiqui, C. Ballatore, C. McGuigan, E. De Clercq and J. Balzarini: J. Med. Chem. *42*, 393 (1999)

36   A.Q. Siddiqui, C. McGuigan, C. Ballatore, F. Zuccotto, I.H. Gilbert, E. De Clercq and J. Balzarini: J. Med. Chem. *42*, 4122 (1999).

37   C. McGuigan, M. Davies, R. Pathirana, N. Mahmood, and A.J. Hay: Antiviral Res. *24*, 69 (1994).

38   G.A. Freeman, S.R. Shaver, J.L. Rideout and S.A. Short: Bioorg. Med. Chem. *3*, 447 (1995).

39   K. Murakami, T. Shirasaka, H. Yoshioka, E. Kojima, S. Aoki, H. Ford Jr., J.S. Driscoll, J.A. Kelley and H. Mitsuya: J. Med. Chem. *34*, 1606 (1991).

40   H. Tanaka, H. Takashima, M. Ubasawa, K. Sekiya, I. Nitta, M. Baba, S. Shigeta, R.T. Walker, E. De Clercq and T. Miyasaka: J. Med. Chem. *35*, 337 (1992).

41   C. Hansch and L. Zhang: Bioorg. Med. Chem. Lett. *2*, 1165 (1992).

42   R. Garg, A. Kurup, and S.P. Gupta: Quant. Struct.-Act. Relat. *16*, 20 (1997).

43   H. Tanaka, S. Takashima, M. Ubasawa, K. Sekiya, I. Nitta, M. Baba, S. Shigeta, R.T. Walker, E. De Clercq and T. Miyasaka: J. Med. Chem. *35*, 4713 (1992).

44   H. Tanaka, H. Takashima, M. Ubasawa, K. Sekiya, N. Inouye, M. Baba, S. Shigeta, R.T. Walker, E. De Clercq and T. Miyasaka: J. Med. Chem. *38*, 2860 (1995).

45   M. Baba, S. Shigeta, H. Tanaka, T. Miyasaka, M. Ubasawa, K. Umezu, R.T. Walker, R. Pauwels and E. De Clercq: Antiviral Res. *17*, 245 (1992).

46   R. Pontkis, R. Benhida, A.-M. Aubertin, D.S. Grierson and C. Monneret: J. Med. Chem. *40*, 1845 (1997)

47   J. Balzarini, M. Baba and E. De Clercq: Antimicrob. Agents Chemother. *39*, 998 (1995).

48   H. Tanaka, M. Baba, H. Hayakawa, T. Sakamaki, T. Miyasaka, M. Ubasawa, H. Takashima, K. Sekiya, I. Nitta, S. Shigeta et al.: J. Med. Chem. *34*, 349 (1991).

49   D.-K. Kim., J. Gam, Y.-W. Kim, J. Lim, H.-T. Kim and K.H. Kim: J. Med. Chem. *40*, 2363 (1997).

50   T. Miyasaka, H. Tanaka, M. Baba, H. Hayakawa, R.T. Walker, J. Balzarini and E. De Clercq: J. Med. Chem. *32*, 2507 (1989).

51   M. Baba, H. Tanaka, E. De Clercq, R. Pauwels, J. Balzarini, D. Schols, H. Nakashima, C.–F. Perno, R.T. Walker and T. Miyasaka: Biochem. Biophys. Res. Commun. *165*, 1375 (1989).

52   M. Tanaka, M. Baba, M. Ubasawa, H. Takashima, K. Sekiya, I. Nitta, S. Shigeta, R.T. Walker, E. De Clercq and T. Miyasaka: J. Med. Chem. *34*, 1394 (1991).

53   H. Tanaka, M. Baba, S. Saito, T. Miyasaka, H. Takashima, K. Sekiya, M. Ubasawa, I. Nitta, R.T. Walker, H. Nakashima et al.: J. Med. Chem. *34*, 1508 (1991).

54   H. Tanaka, M. Baba, M. Ubaswa, H. Takashima, K. Sekiya, T. Miyasaka, I. Nitta, R.T. Walker and E. De Clercq: Collec. Czech. Chem. Commun. *55*, 89 (1990).

55   H. Tanaka, M. Baba, H. Hayakawa, K. Haraguchi, T. Miyasaka, M. Ubasawa, H. Takashima, K. Sekiya, I. Nitta, R.T. Walker et al.: Nucleosides Nucleotides *10*, 397 (1991).

56   J. M. Luco and F.H. Ferretti: J. Chem. Inf. Comput. Sci. *37*, 392 (1997).

57   A.L. Hopkins, J. Ren., R.M. Esnouf, B.E. Willcox, E.Y. Jones, C. Ross, T. Miyasaka, R.T. Walker, H. Tanaka, D.K. Stammers et al.: J. Med. Chem. *39*, 1589 (1996).

58   D.B. Kireev, J.R. Chrétien, D.S. Grierson and C. Monneret: J. Med. Chem. *40*, 4257 (1997).

59   L. Lawtrakul, S. Hannongbua, A. Beyer and P. Wolschann: Biol. Chem. *380*, 265 (1999).

60   L. Lawtrakul, S, Hannongbua, A. Beyer and P. Wolschann: Monatsch. Chem. *130*, 1347 (1999).

61   S. Hannongbua, L. Lawtrakul and J. Limtrakul: J. Comput.-Aided Mol. Design *10*, 145 (1996).

62   S. Hannongbua, L. Lawtrakul, C.A. Sotriffer and B.M. Rode: Quant. Struct.-Act. Relat. *15*, 389 (1996).

63   S. Hannongbua, K. Nivesanond, L. Lawtrakul, P. Pungpo, and P. Wolschann: J. Chem. Inf. Comput. Sci. *41*, 848 (2001).

64   L. Lawtrakul and S. Hannongbua: Sci. Pharm. *67*, 43 (1999).

65   M. Jalali-Heravi and F. Parastar: J. Chem. Inf. Comput. Sci. *40*, 147 (2000).

66   S. Pauwels, K. Andries, J. Desmyter, D. Schols, M. Kukla, H. Breslin, A. Raemaekers, J. Van Gelder, R. Woestenborghs, J. Heykants et al.: Nature (London) *343*, 470 (1990).

67   M. Kukla, H. Breslin, R. Pauwels, C. Fedde, M. Miranda, M. Scott, R. Sherril, A. Raemaekers, J. Van Gelder, K. Andries et al.: J. Med. Chem. *34*, 746 (1991).

68   M. Kukla, H. Breslin, C. Diamond, P. Grous, C.Y. Ho, M. Miranda, J. Rodgers, R. Sherril, E. De Clercq, R. Pauwels et al.: J. Med. Chem. *34*, 3187 (1991).

69   H.J. Breslin, M.J. Kukla, D.W. Ludovici, R. Mohrbacher, W. Ho, M. Miranda, J.D. Rodgers, T.K.Hitchens, G. Leo, D.A. Gauthier et al.: J. Med. Chem. *38*, 771 (1995).

70   W. Ho, M.J. Kukla, H.J. Breslin, D.W. Ludovici, P.P. Grows, C.J. Diamond, M. Miranda, D.W. Rodgers, C.Y. Ho, E. De Clercq et al.: J. Med. Chem. *38*, 794 (1995).

71   S.P. Gupta and R. Garg: J. Enzyme Inhibn. *11*, 23 (1996).

72   R. Pauwels, K. Andries, Z. Debyser, M.J. Kukla, D. Schols, H.J. Breslin, R. Woesternborghs, J. Desmyter, M.A.C. Janssen, E. De Clercq et al.: Antimicrob. Agents Chemother. *38*, 2863 (1994).

73   S. Hannongbua, P. Pungpo, J. Limtrakul and P. Wolschann: J. Comput.-Aided Mol. Design *13*, 563 (1999).

74   T.A. Kelly, J.R. Proudfoot, D.W. McNeil, U.R. Patel, E. David, K.D. Hargrave, P.M. Grob, M. Cardozo, A. Agarwal and J. Adams: J. Med. Chem. *38*, 4839 (1995).

75   K.D. Hargrave, J.R. Proudfoot, K.G. Grozinger, E. Cullen, S.R. Kapadia, U.R. Patel, V.U. Fuchs, S.C. Mauldin, J. Vitous, M.L. Behnke et al.: J. Med. Chem. *34*, 2231 (1991).

76   J.M. Klunder, K.D. Hargrave, M.A. West, E. Kullen, K. Pal, M.L.Behnke, S.R. Kapadia, D.W. McNeil, J.C. Wu, G.C. Chow et al.: J. Med. Chem. *35*, 1887 (1992).

77   T.A. Kelly, D.W. McNeil, J.M. Rose, E. David, C.K. Shih and P.M. Grob: J. Med. Chem. *40*, 2430 (1997).

78   J.R. Proudfoot, K.D. Hargrave, S.R. Kapadia, U.R. Patel, K.G. Grozinger, D.W. McNeil, E. Cullen, M. Cardozo, L. Tong, T.A. Kelly et al.: J. Med. Chem. *38*, 4830 (1995).

79   P. Pungpo and S. Hannongbua: J. Mol. Graph. Model. *18*, 581 (2000).

80   R. Garg and S.P. Gupta: J. Enzyme Inhibn. *12*, 1 (1997).

81   W.S. Saari, J.M. Hoffman, J.S. Wai, T.E. Fischer, C.S. Rooney, A.M. Smith, C.M. Thomas, M.E. Goldman, J.A. O'Brien, J.H. Nurnberg et al.: J. Med. Chem. *34*, 2922 (1991).

82   J.M. Hoffman, J.S. Wai, C.M. Thomas, R.B. Levin, J.A. O'Brien and M.E. Goldman: J. Med. Chem. *35*, 3784 (1992).

83   W.S. Saari, J.S. Wai, T.E. Fisher, C.M. Thomas, J.M. Hoffman, C.S. Rooney, A.M. Smith, J.H. Jones, D.L. Bamberger, M.E. Goldman et al.: J. Med. Chem. *35*, 3792 (1992).

84   J.M. Hoffman, A.M. Smith, C.S. Rooney, T.E. Fisher, J.S. Wai, C.M. Thomas, D.L. Bamberger, J.L. Barnes, T.M. William, J.H. Jones et al.: J. Med. Chem. *36*, 953 (1993).

85   R. Garg and S.P. Gupta: J. Enzyme Inhibn. *11*, 171 (1997).

86   M.J. Camarasa, M.J. Péréz-Péréz, A. San-Felix, J. Balzarini and E. De Clercq: J. Med. Chem. *35*, 2721 (1992).

87   M.J. Péréz-Péréz, A. San-Felix, J. Balzarini, E. De Clercq and M.J. Camarasa: J. Med. Chem. *35*, 2988 (1992).

88   A. San-Felix, V. Sonsoles, M.J. Péréz-Péréz , J. Balzarini, E. De Clercq and M.J. Camarasa: J. Med. Chem. *37*, 453 (1994).

89   J. Balzarini, M.J. Péréz-Péréz, A. San-Felix, D. Schols, C.-F. Perno, A.-M. Vandamme, M.J. Camarasa and E. De Clercq: Proc. Natl. Acad. Sci. USA *89*, 4392 (1992).

90   R. Alvarez, S. Velazquez, A. San-Felix, S. Aquaro, E. De Clercq, C.–F. Perno, A. Karlsson, J. Balzarini and M.J. Camarasa: J. Med. Chem. *37*, 4185 (1994).

91   R.Pauwels, K. Andries, Z. Debyser, P.V. Daele, D. Schols, P. Stoffels, K. De Vreese, R. Woestenborghs, A.M. Vandamme, C.G.M. Janssen et al.: Proc. Natl. Acad. Sci. USA *90*, 1711 (1993).

92   J. Ren, R. Esnouf, E. Garman, D. Somers, C. Ross, I. Kirby, J. Keeling, G. Darby, Y. Jones, D. Stuart et al.: Struct. Biol. *2*, 293 (1995).

93   R. Esnouf, J. Ren, C. Ross, Y. Jones, D. Stammers and D. Stuart: Struct. Biol. *2*, 303 (1995).

94   P.W. Mui, S.P. Jacober, K.D. Hargrave and J. Adams: J. Med. Chem. *35*, 201 (1992).

95   W. Schafer, W.-G. Friebe, H. Leinert, A. Mertens, T. Poll, W. Von de Saal, H. Zilch, B. Nuber and M.L. Zeigler: J. Med. Chem. *36*, 726 (1993).

96   J. Ding, K. Das, H. Moereels, L. Koymans, K. Andries, P.A.J. Janssen, S.H. Hughes and E. Arnold: Struct. Biol. *2*, 407 (1995)

97   P.P. Mager, E. De Clercq, H. Takashima, M. Ubasawa, K. Sekiya, M. Baba and H. Walther: Eur. J. Med. Chem. *31*, 701 (1996).

98   P.P. Mager: Drug Des. Discovery *14*, 241 (1996).

Index Vol. 58

Index of titles
Vol. 1–58 (1959–2002)

Author and paper index
Vol. 1–58 (1959–2002)

Pertussis agglutinins and complement fixing antibodies in whooping cough *19*, 178 (1975)	K. C. Agarwal M. Ray N. L. Chitkara
Pharmacology of clinically useful beta-adrenergic blocking drugs *15*, 103 (1971)	R. P. Ahlquist A. M. Karow, Jr. M. W. Riley
Adrenergic beta blocking agents *20*, 27 (1976)	R. P. Ahlquist
Trial of a new anthelmintic (bitoscanate) in ankylostomiasis in children *19*, 2 (1975)	S. H. Ahmed S. Vaishnava
Development of antibacterial agents of the nalidixic acid type *21*, 9 (1977)	R. Albrecht
The mode of action of anti-rheumatic drugs. Anti-inflammatory and immunosuppressive effects of glucocorticoids *33*, 63 (1989)	Anthony C. Allison Simon W. Lee
Biological activity in the quinazolone series *14*, 218 (1970)	A. H. Amin D. R. Mehta S. S. Samarth
Enhancement and inhibition of microsomal drug metabolism *17*, 11 (1973)	M. W. Anders
Reactivity of rat and man to egg-white *13*, 340 (1969)	S. I. Ankier
Enzyme inhibitors of the renin-angiotensin system *31*, 161 (1987)	Michael J. Antonaccio John J. Wright
Narcotic antagonists *8*, 261 (1965)	S. Archer L. S. Harris

Recent developments in the chemo-therapy of schistosomiasis *16*, 11 (1972)	S. Archer A. Yarinsky
Recent progress in the chemotherapy of schistosomiasis *18*, 15 (1974) Recent progress in research on narcotic antagonists *20*, 45 (1976)	S. Archer
Molecular geometry and mechanism of action of chemical carcinogens *4*, 407 (1962)	J. C. Arcos
Cell-kinetic and pharmacokinetic aspects in the use and further development of cancerostatic drugs *20*, 521 (1976)	M. von Ardenne
Molecular pharmacology, a basis for drug design *10*, 429 (1966) Reduction of drug action by drug combination *14*, 11 (1970)	E. J. Ariëns
Stereoselectivity and affinity in molecular pharmacology *20*, 101 (1976)	E. J. Ariëns J. F. Rodrigues de Miranda P. A. Lehmann
The pharmacology of caffeine *31*, 273 (1987)	M. J. Arnaud
Recent advances in central 5-hydroxytryptamine receptor agonists and antagonists *30*, 365 (1986)	Lars-Erik Arvidsson Uli Hacksell Richard A. Glennon
Drugs affecting the renin-angiotensin system *26*, 207 (1982)	R. W. Ashworth
Tetanus neonatorum *19*, 189 (1975) Tetanus in children *19*, 209 (1975)	V. B. Athavale P. N. Pai A. Fernandez P. N. Patnekar Y. S. Acharya
Toxicity of propellants *18*, 365 (1974)	D. M. Aviado
Polyamines as markers of malignancy *39*, 9 (1992)	Uriel Bachrach
Neuere Aspekte der chemischen Anthelminticaforschung *1*, 243 (1959)	J. Bally

Wert und Bewertung der Arzneimittel *10*, 90 (1966)	J. Büchi
Cyclopropane compounds of biological interest *15*, 227 (1971) The state of medicinal science *20*, 9 (1976) Isosterism and bioisosterism in drug design *37*, 287 (1991)	A. Burger
Human and veterinary anthelmintics (1965–1971) *17*, 108 (1973)	R. B. Burrows
The antibody basis of local immunity to experimental cholera infection in the rabbit ileal loop *19*, 471 (1975)	W. Burrows J. Kaur
Les dérivés organiques du fluor d'intérêt pharmacologique *3*, 9 (1961)	N. P. Buu-Hoï
Teaching tropical medicine *18*, 35 (1974)	K. M. Cahill
Anabolic steroids *2*, 71 (1960)	B. Camerino G. Sala
Immunosuppression agents, procedures, speculations and prognosis *16*, 67 (1972)	G. W. Camiener W. J. Wechter
Dopamine agonists: Structure-activity relationships *29*, 303 (1985)	Joseph G. Cannon
Therapeutic applications of cytokines for immunostimulation and immuno- suppression: An update *47*, 211 (1996)	Gaetano Cardi Thomas L. Ciardelli Marc S. Ernstoff
Analgesics and their antagonists: Recent developments *22*, 149 (1978)	A. F. Casy
Chemical nature and pharmacological actions of quaternary ammonium salts *2*, 135 (1960)	C. J. Cavallito A. P. Gray
Contributions of medicinal chemistry to medicine – from 1935 *12*, 11 (1968) Changing influences on goals and incentives in drug research and development *20*, 159 (1976) Quaternary ammonium salts – advances in chemistry and pharmacology since 1960 *24*, 267 (1980)	C. J. Cavallito

Studies on *Vibrio parahaemolyticus* infection in Calcutta as compared to cholera infection *19*, 490 (1975)	B. C. Deb
Biochemical effects of drugs acting on the central nervous system *8*, 53 (1965)	L. Decsi
Some reflections on the chemotherapy of tropical diseases: Past, present and future *26*, 343 (1982)	E. W. J. de Maar
Drug research – whence and whither *10*, 11 (1966)	R. G. Denkewalter M. Tishler
Immunization of a village, a new approach to herd immunity *19*, 252 (1975)	N. S. Deodhar
Profiles of tuberculosis in rural areas of Maharashtra *18*, 91 (1974)	M. D. Deshmukh K. G. Kulkarni S. S. Virdi B. B. Yodh
The interface between drug research, marketing, management, and social, political and regulatory forces *20*, 181 (1976) Medicinal research: Retrospectives and perspectives *29*, 97 (1985) Serendipity and structured research in drug discovery *30*, 189 (1986) Medicinal chemistry: A support or a driving force in drug research? *34*, 343 (1990) Heterocyclic diversity: The road to biological activity *44*, 9 (1995)	G. deStevens
Hypolipidemic agents *13*, 217 (1969)	G. deStevens W. L. Bencze R. Hess
Antihypertensive agents *20*, 197 (1976)	G. deStevens M. Wilhelm
RNA virus evolution and the control of viral disease *33*, 93 (1989)	Esteban Domingo

Host factors in the response to immunization *19*, 263 (1975)	G. Edsall M. A. Belsey R. Le Blanc L. Levine
Recent advances in potassium channel modulation *49*, 93 (1997) Endothelium-derived hyperpolarizing factor – a critical appraisal *50*, 107 (1998)	Gillian Edwards Arthur H. Weston
5-Hydroxytryptamine (5-HT)$_4$ receptors and central nervous system function: An update *49*, 9 (1997)	Richard M. Eglen
Drug-macromolecular interactions: Implications for pharmacological activity *14*, 59 (1970)	S. Ehrenpreis
Betrachtungen zur Entwicklung von Heilmitteln *10*, 33 (1966)	G. Ehrhart
Progress in malaria chemotherapy, Part I. Repository antimalarial drugs *13*, 170 (1969) New perspectives on the chemotherapy of malaria, filariasis and leprosy *18*, 99 (1974)	E. F. Elslager
Recent research in the field of 5-hydroxytryptamine and related indolealkylamines *3*, 151 (1961)	V. Erspamer
Recent advances in erythropoietin research *41*, 293 (1993)	James W. Fisher
The chemistry of DNA modification by antitumor antibiotics *32*, 411 (1988)	Jed. F. Fisher Paul A. Aristoff
Potassium channels: Gene family, therapeutic relevance, high throughput screening technologies and drug discovery *58*, 133 (2002)	John W. Ford Edward B. Stevens J. Mark Treherne Jeremy Packer Mark Bushfield
Toward peptide receptor ligand drugs: Progress on nonpeptides *40*, 33 (1993)	Roger M. Freidinger
Transfer factor 1993: New frontiers *42*, 309 (1994)	H. Hugh Fudenberg Giancarlo Pizza

Epidemiology of diphtheria *19*, 336 (1975)	L. G. Marquis
Biological activity of the terpenoids and their derivatives *6*, 279 (1963)	M. Martin-Smith T. Khatoon
Biological activity of the terpenoids and their derivatives – recent advances *13*, 11 (1969)	M. Martin-Smith W. E. Sneader
Antihypertensive agents 1962–1968 *13*, 101 (1969) Fundamental structures in drug research – Part I *20*, 385 (1976) Fundamental structures in drug research – Part II *22*, 27 (1978) Antihypertensive agents 1969–1980 *25*, 9 (1981)	A. Marxer O. Schier
Relationships between the chemical structure and pharmacological activity in a series of synthetic quinuclidine derivatives *13*, 293 (1969)	M. D. Mashkovsky L. N. Yakhontov
Further developments in research on the chemistry and pharmacology of synthetic quinuclidine derivatives *27*, 9 (1983)	M. D. Mashkovsky L. N. Yakhontov M. E. Kaminka E. E. Mikhlina S. Ordzhonikidze
Role of neutrotransmitters in the central regulation of the cardiovascular system *35*, 25 (1990) Neurotransmitters involved in the central regulation of the cardiovascular system *46*, 43 (1996)	Robert B. McCall
On the understanding of drug potency *13*, 123 (1971) The chemotherapy of intestinal nematodes *16*, 157 (1972)	J. W. McFarland
Non-steroidal menses-regulating agents: The present status *44*, 159 (1995)	P.K. Mehrotra Sanjay Batra A.P. Bhaduri
Zur Beeinflussung der Strahlen- empfindlichkeit von Säugetieren durch chemische Substanzen *9*, 11 (1966)	H.-J. Melching C. Streffer
Analgesia and addiction *5*, 155 (1963)	L. B. Mellett L. A. Woods

Comparative drug metabolism *13*, 136 (1969)	L. B. Mellett
Prostate cancer and the androgen receptor: Strategies for the development of novel therapeutics *55*, 213 (2000)	Laurane G. Mendelsohn
The oral antiarrhythmic drugs *35*, 151 (1990)	Lisa Mendes Scott L. Beau John S. Wilson Philip J. Podrid
Mechanism of action of anxiolytic drugs *31*, 315 (1987)	T. Mennini S. Caccia S. Garattini
Pathogenesis of amebic disease *18*, 225 (1974) Protozoan and helminth parasites – a review of current treatment *20*, 433 (1976)	M. J. Miller
Medicinal agents incorporating the 1,2-diamine functionality *33*, 135 (1989)	Erik T. Michalson Jacob Szmuszkovicz
Fluorinated quinolones-new quinolone antimicrobials *38*, 9 (1992)	S. Mitsuhashi (Editor) T. Kojima, N. Nakanishi, T. Fujimoto, S. Goto, S. Miyusaki, T. Uematsu, M. Nakashima, Y. Asahina, T. Ishisaki, S. Susue, K. Hirai, K. Sato, K. Hoshino, J. Shimada, S. Hori
Synopsis der Rheumatherapie *12*, 165 (1968)	W. Moll
On the chemotherapy of cancer *8*, 431 (1965) The relationship of the metabolism of anticancer agents to their activity *17*, 320 (1973) The current status of cancer chemotherapy *20*, 465 (1976)	J. A. Montgomery
Present status of Leishmaniasis *34*, 447 (1990)	Anita Mukherjee Manju Seth A. P. Bhaduri
The significance of DNA technology in medicine *33*, 397 (1989)	Hansjakob Müller
Der Einfluß der Formgebung auf die Wirkung eines Arzneimittels *10*, 204 (1966)	K. Münzel

Experience with bitoscanate in adults *19*, 90 (1975)	A. H. Patricia U. Prabakar Rao R. Subramaniam N. Madanagopalan
The impact of state and society on medical research *35*, 9 (1990)	C. R. Pfaltz
Transfer factor in malignancy *42*, 401 (1994)	Giancarlo Pizza Caterina De Vinci H. Hugh Fudenberg
Monoaminoxydase-Hemmer *2*, 417 (1960)	A. Pletscher K. F. Gey P. Zeller
Antifungal therapy: Are we winning? *37*, 183 (1991)	A. Polak P. G. Hartman
Antifungal therapy, an everlasting battle *49*, 219 (1997)	A. Polak
Neuropeptides in drug research *54*, 161 (2000)	David Poyner Helen Cox Mark Bushfield J. Mark Treherne Melissa K. Demetrikopoulos
What makes a good pertussis vaccine? *19*, 341 (1975) Vaccine composition in relation to antigenic variation of the microbe: Is pertussis unique? *19*, 347 (1975) Some unsolved problems with vaccines *23*, 9 (1979) Eradication by vaccination: The memorial to smallpox could be surrounded by others *41*, 151 (1993)	N. W. Preston
Peptide drug delivery into the central nervous system *51*, 95 (1998)	Laszlo Prokai
Antibiotics in the chemotherapy of malaria *26*, 167 (1982)	S. K. Puri G. P. Dutta
Potassium channel openers: Airway pharma- cology and clinical possibilities in asthma *37*, 161 (1991)	David Raeburn Jan-Anders Karlsson
Isozyme-selective cyclic nucleotide phosphodiesterase inhibitors: Biochemistry, pharmacology and therapeutic potential in asthma *40*, 9 (1993)	David Raeburn John E. Souness Adrian Tomkinson Jan-Anders Karlsson
Clinical study of diphtheria, tetanus and pertussis *19*, 356 (1975)	V. B. Raju V. R. Parvathi

Isoprenoids biosynthesis via the mevalonate-independent route, a novel target for antibacterial drugs? *50*, 135 (1998)	Michel Rohmer
Tetrahydroisoquinolines and β-carbolines: Putative natural substances in plants and animals *29*, 415 (1985)	H. Rommelspacher R. Susilo
Functional significance of the various components of the influenza virus *18*, 253 (1974)	R. Rott
Drug receptors and control of the cardiovascular system: Recent advances *36*, 117 (1991)	Robert R. Ruffolo Jr J. Paul Hieble David P. Brooks Giora Z. Feuerstein Andrew J. Nichols
Behavioral correlates of presynaptic events in the cholinergic neurotransmitter system *32*, 43 (1988)	Roger W. Russell
Epidemiology of pertussis *19*, 257 (1975)	J. A. Sa
Surgical amoebiasis *18*, 77 (1974)	A. E. de Sa
Role of beta-adrenergic blocking drug propranolol in severe tetanus *19*, 361 (1975)	G. S. Sainani K. L. Jain V. R. D. Deshpande A. B. Balsara S. A. Iyer
Studies on *Vibrio parahaemolyticus* in Bombay *19*, 586 (1975)	F. L. Saldanha A. K. Patil M. V. Sant
Leukotriene antagonists and inhibitors of leukotriene biosynthesis as potential therapeutic agents *37*, 9 (1991)	John A. Salmon Lawrence G. Garland
Pharmacology and toxicology of axoplasmic transport *28*, 53 (1984)	Fred Samson Ralph L. Smith J. Alejandro Donoso
Clinical experience with bitoscanate *19*, 96 (1975)	M. R. Samuel
Tetanus: Situational clinical trials and therapeutics *19*, 367 (1975)	R. K. M. Sanders M. L. Peacock B. Martyn B. D. Shende

The benzimidazole anthelmitics chemistry and biological activity *27*, 85 (1983) Treatment of helminth diseases, challenges and achievements *31*, 9 (1987) Vector-borne diseases *35*, 365 (1990)	Satyavan Sharma
Chemotherapy of cestode infections *24*, 217 (1980)	Satyavan Sharma S. K. Dubey R. N. Iyer
Chemotherapy of hookworm infections *26*, 9 (1982)	Satyavan Sharma Elizabeth S. Charles
Ayurvedic medicine – past and present *15*, 11 (1971)	Shiv Sharma
Mechanisms of anthelmintic action *19*, 147 (1975)	U. K. Sheth
Aspirin as an antithrombotic agent *33*, 43 (1989)	Melvin J. Silver Giovanni Di Minno
Immunopharmacological approach to the study of chronic brain disorders *30*, 345 (1986) Implications of immunomodulant therapy in Alzheimer's disease *32*, 21 (1988)	Vijendra K. Singh H. Hugh Fudenberg
Neuroimmune axis as a basis of therapy in Alzheimer's disease *34*, 383 (1990) Immunoregulatory role of neuropeptides *38*, 149 (1992) Neuropeptides as native immune modulators *45*, 9 (1995) Immunotherapy for brain diseases and mental illnesses *48*, 129 (1997)	Vijendra K. Singh
Natural products as anticancer agents *42*, 53 (1994)	Shradha Sinha Sudha Jain
Biologically active quinazolones *43*, 143 (1994)	Shradha Sinha Mukta Srivastava
The impact of multiple drug resistance proteins on chemotherapy and drug discovery *58*, 99 (2002)	Paul L. Skatrud
Some often neglected factors in the control and prevention of communicable diseases *18*, 277 (1974)	C. E. G. Smith
Tetanus and its prevention *19*, 391 (1975)	J. W. G. Smith

Immunotherapy for leprosy and tuberculosis *33*, 415 (1989)	J. L. Stanford
The leishmaniasis *18*, 289 (1974)	E. A. Steck
The benzodiazepine story *22*, 229 (1978)	L. H. Sternbach
Immunostimulation with peptidoglycan or its synthetic derivatives *32*, 305 (1988)	Duncan E. S. Stewart-Tull
Hypertension: Relating drug therapy to pathogenic mechanisms *32*, 175 (1988)	David H. P. Streeten Gunnar H. Anderson Jr
Progress in sulfonamide research *12*, 389 (1968) Problems of medical practice and of medical-pharmaceutical research *20*, 491 (1976)	Th. Struller
Bacterial resistance to β-lactam antibiotics: Problems and solutions *41*, 95 (1993)	R. Sutherland
Antiviral agents *22*, 267 (1978) Antiviral agents 1978–1983 *28*, 127 (1984)	D. L. Swallow
Ketoconazole, a new step in the management of fungal disease *27*, 63 (1983)	J. Symoens G. Cauwenbergh
Antiarrhythmic compounds *12*, 292 (1968)	L. Szekeres J. G. Papp
U-50,488 and the κ receptor: a personalized account covering the period 1973–1990 *52*, 167 (1999) U-50,488 fand the κ receptor. Part II: 1991–1998 *53*, 1 (1999)	Jacob Szmuszkovicz
Practically applicable results of twenty years of research in endocrinology *12*, 137 (1968)	M. Tausk
Stereoselective drug metabolism and its significance in drug research *32*, 249 (1988)	Bernard Testa Joachim M. Mayer
Age profile of diphtheria in Bombay *19*, 412 (1975)	N. S. Tibrewala R. D. Potdar S. B. Talathi M. A. Ramnathkar A. D. Katdare

The effect and usefulness of early intravenous beta blockade in acute myocardial infarction *30*, 71 (1986)	Anders Vedin Claes Wilhelmsson
Methods of monitoring adverse reactions to drugs *21*, 231 (1977) Aspects of social pharmacology *22*, 9 (1978)	J. Venulet
The current status of cholera toxoid research in the United States *19*, 602 (1975)	W. F. Verwey J. C. Guckian J. Craig N. Pierce J. Peterson H. Williams Jr
Current and potential therapies for the treatment of herpesvirus infections *56*, 77 (2001)	Elcira C. Villarreal
Systemic cancer therapy: Four decades of progress and some personal perspectives *34*, 76 (1990)	Charles L. Vogel
Abnormalities of protein kinases in neurodegenerative diseases *51*, 133 (1998)	Ravenska T. E. Wagey Charles Krieger
The problem of diphtheria as seen in Bombay *19*, 452 (1975)	M. M. Wagle R. R. Sanzgiri Y. K. Amdekar
Drug nephrotoxicity – The significance of cellular mechanisms *41*, 51 (1993)	Robert J. Walker J. Paul Fawcett
Protease inhibitors as potential antiviral agents for the treatment of picornaviral infections *52*, 197 (1999)	Q. May Wang
Recent advances in prevention and treatment of hepatitis C virus infection *55*, 1 (2000)	Q. May Wang Beverly A. Heinz
Nicotine: An addictive substance or a therapeutic agent? *33*, 9 (1989)	David M. Warburton
Cell-wall antigens of *Vibrio cholerae* and their implication in cholera immunity *19*, 612 (1975)	Y. Watanabe R. Ganguly
Steroidogenic capacity in the adrenal cortex and its regulation *34*, 359 (1990)	Michael R. Watermann Evan R. Simpson
Antigen-specific T-cell factors and drug research *32*, 9 (1988)	David R. Webb

Backlist

Vol. 1–48 available

Vol. 49, 1997, 373 pp. ISBN 3-7643-5672-3
Richard M. Eglen: 5-Hydroxytryptamine (5-HT)4 receptors and central nervous system function: An update
Mont R. Juchau: Chemical teratogenesis in humans: Biochemical and molecular mechanisms
Gillian Edwards and Arthur H. Weston: Recent advances in potassium channel modulation
Helen Wise: Neuronal prostacyclin receptors
M.D. Murray and D. Craig Brater: Effects of NSAIDs on the kidney
Olivier Valdenaire and Philippe Vernier: G protein coupled receptors as modules of interacting proteins: A family meeting
Annemarie Polak: Antifungal therapy, an everlasting battle

Vol. 50, 1998, 373 pp. ISBN 3-7643-5821-1
P.N. Kaul: Drug discovery: Past, present and future
G. Edwards and A.H. Weston: Endothelium-derived hyperpolarizing factor – a critical appraisal
M. Rohmer: Isoprenoid biosynthesis via the mevalonate-independent route, a novel target for antibacterial drugs
R.W. Rockhold: Glutamatergic involvement in psychomotor stimulant action
T.D. Johnson: Polyamines and cerebral ischemia
J.M. Colacino and K.A. Staschke: The identification and development of antiviral agents for the treatment of chronic hepatitis B virus infection

Vol. 51, 1998, 330 pp. ISBN 3-7643-5822-X
Shijun Ren and Eric J. Lien: Development of HIV protease inhibitors: A survey
Nicholas C. Turner and John C. Clapham: Insulin resistance, impaired glucose tolerance and non-insulin-dependent diabetes, pathologic mechanisms and treatment: Current status and therapeutic possibilities
P.N. Kaul: Drug discovery: Past, present and future

G. Edwards and A.H. Weston: Endothelium-derived hyperpolarizing factor – a critical appraisal
M. Rohmer: Isoprenoid biosynthesis via the mevalonate-independent route, a novel target for antibacterial drugs
R.W. Rockhold: Glutamatergic involvement in psychomotor stimulant action
T.D. Johnson: Polyamines and cerebral ischemia
J.M. Colacino and K.A. Staschke: The identification and development of antiviral agents for the treatment of chronic hepatitis B virus infection

Vol. 52, 1999, 280 pp. ISBN 3-7643-5979-X
Bijoy Kundu and Sanjay K. Khare: Recenc advances in immunosuppressants
Vishnu J. Ram and Atul Goel: Present status of hepatoprotectants
Berend Olivier, Willem Soudijn and Ineke van Wijngarden: The $5HT_{1A}$ receptor and its ligands: structure and function
Jacob Szmuszkovicz: U-50,488 and the κ receptor: A personalized account covering the period of 1973–1990
Q. May Wang: Protease inhibitors as potential antiviral agents for the treatment of picornaviral infections

Vol. 53, 1999, 290 pp. ISBN 3-7643-6028-3
Jacob Szmuszkovicz: U-50,488 and the κ receptor: Part II: 1991–1998
Satya P. Gupta: Quantitative structure-activity relationships of antihypertensive agents
Bijoy Kundu, Sanjay K. Khare and Shiva K. Rastogi: Combinatorial chemistry: Polymer supported synthesis of peptide and nonpeptide libraries
Paul Spence: From genome to drug – optimising the drug discovery process
Mary S. Barnette: Phosphodiesterase 4 (PDE4) inhibitors in asthma and chronic obstructive pulmonary disease (COPD)

Vol. 54, 2000, 320 pp. ISBN 3-7643-6113-1
Shijun Ren and Eric J. Lien: Caco-2 cell permeability vs human gastrointestinal absorption: QSPR analysis

Jason C.G. Halford and John E. Blundell: Pharmacology of appetite suppression

Berend Olivier, Willem Soudijn and Ineke van Wijngaarden: Serotonin, dopamine and norepinephrine transporters in the central nervous system and their inhibitors

David Poyner, Helen Cox, Mark Bushfield, J. Mark Treherne and Melissa K. Demetrikopoulos: Neuropeptides in drug research

Meena Kumari and Maharaj K. Ticku: Regulation of NMDA receptors by ethanol

Hiroyoshi Horikoshi, Toshihiko Hashimoto and Toshihiko Fujiwara: Troglitazone and emerging glitazones: New avenues for potential therapeutic benefits beyond glycemic control

Rosamund C. Smith and Simon J. Rhodes: Applications of developmental biology to medicine and animal agriculture

Vol. 55, 2000, 344 pp. ISBN 3-7643-6193-X

Q. May Wang and Beverly A. Heinz: Recent advances in prevention and treatment of hepatitis C virus infections

Jay A. Glasel: The effects of morphine on cell proliferation

Gerlie C. de los Reyes, Robert T. Koda and Eric J. Lien: Glucosamine and chondroitin sulfates in the treatment of osteoarthritis: a survey

Angelo Vedani and Max Dobler: Multidimensional QSAR in drug research

Paul A. Keifer: NMR spectroscopy in drug discovery: Tools for combinatorial chemistry, natural products, and metabolism research

Laurane G. Mendelsohn: Prostate cancer and the androgen receptor: Strategies for the development of novel therapeutics

Satya P. Gupta: Quantitative structure-activity relationships of cardiotonic agents

Vol. 56, 2001, 300 pp. ISBN 3-7643-6265-0

Balawant S. Joshi and Pushkar N. Kaul: Alternative medicine: Herbal drugs and their critical appraisal – Part I

Elcira C. Villarreal: Current and potential therapies for the treatment of herpesvirus infections

Satya P. Gupta: Quantitiative structure-activity relationships of antianginal drugs

Allen D. Lee, Shijun Ren and Eric J. Lien: Purine analogs as CDK enzyme inhibitory agents: A survey and QSAR analysis

Noel A. Roberts: Anti-influenza drugs and neuraminidase inhibitors

Vol. 57, 2001, 310 pp. ISBN 3-7643-6266-9

Pushkar N. Kaul and Balawant S. Joshi: Alternative medicine: Herbal drugs and their critical appraisal – Part II

Esteban Domingo, Antonio Mas, Eloisa Yuste, Nonia Pariente, Saleta Sierra, Mónica Gutiérrez-Rivas and Luis Menéndez-Arias: Virus population dynamics, fitness variations and the control of viral disease: an update

Doreen Ma: Applications of yeast in drug discovery

Chaman Lal Kaul and Poduri Ramarao: Sympathetic nervous system and experimental diabetes: role of adrenal medullary hormones

Jay A. Glasel: From outer to inner space: Traveling along a scientific career from astrochemistry to drug research